Orthodontic Evidence

Samer Mheissen · Haris Khan

Orthodontic Evidence

A Q&A Handbook

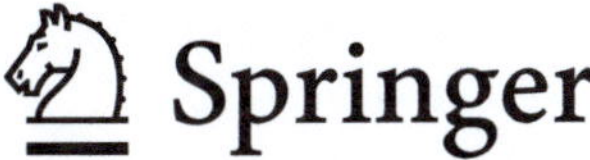
Springer

Samer Mheissen
DDS, SBO, Specialist Orthodontist
Damascus, Syrian Arab Republic

Haris Khan
BDS, FCPS, FFDRCSI
Professor of Orthodontics
Lahore, Pakistan

ISBN 978-3-031-24424-7   ISBN 978-3-031-24422-3   (eBook)
https://doi.org/10.1007/978-3-031-24422-3

This Springer imprint is published by the registered company Springer Nature Switzerland AG
The registered company address is: Gewerbestrasse 11, 6330 Cham, Switzerland

Preface

Orthodontics, like all other domains of human health sciences, has entered the era of evidence-based treatment. This approach starts by finding evidence, critically appraising it, and then applying it in the daily practice. The problem, that most of our fellow orthodontists and postgraduate students encounter, is that hundreds of research papers are published yearly, many of them addressing the same topic and sometimes with contradictory findings. That brings the dilemma of judging the research quality of these papers, for which some of us do not have sufficient time, and others lack the necessary training. So many clinicians buy the author's conclusion rather than judging the quality of the evidence themselves.

Keeping these time and training constraints in mind, we have written this handbook to provide evidence-based answers to most asked questions in orthodontics clinical practice and exams. Our aim was that after reading this book, clinicians could align their practice on evidence-based treatment, and answer relevant questions to their patients. Also, our extensive interaction with students appearing in specialty exams helped us to include many questions routinely asked during exams, both for seen and unseen cases.

We used a systematic approach to answer each question to make both ends meet. An electronic search in PubMed and Cochrane library was undertaken to resource the most recent and relevant evidence to the questions. We followed the hierarchy of evidence in reporting the evidence to answer the questions. Then we summarized the available evidence to provide a concise and focused answer. A brief description of the methodology for each study was given, along with the results in terms of P-value and confidence interval. This section was followed by evidence interpretation in plain language. Finally, a viewpoint was made to appraise the evidence critically and provide some comments on the generalizability and quality. The viewpoint represents the most likely shortcomings in the evidence design, methodology, reporting, and statistical analyses, which may help the readers criticize similar studies. However, no comprehensive assessment of the included evidence was performed as this is out of the scope of this book. At the end of each chapter, recommendations were given as a take-home message.

We have done our best to provide the readers with evidence-based, concise answers in plain language. We hope that the content of this book will solve many problems and give a better understanding of evidence-based treatment for clinicians and students.

Damascus, Syrian Arab Republic   Samer Mheissen
Lahore, Pakistan   Haris Khan

Acknowledgments

This book was not possible without the support of our families. We thank our teachers, colleagues, and students for improving our understanding of evidence-based orthodontics. We are incredibly thankful to our friend Dr. Mohammed Almuzian for encouraging us in orthodontic research. We also want to thank Prof. Nikolaos Pandis for supervising some of our research, which helped us better understand statistics. We feel indebted to Prof. Kevin O'Brien for his contribution to evidence-based orthodontics through his blogs, which inspired us on this subject.

At the end, we want to thank our publisher Springer Nature, project editor Alison Wolf and project coordinator, Shirly Christina, for their continuous support and guidance during this project.

Contents

Evidence-Based Practice

1

Contents

Evidence-based practice (EBP) is the appropriate use of the best available evidence to make the best decisions for improving the healthcare practice based on the values and preferences of the patients. EBP results from the integration of three components: the best available evidence, patients' preferences, and resources, including practitioner experience (Fig. 1.1) [1]. EBP enables practitioners to develop an informed treatment plan, minimize the adverse treatment effects, build up evidence-based experience with more confidence, and avoid legal concerns, as lack of evidence may lead to legal complications.

For example, in Brimm's case against her orthodontist in the United States in 1987, the jury found that the orthodontic treatment involving premolars extraction caused her TMJ disorders and awarded her 850,000 $ [2]. At that time, no proper evidence was present about this aspect of orthodontic treatment, and it was a widely held belief that extraction causes TMJ problems, and the expert orthodontist who was called by the jury agreed with this belief. But it would not have happened if the evidence was present at that time.

© The Author(s), under exclusive license to Springer Nature Switzerland AG 2023   1
S. Mheissen, H. Khan, *Orthodontic Evidence*,
https://doi.org/10.1007/978-3-031-24422-3_1

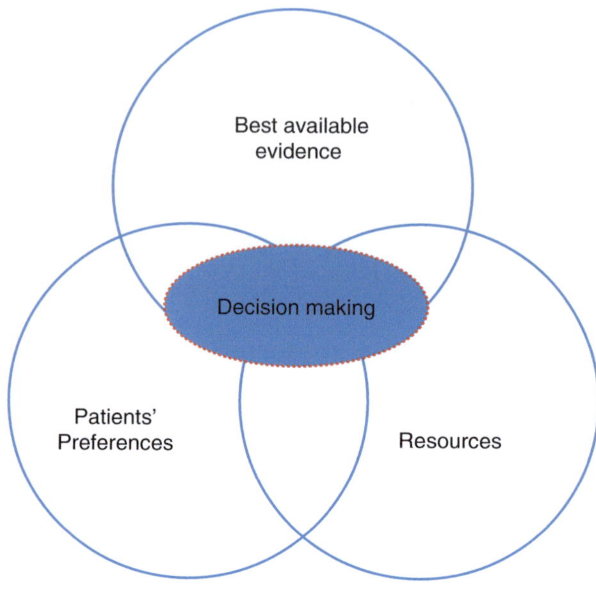

Fig. 1.1 Different EBP components which help in evidence-based clinical decision

Best Available Evidence

Evidence refers to research findings derived from data collection through observation and experiment in response to a research question [3, 4]. The best evidence should be valid and reliable as different researches have different designs and different levels of quality.

Systematic reviews and meta-analyses are at the top of the evidence pyramid since they gather a large number of primary studies and evaluate their internal validity (risk of bias and confounding factors) to provide solid evidence regarding the outcome of interest. Systematic reviews use the Grading of Recommendations Assessment, Development, and Evaluation approach(GRADE) to assess the evidence certainty considering different factors such as imprecision, inconsistency, and indirectness [5].

Patients' Values and Circumstances

Evidence-based healthcare practice is built on including patients in treatment decisions through an informed model of care, which allows patients to decide their treatment plan based on their needs and preferences with the assistance of the clinician who takes into account their individual attributes and history of treatment.

Patients' values refer to the unique preferences, expectations, and concerns that the patient expresses in the first encounter, which must be integrated into shared clinical decisions if they serve the patient.

Resources

This refers to the required infrastructure and skills to provide EBP. These recourses include physical, technical, and financial recourses [3].

The practitioner should have the skills to define the problem and ask an answerable question. Then the practitioner should have skills to acquire and appraise the quality and relevance of the available evidence and apply it in his clinical practice.

Evidence-Based Practice

To apply EBP in daily practice, we need to follow five steps (5As) [3]:

1 ASK a well-formulated and patient-oriented question regarding a health issue.
2 ACQUIRE the best available research evidence to answer this question.
3 APPRAISE the evidence critically to figure out the validity and the applicability of the research evidence.
4 APPLY the evidence according to the available resources and take patients' preferences in making a treatment decision.
5 ANALYZE the new practice and modify your practice according to the results, and assess the implication to the future interventions.

Clinical Scenario

A 10-year-old child visited your clinic along with his mother. The lady was concerned about her son's upper prominent teeth. She told the clinician that her child has bullying issues at school because of his appearance as well as he had suffered from a fracture on one of his upper anterior teeth.

On clinical examination, it was noticed that the child has a Class II skeletal and dental relationship with a severe overjet of 10 mm. Also, it was noticed by the clinician that the child is easily distracted, impulsive, and hyperactive.

His mother was willing to start the treatment as soon as possible and asked the clinician what was the best time for the treatment?

So, what would be your answer?

Your answer would be based upon the available evidence. According to a Cochrane systematic review [6], there is no difference between early and late treatments for Class II malocclusion in terms of ANB angle and the overjet. However, the early treatment enhances the self-esteem and decreases the incisal trauma at a higher cost and for a longer treatment time than late treatment.

So, for the orthodontist, the most evidence-based answer would be that as the child has bullying issues so early treatment will be useful for the child's self-esteem and his social development at this critical stage.

- How do you deal with the evidence if you find more than one research paper answering the same question? For instance, during the search process, to answer the first question asked by the patient's mother, the clinician found a systematic review with four included RCTs and one additional RCT, which was not a part of this review.

  He should follow the hierarchy of evidence and rely on the systematic review, and should assess the evidence presented by the RCT.

- Based on the best available evidence, what would be the choice of your appliance in this case? Do you prefer fixed or removable appliance here?

  A Cochrane systematic review [6] found that the removable functional appliances are better than fixed functional appliances in the reduction of ANB while the fixed functional appliances are better than removable functional appliances in the reduction of overjet.

  As this child has a hypermobility issue, one can expect that his cooperation would be poor, and according to the evidence, there is a little clinical difference between the two appliances, so I will treat this patient with a fixed functional appliance.

- Do you figure out flaws in this evidence? If yes, what are they?

  Yes, there is a limitation in the quality of evidence in this case. In the included Cochrane systematic review [6] most of the included studies were graded as low to moderate evidence. While in one included trial, there was high risk of bias due to loss to follow up, and the authors did not apply intention to treat analysis to minimize bias.

- Do these flaws in evidence affect your treatment plan?

  The quality of evidence is low to moderate which means we are confident in the effect estimate but not to a high level. However, the clinician should take into account the missing data and its reason while interpreting the findings, as lack of compliance may decrease the success rate.

- Is this evidence applicable here?

  Since this form of treatment is not affected by ethnicity, and most of these studies were conducted on school children using popular appliances, so we can use this evidence for our patient. But, the clinician should also take in consideration the high number of loss to follow up in early treatment group [7] and the other factors that may play a role in treatment success.

Research Design

Evidence is defined as the systematic collection and analysis of data. Not all evidence is the same, and for this point, we follow the hierarchy of evidence (Fig. 1.2) which depends on research design.

There are two main categories of study design: experimental and observational, based on assigning the exposure or not (Fig. 1.3). Experimental trials are divided into randomized and non-randomized trials according to the random allocation:

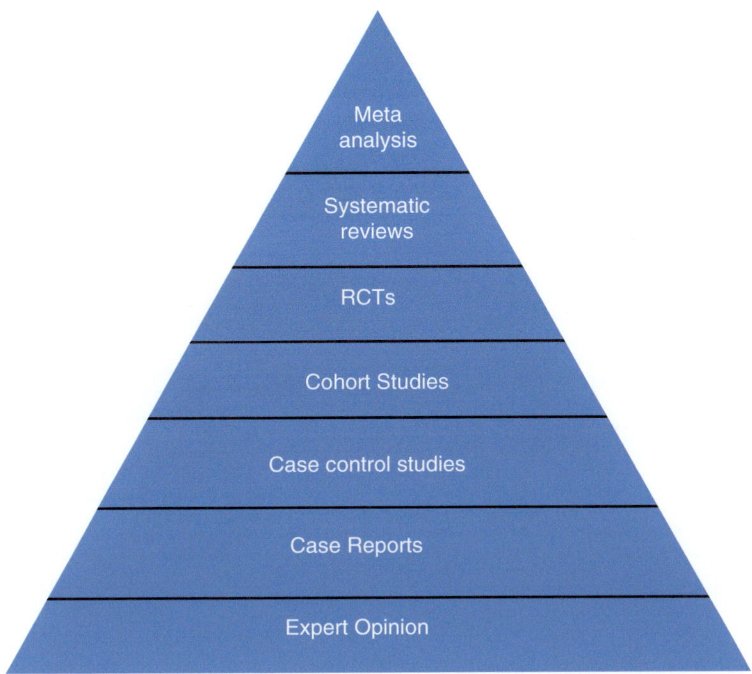

Fig. 1.2 Pyramid of evidence

- Randomized controlled trial (RCT) is the gold standard design in primary research. It randomizes participants into control and intervention groups to eliminate the bias and confounding factors. The assignment of the subjects is purely by the play of chance.

  However, the blinding of the participants and the operator minimizes the bias in measuring the outcome. On the other hand, the external validity of the RCT is limited to the eligible participants, and exposing the patients to a harmful intervention is unethical. Example of RCT includes the random allocation of orthodontic patients into a conventional orthodontic group (control) and orthodontic with piezocision surgery (experimental) to measure the acceleration of orthodontic tooth movement.

- Non-randomized clinical trial is a trial in which participants are assigned to one of the two groups without randomization or allocation concealment. This might increase the selection bias because the research team can select the more responding patients to the intervention group. In the previously given example of RCT for piezocision, if the researcher assigns the conventional orthodontic to one group and orthodontic with piezocision surgery to another group without randomization, the study will be a non-randomized clinical trial.

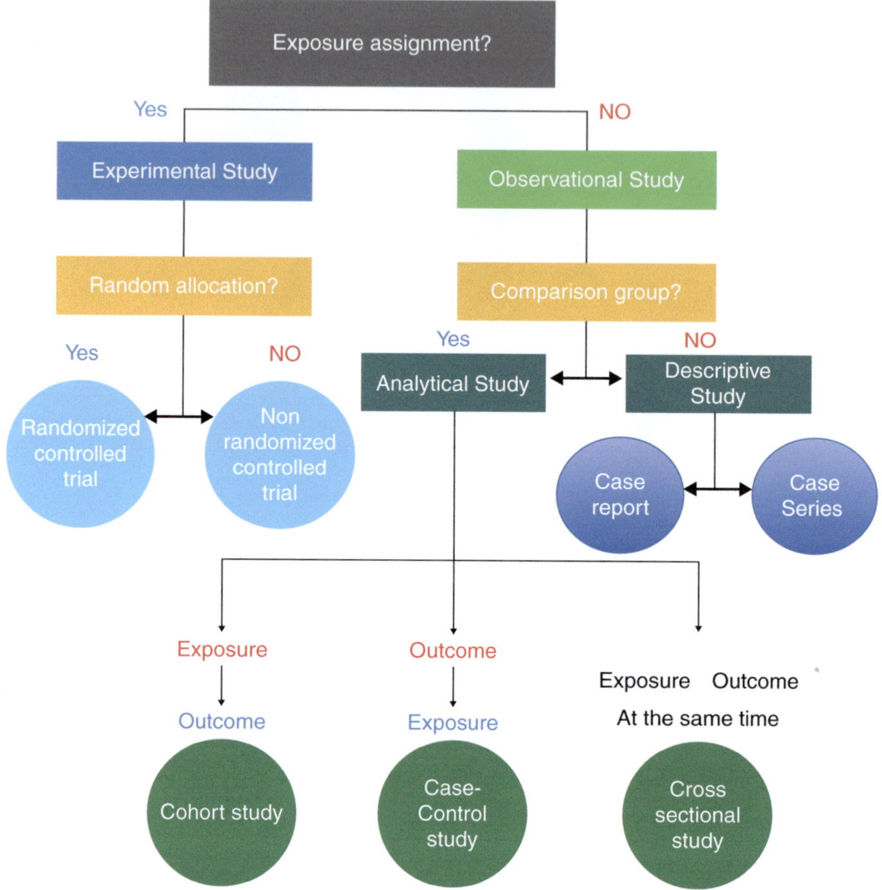

Fig. 1.3 Study design diagram

Observational studies are classified into two groups: analytical and descriptive designs, depending on whether they used a comparison group or not.

Analytical studies are subdivided into three types:

- Cross-sectional study: It is called a survey or prevalence study. This design is similar to taking a snapshot of the sample at one time. For example, a survey of the fifth year dental students to estimate the prevalence of missing teeth among them.
- Case Control study: This design is appropriate for rare diseases. In this study design, there are two groups: one with the disease and one without the disease. The researchers start from the outcome and look for the exposure to a risk factor and its role in both groups. The main investigation is whether the exposure to the risk factor is causing or increasing the incidence of disease or not. For example, correlation between smoking during pregnancy and the incidence of cleft lip and palate. Both cleft and non-cleft children would be enrolled in the study and then interviews

would be undertaken with their mothers to determine whether they were smokers or non-smokers during their pregnancy. After collecting the data, the authors will assess the association between mothers' smoking and newborns' clefts.
- Cohort study: It depends on moving forward from the exposure to the outcome in a logical sequence. Cohort studies compare two groups one is exposed to a risk factor and the other is non-exposed and follow them forward in time. If the exposed group developed more incidence of the outcome, then there is more association between the risk factor and exposure.

Cohort studies have three types according to the time of exposure and the outcome. If the groups followed backward to determine the exposed and non-exposed participants, then they were tracked to detect who developed the outcome, the design is called a retrospective, while if both groups were followed up forward in time, the study is prospective, and if the study has two directions of follow up, it will be ambidirectional cohort study. For example, the collection of orthopantomograms (OPG) radiographs taken 5 years ago in the orthodontic department to determine the canine alpha angle in children, and then reviewing their recent records to assess the upper canine impaction is called a retrospective study. While if researchers collected a number of participants with age range (8–10) and measured the alpha angle in their OPGs, and then they followed them for 5 years to assess the correlation between alpha angle and canine impaction, the study would be from prospective design. However, if the researchers collected alpha angle data from previous OPGs taken 2 years ago, and followed the patients for the next 2 years, the design would be ambidirectional.

Critical Appraisal

Critical appraisal is the prescription to recognize the strength and weaknesses of the evidence. Researchers have developed many tools [8] to critically appraise the evidence. However, RVRA is a simply suggested acronym to critically appraise evidence:

- Relevance: The question here, is the evidence clinically relevant to the patient's case? The relevance of the evidence mainly depends on the practitioner/clinician's knowledge. For instance, a 13-year-old child with a buccally displaced canine presented to an orthodontic clinic. The clinician conducted an extensive search and found Naoumova's study [9] on interceptive treatment in children with palatally displaced canines. Is the study relevant to the patient's case? No, this trial investigated the association between the primary canine extraction and the risk of displaced palatal NOT buccal canine.
- Validity: The extent to which the study is well conducted, including the reliability and the accuracy of the methodology. The risk of bias and confounding factors have a crucial impact on the validity of the evidence. For example, if in RCTs there was a difference in participants' characteristics between groups at the baseline before treatment, this may suggest a problem in the randomization process and it can increase the risk of bias (selection bias) that diminishes the validity of the evidence.

- Results: Refer to the clinical importance of the results and how the clinician can understand the findings. The interpretation and assessment of the results need an understanding of the statistical measures. For instance, a wider confidence interval indicates less precision in the results. On the other hand, some studies interpret their results in a way to let the reader feel a large effect size in so-called spin [10]; for example, some studies concluded that decortication or other surgical adjunctive procedures (SAPs) accelerate orthodontic tooth movement by 300% and decrease the treatment time by 60–70% rather than reporting well-defined measures. At this point, we should have a personal interpretation of the studies' results. For instance, the canine retraction rate was 1.5 mm for the first month and 2 mm for the second month after the surgical intervention, while it was 1 mm/month for the control group. Hence, some authors will divide (1.5/1 and 2/1) and they will conclude that "SAPs increase the tooth movement by (150–200%) that may enlarge the effect in the reader's mind while it is only an additional 1.5 mm for the two months and mostly the effect of SAPs lasts for 2–3 months according to many systematic reviews [11, 12].
- Applicability: The extent to which the valid study results can be applied to cases in real-life settings, in other words, the evidence generalizability. Like in the Naoumova study [9] which randomly assigned 67 patients having palatally displaced canine (PDC) with an age range 10–13 years, into two groups with and without primary canine extraction and they found more spontaneous eruptions of the PDCs in the extraction group (EG) than in the control group (CG), with rates of 69% and 39%, respectively. As such when we generalize the results of this study, to children aged 10–13 years, there is an increase of 30% in PDCs spontaneous eruption after extraction of primary canines compared to non-extraction. A related point to consider is that some factors such as ethnicity, age, trial settings, and study design, may hinder the applicability.

Effect Measures

It is the statistical paradigm that compares outcome data between two groups to help understanding different effects.

Mean difference (MD):

It is the absolute difference in mean values of two groups in the case of continuous data. It is historically called "weighted mean difference" (WMD).

Standardized mean difference (SMD):

It is a tool to measure the effect in meta-analysis for outcomes measured in different scales. SMD is equal to the mean difference divided by the standard deviation.

$$SMD = \frac{MD}{SD}$$

Relative Risk (RR): It is the incidence ratio between the exposed group to the non-exposed group, and it is used for cohort studies.

$$RR = \frac{EER}{CER}$$

EER: Event rate in the exposed group

$$EER = a/(a+b)$$

CER: Event rate in the non-exposed group

$$CER = c/(c+d)$$

From the example in Table 1.1, the rate of dental trauma is EER = 7.5% for the exposed group and it is CER = 13.8% for non-exposed group then RR = 0.075/0.138 = 0.54, which means exposed group is 54% times less likely to have dental trauma than non-exposed group.

Odds Ratio (OR): It is the odds of an exposed person having the disease divided by the odds of a non-exposed person having the disease. OR is mostly used in case control studies.

$$OR = (a/b)/(c/d)$$

For the same example according to Table 1.1, odds of dental trauma are 2/25 = 8% for Class II division 1 patients in early treatment group and odds of dental trauma are 4/25 = 16% for Class II division 1 patients in the late treatment group, so OR = 8%/16% = 0.5 means early treated patients are less likely to have a dental trauma by 50% when compared to the lately treated patients.

Probability (P) Value

P value tells whether the results you have obtained after applying a statistical test are significant or not. In most of the studies, an arbitrary P value of 0.05 (type I error) is taken as an indicator for a statistically significant effect/difference. Hence, the P value less than 0.05 mean that the result is statistically significant and vice versa.

Table 1.1 Dental trauma in early and late treatment groups

	Outcome dental trauma		
	Yes	No	Total
Exposed (early treatment)	A = 2	B = 25	27
Non-exposed (late treatment)	C = 4	D = 25	29

Confidence Interval (CI)

CI is a range around a single value, mean from a single sample in which we can be certain that the mean of a population lies. The confidence interval reflects the uncertainty regarding the population mean.

The confidence interval width gives us additional information about the variability of the estimate.

As the confidence interval represents the normal distribution, which is infinity range, so we could not construct a 100% CI but pretty close, which is usually set as 95% of CI. Another benefit of the CI is deciding if the difference in the results between two groups is statistically significant or not, and how big or small the difference is? When the effect measure is an absolute scale (mean difference MD), the CI should not contain the value of 0 (no effect) for significant difference otherwise, there is no difference between groups. On the other hand, if the effect measure is a relative scale (risk or odds ratio) then the confidence interval should not contain the value of 1 (no effect) to have a significant effect.

To understand the concept of CI let us review a research paper:

Authors measured the overjet reduction after using twin block appliance in one group and leaving the other group as control without treatment. They found more overjet reduction in the twin block group by (MD = 5 mm, 95%CI [2–8]).

The result is statistically significant as the CI range does not include the null value in this continuous data. On average, the overjet reduction was greater by 5 mm in the treated group than the control group, but this difference could be as low as 2 mm or as high as 8 mm. However, with a narrower CI such as [3.5–6.5] we would be more confident in terms of the outcome difference. While if the findings were (MD; 5, 95%CI [−1 to 10]), the difference would not be statistically significant because the CI range contains the null value.

Another research paper: The authors investigated the incisors' trauma between early and late Class II treatment groups, and found that the (OR=0.7, 95%CI [0.4 to 1.2]) favored the early treatment group.

Though there is a less likely chances to have trauma in the early treatment group by 30% (1–0.7 = 0.3), but this was not statistically significant as the CI includes the value of 1 in this relative scale effect measure.

References

1. Mayer D. Essential evidence-based medicine. Second Edition, Cambridge University Press, New York, 2010.
2. Pollack B. Michigan jury awards $850,000 in ortho case: a tempest in a teapot. Am J Orthod Dentofac Orthop. 1988;94(4):358–60.
3. Steglitz J, Warnick JL, Hoffman SA, Johnston W, Spring B. Evidence-based practice. International Encyclopedia of the Social & Behavioral Sciences. 2015;8:332–8.
4. Grimes DA, Schulz KF. An overview of clinical research: the lay of the land. Lancet. 2002;359(9300):57–61. https://doi.org/10.1016/s0140-6736(02)07283-5.

5. Murad MH, Asi N, Alsawas M, Alahdab F. New evidence pyramid. Evid Based Med. 2016;21(4):125–7. https://doi.org/10.1136/ebmed.

6. Batista KB, Thiruvenkatachari B, Harrison JE, O'Brien KD. Orthodontic treatment for prominent upper front teeth (class II malocclusion) in children and adolescents. Cochrane Database Syst Rev. 2018;3:CD003452. https://doi.org/10.1002/14651858.CD003452.pub4.

7. Tulloch JFC, Proffit WR, Phillips C. Outcomes in a 2-phase randomized clinical trial of early class II treatment. Am J Orthod Dentofac Orthop. 2004;125(6):657–67. https://doi.org/10.1016/j.ajodo.2004.02.008.

8. Katrak P, Bialocerkowski AE, Massy-Westropp N, Kumar S, Grimmer KA. A systematic review of the content of critical appraisal tools. BMC Med Res Methodol. 2004;4:22. https://doi.org/10.1186/1471-2288-4-22.

9. Naoumova J, Kurol J, Kjellberg H. Extraction of the deciduous canine as an interceptive treatment in children with palatal displaced canines - part I: shall we extract the deciduous canine or not? Eur J Orthod. 2015;37(2):209–18. https://doi.org/10.1093/ejo/cju040.

10. Eleftheriadi I, Ioannou T, Pandis N. Extent and prevalence of spin in randomized controlled trials in dentistry. J Dent. 2020;100:103433. https://doi.org/10.1016/j.jdent.2020.103433.

11. Mheissen S, Khan H, Alsafadi AS, Almuzian M. The effectiveness of surgical adjunctive procedures in the acceleration of orthodontic tooth movement: a systematic review of systematic reviews and meta-analysis. J Orthod. 2021;48(2):1465312520988735. https://doi.org/10.1177/1465312520988735.

12. Mheissen S, Khan H, Samawi S. Is Piezocision effective in accelerating orthodontic tooth movement: a systematic review and meta-analysis. PLoS One. 2020;15(4):e0231492. https://doi.org/10.1371/journal.pone.0231492.

Maxillary Molar Distalization

2

Contents

© The Author(s), under exclusive license to Springer Nature Switzerland AG 2023   13
S. Mheissen, H. Khan, *Orthodontic Evidence*,
https://doi.org/10.1007/978-3-031-24422-3_2

Abbreviations

BAPA	Bone anchored pendulum appliance
EOA	Extraoral appliances
FA	Frog appliance
FA/HG	Frog appliance combed with a high pull headgear
HG	Headgear
IOA	Intraoral appliances
JJA	Jones jig appliance
MI	Miniscrew
MIs	Miniscrews
MPs	Mini-plates
MTTMS	Moving teeth through the maxillary sinus
RCT	Randomized Controlled Trial
TSADs	Temporary skeletal anchorage devises
URA	Upper removable appliance

Introduction

Non-extraction treatments are gaining popularity in contemporary orthodontics. One treatment option for dental correction of Class II molar relationship and relief of crowding is the maxillary molar distalization. The concept of distalization by extraoral appliance was first introduced by Kingsley [1] in 1892. The early distalization appliances used for molar distalization were extraoral, but over a period of time, intraoral appliances became more popular, especially after introducing temporary skeletal anchorage devices (TSADs or TADs) such as mini-implants (MIs) and mini-plates (MPs).

Force application system in distalization depends on the design of the appliance; for extraoral appliances, the force is typically applied from the buccal side, while for intraoral appliances the force can be applied from the buccal side, the palatal side, or both sides.

Many distalization appliances are used in clinical orthodontics. These appliances differ in terms of design, biomechanics, anchorage, patient compliance, and appliance location. Distalization appliances can be classified either according to the type of fixation or mode of working. For the type of fixation distalization appliances can be removable or fixed, while according to the mode of working, these appliances can be frictionless or frictional appliances.

Removable appliances: These appliances can be removed by the patient, and their success is completely dependent on the patient's compliance. These include removable intraoral appliances and all extraoral appliances.

Fixed appliances are generally bonded/banded or ligated to the teeth with no dependence on the patient. The success of the treatment depends on the appliance design and selection of the proper case.

Frictionless appliances: The biomechanics of these appliances do not involve any friction while distalization. Forces are mostly generated from loops, screws, or from some extraoral sources. The most commonly used frictionless intraoral appliances are Pendulum and Frog appliances.

Frictional appliances: These are mostly based on sliding mechanics and encounter friction in their force system. These appliances include Jones Jig, distal jet, first class appliance, and Keles slider.

All distalization appliances need anchorage while distalizing the molars. The conventional anchorage is usually prepared using the other teeth and the hard palate in the intraoral appliances and the skeletal structures in case of headgear. Appliance anchorage parts are the base plate of removable appliances, Nance buttons, and teeth in case of conventional fixed distalization appliances. In the last 10 years, TSADs have gained tremendous use in providing anchorage for molar distalization in different ways. TSADs were used either to apply the push/pull force directly to the tooth or to support and anchor the appliance [2–6].

Effectiveness of Maxillary Molar Distalization

Clinical Question 1: How Much Maxillary Molars Can Be Distalized?

Evidence

Systematic Reviews and Meta-Analyses
Jambi/2013 [4]
This is a Cochrane systematic review that included 10 randomized controlled trials (RCTs) in the qualitative synthesis and four RCTs in meta-analysis to compare the effectiveness of distalizing with intra versus extraoral appliances. The authors concluded that the intraoral appliances (IOA) provide an average distal molar movement of 2.2 mm with a range of 1.6–4.04 mm. While the extraoral appliances (headgear) attain a mean distal molar movement of 1.04 mm. In other words, the average amount of distal molar movement was 1.04 and 2.2 mm, using headgear and intraoral distalization appliances, respectively. The author found this evidence of a very low quality.

Grec RH/2013 [7]

This systematic review included 40 studies in the qualitative synthesis and six trials in meta-analysis investigating the amount of molar distalization. Mostly pendulum appliance was used (22 trials) followed by the distal jet (7 trials) and the Jones jig appliance (JJA) (6 trials) with a conventional anchorage using Nance appliance in 34 trials and MIs in 6 trials. The meta-analysis showed that the average amount of molar distal movement was 3.34 mm (95% CI; 2.73–4.29, $p < 0.01$, $I^2 = 0\%$, 3 trials) using conventional anchorage and 5.10 mm (95% CI;4.11–6.09, $I^2 = 82\%$, 4 trials) using MIs.

Systematic Reviews
Atherton/2002 [8]

This systematic review included 58 studies with different study designs; 18 case series, 6 comparisons of case series, 23 cohort retrospective studies, 8 controlled trials, and 3 RCTs. The included controlled clinical trials indicated that the Ni-Ti coil springs could produce the most distal movement (3.8 mm), while acrylic splint Herbst produced the least distal movement (0.5 mm). Cohort studies included in the review found that some fixed Class II correctors like Herbst can produce the most distal movement (2.7 mm). The included case-control studies concluded that the most efficient appliance was an en-mass appliance with headgear that produced 5.7 mm of distal maxillary molar movement, while the cervical headgear reported the least molar distalization. The review found that for most of the patients no more than half-cusp maxillary molar distalization can be done. The authors found that the level of evidence in this systematic review was low.

Fudalej/2011 [9]

This systematic review included 12 studies; 9 were from a retrospective design and 3 were from a prospective design. The authors aimed to investigate the effectiveness of TSADs in distalization the maxillary molar. The mean age at the start of the treatment ranged from 13 to 27.3 years as six trials recruited teenagers, three comprised adults, while the rest included both. Six trials used palatal TSADs, two used infrazygomatic crest TSADs, and one used the anterior margin of the mandibular ramus. For molar distalization, MIs were mostly used with Pendulum appliances, while MPs were used with power chain elastics. As a result, the mean distal movement of the maxillary molars using TSADs ranged from 3.5 to 6.4 mm, with associated distal tipping ranging from 0.8° to 12.20°. The overall quality of evidence for this review was low.

Evidence Summary

The collective evidence [4, 8] supports that the most distal movement of the molars that could be achieved is not more than half a unit by using traditional appliances. If more than half-cusp molar correction is required, then either the mesial movement of a lower molar or the skeletal anchorage devices would be required. The amount of molar distalization that can be attained by skeletal anchorage devices is in the range of 5.1–6.4 mm.

Evidence Interpretation

Distalization is an effective procedure in orthodontic correction of Class II molar relationship. In patients with up to half unit Class II molar relationship, conventional distalization appliances can be used successfully. But if a greater amount of distalization (5–6 mm) is required, skeletal anchorage devices are effective means to do the task.

The quality of evidence for this question is low or very low; the clinician's skills, patient cooperation, and available resources can affect the final outcome.

Viewpoint

According to the GRADE approach, all trials included in Jambi [4] systematic review were downgraded due to low numbers of participants and the high risk of bias. The heterogeneity was substantial in the meta-analysis, which may be due to the different intraoral appliances used, different participants, or the applied force. Hence, these trials are assessed as very low to low quality, leaving the evidence inconclusive.

Grec review [7] is a well-conducted review. However, there was a potential language bias due to English language restriction and publication bias due to published studies' search. Most of the included studies were of moderate quality from non-randomized design. Two trials were classified as high quality, 27 as medium quality, and 11 as low quality based on sampling, statistical analysis, and study design. The sample description in most included studies was not clear. Also, the authors used a random effect model in the meta-analysis, but it was better to use a fixed-effect model in conventional devices as there were only few studies with no statistical heterogeneity. The statistical heterogeneity was high ($I^2 = 82\%$) in the skeletal anchorage device forest plot, which may lead to misleading results. So, the aforementioned issues can affect the interpretation of results and reduce the quality of the evidence.

There was a lack of high-quality evidence for this answer in the Atherton [8] review as 70% of the included studies were observational (mostly retrospective and case series), which have different control samples in their methodology. Also, most of the included trials were generally of low quality as there was no risk of bias assessment. The authors did not follow rigorous guidelines in conducting their review that may reduce the quality of the evidence. As a result, there is a demand for good quality research to build our clinical decisions.

In Fudalej [9] review, eight of the included studies were assessed as low quality, and four studies were assessed as medium quality. These studies were from retrospective or prospective designs, indicating compromised methodological soundness. Likewise, most of those studies were having inadequate and low sample sizes (fewer than 20 patients) and lacking the method error analysis. As such, the review provides low-quality evidence.

Distalization in Adolescent Patients

Clinical Question 2: What Should Be the Appliance of Choice in Adolescents' Patients (Intra versus Extraoral)?

Evidence

Systematic Review and Meta-Analysis
Jambi/2013 [4]

As discussed before, this Cochrane review compared distalizing intra and extraoral appliances' effectiveness in adolescents with an age range of 11.45–14.75 years. This review found that all appliances provide some degree of distal movement. Four included trials were pooled in a meta-analysis, which concluded that the intraoral appliances (IOA) were more effective than extraoral appliances (EOA) in distalizing the maxillary first molar by 1.45 mm (95%CI;0.15–2.74, $p = 0.03$, $I^2 = 73\%$, participants = 150, 4 trials, very low quality). However, IOA were associated with loss of anterior anchorage. The difference in mean mesial upper incisor movement was statistically significant (MD;1.82 mm, 95%CI;1.27–2.65, $p < 0.001$, 4 RCTs, low quality) and overjet (MD; 1.64 mm,95%CI;1.26–2.02, $p < 0.001$, 2 RCTs, low quality) favoring headgear indicating a less loss of anterior anchorage with headgear.

No study reported the adverse effects (harm or injury), or the failure rate (broken appliance).

Randomized Controlled Trials
Bondemark/2005 [10]

This RCT was also included in Jambi et al. review [4], and it was a low-biased trial. The authors randomized 40 patients into two groups to compare EOA with IOA. The EOA group received the Kloehn cervical headgear, while the IOA group received an appliance consisting of a bilateral NI-Ti coil spring that generates 180–200 g of force between the first molar and second premolar supported by the Nance appliance. The mean age was 11.4 years and 11.5 years in IOA and EOA groups, respectively. It is worth mentioning that the mean wearing time of HG was 10.8 hours/day. The study found that the molar distalization time was significantly shorter ($p < 0.01$) in the IOA group (5.2 months) than EOA group (6.4 months), and the average amount of the molar distalization was significantly greater in the IOA group (3 mm) than in the EOA group (1.7 mm). The molar relation correction was also significantly higher ($p < 0.001$) in IOA group (3.3 mm) than EOA group (2.4 mm). Interestingly, the maxillary incisors, in the IOA group, proclined labially and moved forward by 0.8 mm, while the maxillary incisors retroclined by 1 mm in EOA group and the overjet decreased by 0.9 mm.

Evidence Summary

Looking into the evidence collectively, the best available evidence supports that more distal movement (2.2 mm [4] or 3.3 mm [10]) of the molars can be achieved by using IOA in comparison with HG (1.04 mm [4] or1.7 mm [10]). But IOA are associated with more anterior anchorage loss than the EOA by 1.82 mm which will result in increased overjet in IOA by 1.64 mm. Interestingly, the total treatment duration provided by an RCT [10] was longer in EOA group than IOA group,6.4 months and 5.2 months, respectively, with a mean wearing time of 10.8 hours/day for EOA.

Evidence Interpretation

Intraoral appliances are more favored in adolescents orthodontic patients as they are more effective in terms of distalization and treatment duration. The shortcomings of intraoral appliances are the anterior anchorage loss, the increased overjet, and the compliance issues in the case of removable appliances. Fixed IOA appliances may overcome the problem of patients' cooperation. But if up to 2 mm of molar distalization is required without increasing the proclination of upper incisors, EOA such as headgear can be used for 6 months and 11 hours per day.

Viewpoint

Jambi [4] systematic review is already being discussed with a small addition; the authors included the molar relationship correction instead of molar distal movement. Bondemark [10] trial was a well-conducted study with some limitations; the authors did not provide enough information about the allocation concealment or operator blinding. There were no clear baseline characteristics regarding the molar relationship between groups.

The mean wearing time of the HG was 10.8 hours/day, and at this wearing time, the authors did not report any correlation between the time of use of the appliance per day and distal molar movement amount, but the value ($r = 0.23$) suggests a small association within the small sample that may be not enough to detect this outcome.

For generalization, the study results of HG are applicable in patients with age (11.4–11.5 years) and with no erupted upper second molars.

Sliding vs. Frictionless Appliance

Clinical Question 3: What Is the Ideal Side of Force Application for Distalization (Buccal or Palatal) in Adolescents?

Evidence

Systematic Review and Meta-Analysis
Antonarakis/2008 [2]

This evidence includes patients with an age range from 11.2 years to 14.9 years. The researchers compared the effectiveness of intramaxillary non-compliance appliances (buccal versus palatal) in distalizing the maxillary molar. This review found that all appliances provided a distal molar movement with a mean of 2.9 mm associated with 5.4° of distal tipping of the molar crown. The meisal movement of the incisors, by these appliances, was 1.8 mm with a mesial tipping of 3.6°, and the premolar mesial movement was 1.7 mm. Also, the incisors and premolars showed some extrusive movement.

The molar distal movement was greater in the palatal acting appliances 3.1 mm(95% CI;2.1–3.8) than the buccal acting appliances 2.6 mm(95% CI;2.1–3), with less molar tipping in the palatal appliance 3.6° than the buccal ones 8.3°. The incisor mesial movement was 1.9 mm with 5° mesial tipping for buccal appliances and 1.8 mm with less mesial tipping 2.9° for palatal appliances. For premolars, there was mesial movement of 2 mm for buccal appliances and 1.3 mm for palatal appliances.

Randomized Controlled Trial
Papadopoulos/2010 [5]

The researchers recruited 27 patients with mixed dentition (11 in the control group and 16 in the distalization group) with a mean age of 9.2 years and 9.7 years for the treatment and control groups, respectively. The authors compared the non-compliance First Class Appliance (FCA) group (combination of palatal and buccal acting force) with the untreated control group. The study found that this appliance can distalize molars by 4 mm, with a total treatment time of 4 months, which leads to 1 mm molar distalization per month. However, the distalization was associated with significant distal tipping of the first molars by 8.56° with anterior anchorage loss and mesial movement of premolars by 1. 86 mm.

Evidence Summary

The best available evidence indicates that palatal appliances like Distal Jet or Pendulum appliances seem to create more distal molar movement(3.1 mm) than buccal appliances such as buccal Ni-Ti coil (2.6 mm). Palatal appliance also provided a less distal tipping 3.6° than the buccal ones 8.3°. Both buccal and palatal appliances were associated with a similar degree of anterior anchorage loss of 1.9 mm and 1.8 mm, respectively, with a slight difference in the mesial tipping; 5° and 2.9° for buccal and palatal appliances, respectively [2]. One RCT [5] that recruited younger patients of 9 years found that FCA is effective in distalizing maxillary molars by 4 mm in nearly 4 months with a similar anchorage loss of 1.8 mm in the first deciduous molars region but with greater buccal tipping of 8.56° in first molar.

Evidence Interpretation

IOA palatal appliances are more effective than buccal appliances in terms of distalization and bodily molar movement with minor differences in anterior anchorage loss. In patients requiring 2–3 mm molar distalization and where proclination of upper incisors is acceptable, buccal acting distalization appliances can be used. Due to tipping of molars, some bite opening can be expected in these appliances. In comparison, palatal acting distalization appliances can attain more distal and bodily movement as forces are applied closer to the center of resistance of the molars. Also, these appliances are more effective if proclination of upper incisors is not desired.

A combination of buccal and palatal acting appliances, the FCA, produces a greater amount of distalization than palatal or buccal acting appliances alone but with more tipping and less rotation of the molars. As this is a single study with low evidence so our confidence in this study is low, and more evidence is needed for the clinician to use such appliances.

Viewpoint

Most of the included studies, in Antonarakis [2] review, were cohort studies and graded as low quality which may reduce the level of the evidence. Papadopoulos's [5] trial was underpowered due to an imbalanced number of patients between groups at the baseline as the authors randomized the patients and then excluded five patients from the control group, which suggests some flaws in the randomization process. Interestingly, the authors mentioned that they had treated three patients with full cusp Class II relationship, and this is a low number of cases to generalize full cusp correction. For generalizability, the authors excluded patients with mobility of the maxillary deciduous second molars, and this means the appliance is limited to patients with stable maxillary deciduous second molars; also, they excluded patients with increase vertical growth patterns.

Sliding vs. Frictionless Appliance

Clinical Question 4: What Should Be the Ideal Mode of Action of a Distalization Appliance, Sliding vs. Frictionless?

Evidence

Non-Randomized Controlled Trial
Patel/ 2007 [11]

In this trial, the authors assigned 40 patients with a Class II malocclusion into two groups: 20 subjects with an average age of 13.17 years (range 10.83–16.24 years) for treatment with the Jones jig appliance (JJA) and 20 subjects with an average age of 13.98 years (range 11.33–17.26 years) for treatment with pendulum appliance (Table 2.1). The endpoint of the treatment was a Class I molar relationship. The study found that the monthly rate of distalization was similar between the two appliances; 0.338 mm/month and 0.263/month for JJA and pendulum appliances, respectively, $p = 0.25$. However, the anchorage loss was significantly greater in the JJA group;

Table 2.1 Characteristics of dental relationship in Patel study

Severity of Class II	Jones jig group	Pendulum group
Full cusp	4	6
Three quarters	1	5
Half-cusp	8	8
One quarter-cusp	7	1

mesial tipping and extrusion of the second premolars were significantly higher in Jones jig group than in the pendulum group, as the angle SN. Mx5 (angle formed by the intersection of the long axis of the maxillary second premolar and the SN line) increased by 9.29° and 2.37° in JJA and pendulum appliances, respectively, $p = 0.002$.

Evidence Summary

The best available evidence suggests that there is no statistically significant difference between frictionless and sliding appliances in the monthly distalization rate of maxillary molars. The monthly distalization rate was 0.338 mm/month in the JJA group and 0.263 mm/month in the pendulum group. On the other hand, JJA yielded a significantly greater mesial tipping and extrusion of the second premolars (SN. Mx5 increased by 9.29°) when compared with the pendulum appliance (SN. Mx5 increased by 2.37°).

Evidence Interpretation

There is no clinically significant difference between frictionless and sliding appliances, and other variables can affect the final outcomes. These include the location of the appliance taking into consideration the patients' preferences, the insertion and the activation of the appliance that is influenced by clinician's skills, and the sources such as the manufacturers' availability and the cost-effectiveness.

Viewpoint

Patel trial [11] provides good information regarding the maxillary molar distalization with some limitations. The lack of randomization may expose the study to selection bias. There were three cases with unerupted second molar in addition to the difference in Class II malocclusion severity that might be considered as confounders. In terms of the generalizability of the results, in Class II malocclusion with all permanent teeth up to the first molars erupted, there were no significant differences between frictionless and sliding mechanics in the monthly rate of distalizing maxillary molars with a low certainty in the available evidence.

Compliant vs. Non-compliant Appliances

Clinical Question 5: For Adolescent's Patients, What Is the Appliance of Choice for Molar Distalization in Terms of Compliance?

Evidence

Systematic Review and Meta-Analysis
Jambi/2013 [4]

As discussed before, this Cochrane review compared the effectiveness of IOA and EOA in maxillary molar distalization. This review found that intraoral appliances (non compliant appliances) were better than extraoral appliances (compliance dependant appliances) in distalizing the maxillary molar by 1.45 mm.

Randomized Controlled Trial
Paul/2002 [12]
This randomized clinical trial compared the effectiveness of two appliances, the upper removable appliance (URA) and JJA. The authors randomized 27 patients for molar distalization; 14 patients in URA group and 13 patients in JJA group. The assessor was blinded and assessed the collected records for only 23 patients after 6 months of treatment in the two groups. The researchers found that there was no statistically significant difference between the URA and JJA in regard to the molar distal movement (1.3 ± 1.34 mm and 1.17 ± 1.94 mm in URA and JJA groups, respectively $= 0.85$), and in regard to patient discomfort on Likert scale (2.8 ± 1.54 in URA group versus 2.39 ± 1 in JJ group, $p = 0.47$).

Evidence Summary
The best available evidence suggest that intraoral non-compliant appliances are better than compliance-dependent appliances like HG by average amount of 1.45 mm [4]. Interestingly, one RCT concluded that the URA (compliance) and the JJA (non-compliance) are equally effective [12] with similar discomfort in both appliances.

Evidence Interpretation
Compliant and non-compliant IOA appliances are equally effective in molar distalization when a small amount of distalization is required. Also, IOA are more effective than EOA. As such, the available evidence is related to a small amount of distalization (less than 1.5 mm), and there is an absence of evidence for a large amount of distalization in terms of patient compliance.

Viewpoint
Jambi systematic review [4] is already discussed. Paul et al. RCT [12] is an ambitious study that addressed a clinically relevant question. The authors used block randomization with no clear description of the allocation concealment. The measurement method was valid, and the authors tried to avoid any effects on the reference landmarks in the two groups. However, there were some limitations in this RCT. There was a lack of blinding for the patients and the operators, and this blinding is sometimes difficult in orthodontic domain. Interestingly, the lost to follow up was more than 20% without treating the missing data by intention to treat analysis and this may lead to bias. The effect size was very low and different from the effect size in the sample size calculation in the study, so this study is underpowered and a large study is needed to be certain about the estimate. The present evidence for this question is low or very low quality.

Combination of Intraoral and Extraoral Appliance

Clinical Question 6: Which Is a Better Appliance for the Molar Distalization in Adolescents (Intraoral Alone or with a Combined Extraoral Appliance)?

Evidence

Randomized Controlled Trial
Burhan/2013 [13]

This study compared the Frog appliance (FA) alone and the Frog appliance in combination with a high pull headgear (FA/HG) for maxillary molars distalization. The authors randomized 50 patients into the two treatment groups; the mean age was 14.5 ± 1.7 years in the FA group and was 14.1 ± 1.8 years in FA/HG group. The ratio of female/male was 13/12 and 11/14 in FA and FA/HG groups, respectively. They found that there was no statistically significant difference between the two groups regarding molar distalization. The mean distal movement was 5.51 ± 2.56 mm in the FA group and 5.93 ± 1.46 mm in the FA/HG group. The tipping was significantly higher in the FA group ($4.96° \pm 1.41$) when compared to the FA/HG group ($1.25° \pm 2.02$) ($p < 0.001$). The mesial movement of the second premolars was significantly higher in the FA group (2.70 ± 1.37 mm) than in the FA/HG group (0.90 ± 1.38 mm) ($p = 0.008$).

Evidence Summary

The best available evidence suggests that there is no statistically significant difference between the intraoral appliance alone or in combination with a high pull headgear regarding the amount of the maxillary molar distalization. The average distal movement was 5.51 ± 2.56 mm and 5.93 ± 1.46 mm in FA and FA/HG groups, respectively. On the other hand, HG decreased the molar tipping during the distalization, which means more translation movement. Also, the use of high-pull HG enhanced the anchorage; the mesial premolar movement was 2.70 ± 1.37 and 0.90 ± 1.38 mm in FA and FA/HG groups, respectively.

Evidence Interpretation

If your patient is cooperative and you want to avoid the distalization side effects like distal tipping of maxillary molars and loss of anterior anchorage, high-pull headgear can be used in combination with an intraoral distalization appliance. This combination may increase the molar bodily movement by decreasing the distal crown tipping.

Viewpoint

Burhan RCT [13] was a well-conducted trial with some limitations; the effect size in the sample size calculation was not clear, so the power of the study is a concern. There was a lack of information regarding the allocation concealment while the authors reported that neither the patients nor the operators were blinded to the procedure, which may increase the bias. Interestingly, the basic characteristics of the malocclusion and the extent of the Class II molar relationship in each group were missing. Likewise, the lack of HG wears duration and the patient's compliance within the group. The aforementioned factors may be considered confounders. For generalizability, the study is applicable to patients with a normal or horizontal growth pattern, having ANB value of almost $5°$, with a sufficient posterior space according to Ricketts analysis, and with erupted second molars. As such, further trials are needed to increase the certainty of the effect estimate, mainly through well-designed trials.

Temporary Skeletal Anchorage Devices and Molars Distalization

Clinical Question 7: Are TSADs Effective for Molar Distalization?

Evidence

Systematic Review and Meta-Analysis
Grec RH/2013 [7]

As discussed before, this meta-analysis found an average amount of distal molar movement of 3.34 mm (95%CI; 2.83 to 3.85 mm, $P < 0.001$, $I^2 = 0\%$, 3 trials) with conventional anchorage and 5.10 mm (95%CI; 4.11–6.09 mm, $P < 0.001$, $I^2 = 82\%$, 4 trials) with skeletal anchorage devices. The premolar has a mesial movement of 2.30 mm (95%CI; 1.73 to 2.86 mm, $P < 0.001$, $I^2 = 0\%$, 3 trials) in the conventional anchorage group, while distal movement of 4.01 mm (95%CI; 3.23 to 4.8 mm, $P < 0.001$, $I^2 = 69\%$, 3 trials) was found in TSADs groups.

Soheilifar/2019 [14]

This systematic review has included five cohort studies in the quantitative analysis. Of those, two were from prospective design, and three were from retrospective design. The review found that the mean molar distalization was 5.35 mm ($8.44°$ tipping) and 4.25 mm ($8.31°$ tipping) in skeletal anchorage devices and conventional anchorage groups, respectively, and this difference was not statistically significant (MD; -0.06, 95%CI; -0.7 to 0.58, $P = 0.85$, $I^2 = 80\%$, 5 trials). Likewise, the molar tipping was similar $8.44°$ and $8.31°$ in TSADs and conventional anchorage groups, respectively, with no statistically significant difference between both groups (MD $= 0.01$, 95%CI; -0.98 to 1.01, $P = 0.98$, $I^2 = 89\%$, 4 trials). The mean premolar movement was distalization of 0.96 mm in the TSADs group and it was mesialization of 2.21 mm in the conventional anchorage group. The difference in premolar movement was statistically significant between the two groups (MD $= 1.84$, 95%CI; 0.59 to 3.10, $P = 0.004$, $I^2 = 93\%$, 5 trials).

Bayome/2021 [15]

This systematic review evaluated the effectiveness of buccally or palatally placed TSADs in maxillary molar distalization. The reviewers included nine trials; two were RCTs and seven were non-RCTs. Two trials used interradicular TSADs, five trials placed TSADs in the infrazygomatic process, and two trials used palatal TSADs. The mean molar distalization using TSADs was 3.957 mm (95%CI: 3.42 to 4.49, $p < 0.001$, $I^2 = 61.95\%$, 9 trials). The average molar tipping during distalization was 3.768° (95%CI: 3.18°–4.36°, $p < 0.001$, $I^2 = 52\%$, 9 trials). Likewise, the molar intrusion was minimal 0.64 mm (95%CI: 0.47 to 0.8 mm, $p < 0.001$, $I^2 = 15\%$, 9 trials).

Systematic Reviews
Fudalej/2011 [9]

As discussed before, this systematic review evaluated the effects of skeletal anchorage on molar distalization. Either MIs or MPs were used for skeletal anchorage. The average age of the subjects ranged from 13 years to 27.3 years with mostly teenagers included in most studies. The placement of the MIs was in the para-median suture in the anterior region of the hard palate in six studies, and anchorage devices, MPs were placed in the infrazygomatic crest in two studies. In one study, MPs were placed in the anterior margin of the mandibular ramus. Most studies used pendulum appliance except when MPs were used, where elastomeric power chains attached to the fixed orthodontic appliance were used. The reviewers found that the mean distal movement of the maxillary molars ranged from 3.5 to 6.4 mm, with a molar tipping of 0.8° to 12.20°. The incisors' position remained stable during distalization, however, two trials reported central incisors' retraction by 1.4 mm [16] and 0.5 mm [17].

Al-Thomali/2017 [18]

This systematic review evaluated the effects of pendulum appliances and modified pendulum appliances. The 25 included studies' quality was varied; 4 studies have high quality and 21 studies have moderate quality. In 14 included trials, the mean of molar distalization was 2 to 6.4 mm, with a distal tipping of 8.36°–14.50° using the Hilgers pendulum appliance. Interestingly, the anchorage loss showed premolar and incisor mesial movement of 1.63–3.6 mm and 0.92–6.5 mm, respectively. Three included trials used bone anchorage pendulum appliance (BAPA) and found more distal movement of 4.8–6.4 mm with distal tipping of 9°–10.9°. The BAPA showed a mean premolar distalization of 1.7–5.4 mm with distal tipping of 6.04°–16.3°.

Mohamed/2018 [19]

This systematic review evaluated the effectiveness of MIs-supported molar distalization appliances in Class II cases. The 14 included articles were cohort studies. The authors assessed seven studies as high quality, three studies as low quality, and four retrospective studies as moderate quality. The mean molar distalization ranged from 1.8 mm [20] to 6.4 mm [21], with distal tipping of 1.65°–11.3°. The mean distal movement of premolars ranged from 1.75 mm to 5.4 mm, and the retraction movement of incisors varied from 0.1 mm to 2.7 mm.

Evidence Summary

Looking at the evidence collectively, the best available evidence support that TSADs are effective for enhancing anchorage during distalization, and yielded a greater amount of distalization; 3.5–6.4 mm according to Fudalej review [9],

5.1 mm according to Grec et al. [7], 4.8–6.4 according to Al-Thomali et al. [18], 1.8–6.4 mm according to Mohamed et al. [19], 5.35 according to Soheilifar et al. [14], and 3.96 mm according to Bayome et al. [15]. All the aforementioned reviews found that the skeletal anchorage distalization moves the premolar distally when compared to conventional anchorage distalization where anterior anchorage loss was present during distalization. The distal movement of the premolars ranged from 1.75 mm to 5.4 mm in Al-Thomali and Mohamed reviews [18, 19], 0.96 mm in Soheilifar review [14], and 4.01 mm in Grec review [7]. Interestingly, there was a difference between the systematic reviews in regard to similar findings. This difference could be due to the difference in the inclusion criteria, search date, language restriction, and data synthesis. Grec et al. [7] and Soheilifar et al. [14] pooled the data in a meta-analysis, however, the most recent study [14] missed some included trials in Grec et al. review [7], so it provided a slightly different estimate.

Evidence Interpretation

MIs-supported appliances are effective in molar distalization with minimal distal tipping and simultaneous premolar distalization without anchorage loss. So, if the patient is not concerned about any invasive procedure, TSADs are superior to conventional anchorage devices in maxillary molar distalization as TSADs can attain more distalization (up to 6 mm) with limited side effects. In addition to that, the simultaneous premolar distalization (not the case in interradicular TSADs) due to en masse retraction or driftodontics may save the time for correction of buccal and anterior segment Class II relationship.

Viewpoint

Fudalej et al. [9] and Grec et al. [7] reviews are already discussed. Al-Thomali et al. [18] review was a well-conducted study. The limitation of this study was: language restriction, which may lead to language bias. The inclusion criteria have no clear description of the study's design. Most of the included studies were from cohort design that may reduce the quality of the evidence. Also, the inter-rater agreement was low at 0.65, which also increases bias in this review. The author did not provide a meta-analysis for their outcomes due to the heterogeneity without clear justification.

Mohamed et al. review [19] was an ambitious study but with the following limitations; The included studies were from a cohort design, and there was language restriction in the search. Also, the authors did not pool the estimate in meta-analysis due to the heterogeneity with no clear justification.

Soheilifar et al. review [14] has the following limitations: The risk of bias was high in the included studies. There was a methodological clinical heterogeneity as the authors included two controlled trials and three retrospective studies that reduced the quality of the evidence. Also, the authors reported that there was a clinical heterogeneity. The meta-analysis showed a high statistical heterogeneity $I^2 \geq 80\%$ that may provide misleading results and misinterpretation.

Bayome et al. review [15] included two RCTs with unclear risk of bias, and seven non-randomized studies of moderate quality that may provide low-quality evidence. However, pooling single-arm studies in a meta-analysis may be questionable due to a potential bias and diversity in study designs. Also, the authors reported that the included studies used different measure methods that may increase the clinical heterogeneity.

The evidence quality of the included studies in these reviews [7, 9, 14, 15, 18, 19], varies from low to high and is mostly downgraded by its design, which may suggest an absence of a high-quality evidence. As such, further research is likely to have an impact on our confidence in the estimate of the effect that may change the future treatment.

TSADs Placement and Distalization

Clinical Question 8: What Should Be the Ideal Location of TSADs during Distalization: Palatal, Buccal, or Infrazygomatic?

Evidence

Systematic Review and Meta-Analysis
Bayome/2021 [15]

This systematic review has been discussed before. Its aim was to evaluate the effectiveness of buccally or palatally placed TSADs in maxillary molar distalization. The reviewers included nine trials; two trials used interradicular MIs, five trials used infrazygomatic TSADs, and two trials used palatal MIs. The average maxillary molar distalization was 4.07 mm (95%CI:3.42–4.72, $p < 0.001$, 2 trials) in palatal bone anchored appliance (pendulum), 4.17 mm (95%CI: 3.02–5.3, $p < 0.001$, 5 trials) using infrazygomatic TSADs, and 2.75 mm (95%CI: 1.07–4.4, $p = 0.001$, 3 trials) using interradicular MIs. The associated distal tipping of the molar was 11.17° (95%CI:9.9°–12.5°, $p < 0.001$,2 trials) in the palatal MIs group, 3.99° (95%CI:1.4°–6.6°, $p < 0.001$, 5 trials) in the infrazygomatic TSADs group, and 1.7° (95%CI:1°–2.4°, $p < 0.001$, 3 trials) using interradicular MIs. The duration of molar distalization was 5.3 months (95%CI:4.7–5.9, one trial) using palatal anchored appliances, 6.7 months (95%CI:4.4–8.9, 4 trials) using infrazygomatic TSADs, and 8.2 months (95%CI: 3.96–12.5, 3 trials) using interradicular MIs.

Systematic Review
Mohamed/2018 [19]

As discussed before, this review included 14 cohort studies to evaluate the effectiveness of MIs-supported molar distalization appliances in Class II cases.

The reviewers found that the molar distalization was greater in palatal MIs-supported pendulum appliance (6.4 ± 1.3 mm, $p = 0.005$, 10 participants) [21] than the distalization using a single interradicular MIs (1.8 mm) [20].

Evidence Summary

The best available evidence suggests that the first molar distalization was 4.17 mm using infrazygomatic TSADs, 4.07 mm using palatal MIs, and 2.75 mm using buccal inter radicular MIs according to Bayome [15]. This distalization was 6.4 mm and 1.8 mm using MIs-supported pendulum appliance and interradicular MIs, respectively, in another qualitative review [19]. The molar tipping was 3.99° in infrazygomatic TSADs studies, 11.17° using palatal MIs, and 1.70° using buccal interradicular MIs. First molar distalization was achieved in 6.7 months using infrazygomatic TSADs, 5.3 months using palatal MIs, and 8.2 months using buccal interradicular MIs.

Evidence Interpretation

Infrazygomatic and palatal TSADs are more effective in molar distalization than interradicular TSADs. The palatal TSADs are associated with decreased treatment duration than Infrazygomatic and interradicular TSADs, but with increased distal molar tipping. For the bodily molar distalization up to half-cusp, Infrazygomatic TSADs can be given. But if some distal tipping of the molar is permissible palatal TSADs are more effective, but on the downside they may be associated with some bite opening. Buccal interradicular MIs can be used for a small amount of distalization, as their position would hinder the simultaneous distal movement of the adjacent teeth.

Viewpoint

The aforementioned reviews have been discussed before. However, Bayome et al. [15] included only a single arm data without comparison between different placed TSADs that may reduce the certainty of the evidence.

Clinical Question 9: Which Is Better One or Two MIs for TSADs Molar Distalization?

Evidence

Randomized Clinical Trial
Bechtold/2013 [20]
This trial investigated the effectiveness of the interradicular MIs number for molar distalization. The authors recruited 25 adult patients with mild to moderate Class II in two groups; 12 participants with a mean age of 23.58 years in single MI group, and 13 participants with mean age of 22.92 years in dual MIs group. Each MI was given approximately 200-gram force in both groups. The molar distalization was statistically greater in the dual MIs group (2.9 ± 0.96 mm) compared to the single MI group (1.29 ± 0.66 mm) $P < 0.001$. The associated molar tipping was greater in single MI group, but not statistically significant 3.19° ± 4.61 and 1.55° ± 1.32 in single and dual MIs groups, respectively. The associated intrusion was statistically greater in dual group 1.4 ± 0.99 mm than single MI group 0.84 ± 1.09 mm ($p < 0.05$). The success rate of MIs was similar between single (87.5%) and dual MIs groups (86.5%).

Evidence Summary

The best available evidence suggests that dual interradicular MIs are more effective in molar distalization (2.9 mm) when compared to single interradicular MI (1.29 mm). Also, the molar tipping was greater in single MI group (3.19°) than the dual MIs group (1.55°), with a greater amount of intrusion in dual MIs group by 0.56 mm. It is noteworthy that a higher force was used in the dual MIs group.

Evidence Interpretation

First of all, it is important to mention that this evidence is for interradicular MIs only as no study till the writing of this book have been done on the ideal number of TADs at other locations. According to the present evidence, dual MIs-supported appliances can achieve greater distalization than placing a single screw.

Though not related to present evidence but depending upon appliance design a single MI has great chance of failure if the line of action of force causes rotation of screw around its axis. This mostly happens when extension arms are directly attached to the MI and their activation causes unscrewing the MIs. However, in dual MIs-supported distalization appliances, the rotation of the appliance or the screw is counteracted by the other screw. In single screw-supported distalization appliance, the rotation of the appliance around the screw can only be prevented by a good-fit analog-type assembly that can be adjusted over the MI head.

Viewpoint

Bechtold et al. trial [20] has some shortcomings which may downgrade the level of the evidence; The lack of information regarding the severity of Class II, the difference in the applied force on each side, and the difference in the amount of force between groups may confound the results. The lack of a sample size calculation may result in an underpowered study. Due to the methodology of the study, this evidence provides low evidence, and it would be more reasonable to take this evidence for force level than two versus single MIs. The conclusion from this study can be 400 grams per side would be more effective than 200 grams per side for en-masse distalization of whole arch. As such, further RCTs are required to increase the certainty of the effect of the estimate.

Molar Distalization and Aligners

Clinical Question 10: Can we Distalize Upper Molars by Using Aligners and Class II Elastics?

Evidence

Retrospective Study
Ravera/2016 [22]
This study investigated molar distalization by using aligners in 20 Caucasian adult patients (9 males, 11 females; mean age of 29.73 ± 6.89). The distalization was

done by sequential distalization of 0.25 mm per stage of aligners with Class II elastics (1/4 in., 4.5 oz) to reinforce the anchorage. The number of required aligners were 42.6 ± 4.4 and 21.4 ± 3.2 for the upper and the lower arch, respectively. The authors reported that the mean treatment time was 24.3 ± 4.2 months, and the first molar distal movement was 2.25 mm without significant tipping or vertical movements. The second molar distal movement was 2.52 mm, without significant tipping or vertical movements.

Evidence Summary

The available evidence suggests that aligner therapy in association with composite attachments and Class II elastics can distalize maxillary first molars by 2.25 mm without significant tipping or vertical movements of the crown. No changes in the facial height were noticed.

Evidence Interpretation

In light of present low-quality evidence, up to 2.25 mm of maxillary molar distalization can be achieved by aligner therapy.

Viewpoint

The study is classified as low-quality evidence. The retrospective study design and the small sample size downgraded the evidence. There was no clear description of the malocclusion itself in the recruited patients, which may increase the mystery regarding the confounder factors. The authors used a t-test, but it was better to use a paired t-test in this study as the data were correlated. For applicability, the study comprised adult patients with half-cusp molar relationship, average divergence pattern (SN/GoGn angle less than 37°), without molar mesial rotation, and with good compliance.

We are uncertain about the estimate. So, further high-quality research is needed, and it is very likely to have a substantial impact on our confidence that may change the estimate.

Molar Distalization Time

Clinical Question 11: How Much Time Duration Is Needed to Distalize Maxillary Molars Using a Non-compliance Intraoral Distalizing Appliance?

Evidence

Systematic Review and MetaAanalysis
Bayome/2021 [15]

This systematic review has been discussed before. The review evaluated the effectiveness of buccally and palatally placed TSADs in maxillary molar distalization. The overall duration for molar distalization was 5.45 months (95%CI: 4.86–6.05, 8 trials). The subgroup analysis indicated that the duration was 5.3 months (95%CI:4.7–5.9, one trial) in palatal TSADs, and 6.7 months (95%CI:4.4–8.9, 4 trials) using infrazygomatic TSADs to correct half-cusp. While it was 8.2 months (95%CI:4–12.5, 3 trials) using interradicular MIs to correct 2.75 mm of molar relationship.

Bellini-Pereira/2019 [23]

A systematic review and meta-analysis included two randomized controlled trials and seven controlled clinical trials. The quality of the included studies ranged from low to high according to the risk of bias assessment. The meta-analysis showed that 8.34 months (95% CI: 6.10, 10.58, p<0.001, $I^2 = 97\%$, 4 trials) are necessary to correct a half-to-full cusp Class II molar relationship in the growing patients (11–14 years) regardless of the type of the anchorage of the appliance. The authors indicated that the amount of molar distalization is directly associated with distalization time; the time for distalization was 6.10 months (95%CI: 4.82–7.38, 3 trials) when the distalization amount was less than 3.5 mm, while it was 11.27 months (95%CI:7.91–14.62, 2 trials) when the amount was more than 3.5 mm, and this difference was statistically significant. The distalization took more time in the palatal MIs 11.27 months (95%CI: 7.91–14.62, 2 trials) when compared to the buccal MIs 7.07 months (95%CI:3.25–10.89, 2 trials).

Soheilifar/2019 [14]

This systematic review compared conventional and skeletal anchorage in maxillary molar distalization and found that the mean treatment time was 7.95 months (4.25 mm distalization) in the conventional group and 8.23 months (5.35 mm distalization) in the skeletal anchorage group. The mean difference between the TSADs and conventional anchorage was 1.12 months (95%CI:0.56–1.69, 4 trials, $p < 0.001$, $I^2 = 84\%$), favoring TSADs with no significant difference in the mean molar distalization.

Grec RH/2013 [7]

This systematic review has studied the effects of skeletal anchorage on molar distalization, which found that the mean treatment time was 6–7 months (3.34 mm distalization) in the conventional anchorage group and 5–7.8 months (5.1 mm distalization) in the skeletal anchorage group.

Systematic Review
Mohamed/2018 [19]

This systematic review evaluated the skeletal anchorage and the maxillary molar distalization. However, the treatment duration varied from 4.6 months to 11.27 months to achieve 1.8–6.4 mm molar distalization.

Evidence Summary

The summary of evidence supports that the correction of a half-to-full cusp Class II molar relationship with intraoral distalization can be achieved in (5–11) months, and the type of anchorage used, whether conventional or skeletal, may not influence the distalization time. The duration of distalization is related to the amount of distalization needed.

Evidence Interpretation

To distalize half-to-full cusp molar Class II relationship in growing patients, you need 9 ± 3 months regardless of the anchorage type. The greater the amount of distalization required, more would be the duration of distalization.

Type of anchorage, though has a little role in the duration of distalization, but it does play a more significant role in the overall duration of treatment. Skeletal anchorage, which does not hinder root movement during distalization, provides the further advantage of simultaneous distal movement of premolars during distalization, thus decreasing the overall treatment duration. Also, there is no anterior anchorage loss during distalization with skeletal anchorage, so there is less round tripping of the incisors.

Viewpoint

Bellini-Pereira [23]review is a well-conducted review. The included studies were graded as low quality due to the high risk of bias in most studies. The seven controlled trials were more prone to selection bias and confounding factors. Finally, the statistical heterogeneity was too high, and this may result in misleading results; thus, the findings of this meta-analysis should be taken with caution. Other reviews for this question are already discussed.

Further high-quality research is needed to increase the robustness of the results, mainly through well-designed studies comparing different types of anchorage.

Growth Pattern and Molar Distalization

Clinical Question 12: Can we Distalize Molars in Increased Vertical Growth Pattern Patients?

Evidence

Systematic Review and Meta-Analysis
Bayome/2021 [15]

This systematic review assessed the molar intrusion during the maxillary molar distalization using TSADs. Meta-analysis concluded that the overall vertical molar movement was an intrusion by 0.6 mm (95%CI:0.47–0.8, 9 trials) using different types of TSADs. The intrusion was 0.64 mm, 0.6 mm, and 0.69 mm using palatal, infrazygomatic, and buccal interradicular TSADs, respectively.

Systematic Review
Al-Thomali/2017 [18]

In this systematic review, the authors found that the vertical movement of the maxillary molars was minimal regardless of the growth pattern, and the Pendulum appliance caused intrusion of 0.10–1.68 mm. Otherwise, some included studies showed extrusion of maxillary molars, and the mean values varied from 0.1 to 1.75 mm.

Mohamed/2018 [19]

This systematic review of cohort studies evaluated MIs-supported appliance effects for maxillary molar distalization in Class II malocclusion regardless of growth pattern. Interestingly, the vertical movement of the maxillary molar was minimal, and the MIs-supported appliances caused both maxillary molar intrusion and extrusion. The mean rate of intrusion varied from 0.1 mm to 1.4 mm while extrusion mean values varied from 0.1 mm to 2.7 mm.

Randomized Controlled Trial
Bondemark/2005 [10]

As discussed before, this trial compared the effectiveness of IOA with the EOA. The trial randomly assigned 40 Class II patients; 20 patients each. The overbite significantly reduced in both groups, with no statistically significant difference between IOA (0.8 ± 0.8 mm) and EOA (0.7 ± 0.72 mm).

Retrospective Cohort Study
Godt/2005 [24]

This is a retrospective analysis of 86 adolescents' cast models before and after treatment. The study found that the distal molar movement using cervical headgear decreased the overbite. The authors reported that the decrease in the overbite was small (0–0.04 mm) and the overbite decreased in average patterns more than in increased vertical patterns. However, this study found that there is no change in the vertical dimension.

Evidence Summary

Looking at the evidence collectively, the best available evidence concluded that the vertical movement during molar distalization is not predictable [18, 19] as there was either decrease or increase in the overbite due to the appliance used. Bayome et al. [15] found associated molar intrusion (0.6 mm) while using different types of TSADs, while there was a decrease in the overbite in both IOA and EOA in one RCT [10].On the other hand, a low-level evidence [25] revealed that there is no change in the vertical dimension during distalization.

Evidence Interpretation

The present evidence is inconclusive regarding the effect of distalization on the vertical dimension, which may depend upon the line action of force and the vertical component of applied force.

From a clinical perspective, if the line of action of force passes below the center of resistance of the molars, it will cause extrusion of the molars along with its distalization. This is usually a case when one does distalization with low-pull headgear. However, if the line of action of the force passes through the center of resistance of the molar it will cause bodily movement. This is usually a case with Nance or implant-supported distal jets where the line of action of the force is at the level of the center of resistance with no vertical force. For appliances where a line of action of force passes above the center of resistance with a vertical component of force, there would be an intrusion of the molars and increase in overbite. Such type of distalization can be done with help of infrazygomatic TSADs.

Viewpoint

All the systematic reviews are previously discussed. Godt [24] study is a retrospective study. This design is more prone to confounders and selection bias. Furthermore, the measurement method was not valid as the authors investigated the molar relationship on the study models to measure the molar distalization capacity. There was a lack of information about the blinding, the baseline patients' characteristics, and the confounding factors in the malocclusion. The unpaired t-test is not the right choice for this study as the researchers compared the change in the same patients, which calls for a paired t-test. As such, the evidence collectively varied from low to high-level quality. There were many retrospective studies without comparison groups, and the available studies did not investigate the relationship between the growth pattern and the molar distalization. So, there is a need for further well-conducted trials as we are very uncertain about the estimate.

The Stage of Second or Third Molar Eruption and the Upper First Molar Distalization

Clinical Question 13: What Is the Effect of the Second or Third Molar Eruption Stage on the Upper First Molar Distalization?

Evidence

Systematic Review
Flores-Mir/2013 [26]
This evidence is based on low-level four studies; three of them were from retrospective design, and one was a prospective study. Three studies found that molar distalization time was not significantly affected by the second or third molar eruption. These studies used the pendulum appliance. On the other hand, one retrospective study [27] used Ni-Ti coil appliance with Nance, and found that the treatment time for the distal molar movement was significantly shorter before the second molar eruption (5.2 months) when compared to the duration after the second molar eruption (6.5 months). Likewise, the same study [27] found that the mean amount of distal molar movement was greater before the second molar eruption, 3.3 mm versus 2.2 mm after the second molar eruption. The anchorage loss was significantly greater after the second molar eruption, 0.82 mm versus 0.27 mm for every 1 mm distal movement before the second molar eruption [27].

Non-Randomized Clinical Trial
Kinzinger/2004 [28]
This clinical trial divided the patinates into three groups; the first group: the second molar has not erupted, the second group: the second molar has erupted, and the third

group: the second molar has erupted, and the authors have done germectomy to the third molar (the extraction of the third molar tooth bud). This study found that the first molar distal tipping was less in patients with erupted second molars ($0.9° \pm 3.43°$) than in those whose second molars were not yet erupted ($5.89° \pm 3.74°$), but the lowest tipping was in the third molar germectomy group ($0.33° \pm 0.58°$).

Also, there was less incisor protrusion in the non-erupted second molar group ($3.28° \pm 1.97°$ and $2.89° \pm 2.17°$ to the palatal plane and anterior cranium floor, respectively) than in other groups ($5.5° \pm 3.33°$ and $6.03° \pm 4.29°$ for the second group, and $5.5° \pm 3.28°$ and $6.67° \pm 3.09°$ for the third group).

Interestingly, the mean first molar distal movement was 3.16 mm in the non-erupted second molar group, 3.21 mm in the erupted second molar group, and 2.70 in the third group, with no statistical difference between groups.

Retrospective Study
Flores-Mir/2013 [29]
This study has evaluated the lateral cephalogram changes in the position of the maxillary first molar based on the eruption of maxillary second molars during distalization with the XBow appliance (fixed functional appliance). The statistical analysis showed that the eruption stage of the second molar did not have a significant effect on the horizontal distalization of the maxillary first molar ($P = 0.16$). In the non-erupted second molar group, the mean molar distalization was 1.7 ± 1.1 mm with $3.1° \pm 2.7$ tipping, while it was 1.6 ± 0.6 mm with $3.1° \pm 2.3$ tipping in the erupted second molar group with no statistically significant difference between groups. Interestingly, there was a significant effect of the Class II severity on the molar distalization (Wilk's lambda = 0.8, eta^2 = 0.19, $p < 0.001$).

Evidence Summary
Looking at the evidence collectively, the best available evidence concluded that the molar distalization is not affected by the second or third molar eruption, and there is no difference in the quantity or quality of distalization in patients with erupted and unerupted maxillary second molars. However, Kinzinger study [28] concluded that the best time to start therapy is before the eruption of the second molars. On the other hand, one retrospective study [27] reported that the molar distalization was greater before the second molar eruption (3.3 mm) versus (2.2 mm) after the second molar eruption. Interestingly, Flores-Mir et al. [29] found that the pre-treatment Class II severity has a significant effect on the maxillary first molar.

Evidence Interpretation
The effect of the second or third molar eruption stage on the upper first molar distalization is negligible, but slightly greater distalization is achieved if the second or third molars have not erupted. As such, in the absence of high quality evidence, the general clinical perception is that more the number of teeth to be distalized more would be the anchorage demand.

Presently there are no studies on whether to extract the second or third molar to make the distalization more effective. So, the clinician should make this decision on their experience, patient expectation, and available circumstances. Also, molar distalization at an early age with the second molar not erupted is usually easier but many times after distalization there is not enough space for the second molar eruptions. The orthodontist must keep these factors into consideration while distalizing the first molars.

Viewpoint

Flores-Mir et al. review [26] was a well-conducted study. As the authors pointed out some limitations in their review that reduce the quality of the evidence. The design of the three studies was retrospective with inadequate reporting for the sample size or intention to treat analysis. The methodological heterogeneity precluded meta-analysis. The baseline differences were confounding factors, especially the sagittal molar relationship, as it is well known that correction of full cusp Class II molar relationship requires more movement and time than correction of cusp-to-cusp relationship and this confounds the effect of second molar eruption on the distalization amount. As such, the included studies have inconsistency and variability in the results. Karlsson study [27] which was a part of the systematic review [26], may have suffered from inadequate statistical analysis and there is a chance of false-positive results. Kinzinger et al. trial [28] was a non-randomized study that may arise selection bias, as the groups were not identical at the baseline. Also, unmeasured confounding may arise regarding the severity of Class II and the crowding which have not been measured at all or not controlled for in the analysis. As a result, these studies are of low quality and further research is very likely to have an important impact on our confidence and is likely to change the estimate.

Flores-Mir study [29] was an ambitious study, which used a fixed functional appliance for distalization. There were gender differences between groups, but the authors did a regression analysis to isolate the effect of this confounder on the outcome. In general, the retrospective design has a limitation related to recall and selection bias, as the patients without full records and good final results were included in the study, and patients who failed to follow up and did not get good final results were excluded from the study. Additionally, the age of patient and the anchorage requirements may be confounding factors in this study. For the applicability, there is no effect of second molar eruption in mild Class II cases with up to 4 mm molar distalization, especially when using the XBow appliance.

Force Level for Molar Distalization

Clinical Question 14: What Is the Optimal Force for Upper Molar Distalization?

Evidence

Systematic Review and Meta-Analysis
Jambi/2013 [4]

As discussed before, this systematic review compared IOA with EOA and concluded that the average amount of distal molar movement was 1.04 and 2.2 mm, using headgear and intraoral distalization appliances, respectively. The force level in IOA was 230 grams for the activated Pendulum appliance in one included RCT [30] for each side. While the force level in EOA was 400 grams [10, 30], 150–300 grams [31], and 500 grams[32] for each side.

Fudalej/2011 [9]

In this systematic review which has been discussed before, the authors investigated the efficacy of using different types of TSADs (MIs and MPs) in maxillary molar distalization. They concluded that the mean molar distalization ranged from 3.5 to 6.4 mm and the included studies used a wide range of force magnitudes (150–300 g) with no related analysis of the force level effect on the distalization.

Systematic Review
Al-Thomali/2017 [18]

This systematic review investigated the effectiveness of the pendulum and modified pendulum appliances in molar distalization. The authors found the mean molar distalization ranged from 2 to 6.4 mm with a wide range of applied force from 180 to 500 grams in the included trials.

Randomized Controlled Trial
Bechtold/2013

In this RCT, the authors compared the efficacy of using one interradicular MI versus two MIs to apply force to the fixed appliance by archwire hook. They used different force levels between groups. The force was 200 grams in the one MI group and 400 grams in the two MIs group. The authors found that the distal movement comprised the whole arch (incisor crown, molar crown, and distal molar root) in both groups. Interestingly, a statistically significant distal movement of the molar was achieved in the two MIs group (2.91 ± 0.96 mm) when compared with the one MI group (1.29 ± 066 mm, $p < 0.001$) in the trial period with a less but not statistically significant tipping in the two MIs group (1.55° ± 1.32 vs. 3.19° ± 4.6, in two and one MIs groups, respectively).

Evidence Summary

The best available evidence suggests that there is a wide range of applied forces for the maxillary molar distalization. The force level ranged from 150 to 500 grams for each side in EOA, [4] 180 to 500 grams [4, 18] in IOA and 150 to 300 grams [9] when TSADs were used. Heavy force (400 g) was associated with greater amount of distalization (2.91 ± 0.96 mm) compared to the lighter force levels of 200 gs (1.29 ± 066 mm).

Evidence Interpretation

As the evidence did not correlate the amount of the distalization with the applied force level, there is no answer for the optimal force that the clinician can use. In addition to that, there is a lack of information regarding the harmful effects of the high force levels or the ineffective force for the maxillary molar distalization.

Viewpoint

All the mentioned studies have been discussed previously.

The Maxillary Sinus and the Upper Molar Distalization

Clinical Question 15: Can we Move the Teeth through the Maxillary Sinus?

Evidence

Systematic Review

Sun/2018 [33] This systematic review found only nine case reports investigating moving teeth through the maxillary sinus (MTTMS), although these reports have a high risk of bias, they remain the best available evidence on this topic till now. These cases showed that the teeth movement through maxillary sinus varied between 0.16 mm and 1.17 mm per month for premolars and 0.05 and 0.16 mm per month for molars. Almost all the authors of the case reports have stated that the overall translation consisted of tipping followed by uprighting with a normal risk of orthodontic-induced root resorption.

Evidence Summary

Low-quality evidence suggests that teeth roots can move through the sinus. But there is no evidence-based protocol that can be recommended to guide MTTMS due to the absence of evidence.

Evidence Interpretation

Teeth sinus relationship should be taken into account while planning for molar distalization. If the roots maxillary first or second molars are in the sinus, avoid tooth distalization, or expect less amount of distalization or more distal tipping in more time. The patient should be made aware of this, and proper informed consent should be taken.

Viewpoint

This conclusion should be interpreted with caution as the current systematic review[33] is based on only very low evidence with inherent bias (case reports), and we are very uncertain about the estimate. Further research with a high-quality design and long-term follow up is needed to be confident about the estimate.

Author's Recommendations

- Molar distalization is an effective method for creating the space in the arch, for relief of crowding and correction of Class II molar relationship.
- Intraoral appliances should be preferred over extraoral appliances. Extraoral appliances can be used when their orthopedic effects are desired.

- Skeletal anchorage is better than conventional anchorage as a greater amount of distalization can be achieved. For skeletal anchorage, use palatal-supported frictionless distalization appliances. These appliances give the added benefit of simultaneous leveling, alignment, and space closure. Infrazygomatic TSADs can also be given for en masse distalization, but their use is limited by racial variations, availability of site, resources, and increased failure rate.

- Clinically presence of an additional distal tooth can add to the anchorage requirement. So, extracting the third molar will help in distalization if a greater amount of distalization is required. If the second molar is not erupted, its position should be monitored during distalization of first molar as it might lead to impaction or deviated path of eruption of second molar.

- When the Class II molar relationship is due to skeletal components, it would be better to use orthopedic or functional appliances in young patients rather than doing distalization.

- The greater the amount of distalization required, the greater would be the distalization time period. If roots of the maxillary molars are within the sinuses, more time would be required to distalize the teeth.

- Aligner with attachments can only be used when a small amount of distalization, ideally up to 2 mm, is required. The force level of intraoral appliances ideally should not exceed 300 grams/side, while for extraoral appliances it should be less than 500 grams.

References

1. Kingsley N. Jumping the bite. Dent Cosmos. 1892;33:788.
2. Antonarakis GS, Kiliaridis S. Maxillary molar distalization with noncompliance intramaxillary appliances in class II malocclusion. A systematic review. Angle Orthod. 2008;78(6):1133–40. https://doi.org/10.2319/101507-406.1.
3. Amasyali M, Sabuncuoglu FA, Oflaz U. Intraoral molar distalization with intraosseous mini screw. Turk J Orthod. 2018;31(1):26–30. https://doi.org/10.5152/TurkJOrthod.2018.17030.
4. Jambi S, Thiruvenkatachari B, O'Brien KD, Walsh T. Orthodontic treatment for distalising upper first molars in children and adolescents. Cochrane Database Syst Rev. 2013;10:CD008375. https://doi.org/10.1002/14651858.CD008375.pub2.
5. Papadopoulos MA, Melkos AB, Athanasiou AE. Noncompliance maxillary molar distalization with the first class appliance: a randomized controlled trial. Am J Orthod Dentofacial Orthop: official publication of the American Association of Orthodontists, its constituent societies, and the American Board of Orthodontics. 2010;137(5):586 e1–e13. https://doi.org/10.1016/j.ajodo.2009.10.033.
6. Keles A. Maxillary unilateral molar distalization with sliding mechanics: a preliminary investigation. Eur J Orthod. 2001;23(5):507–15.
7. Grec RH, Janson G, Branco NC, Moura-Grec PG, Patel MP, Castanha Henriques JF. Intraoral distalizer effects with conventional and skeletal anchorage: a meta-analysis. Am J Orthod Dentofacial Orthop: official publication of the American Association of Orthodontists, its constituent societies, and the American Board of Orthodontics. 2013;143(5):602–15. https://doi.org/10.1016/j.ajodo.2012.11.024.
8. Atherton GJ, Glenny AM, O'Brien K. Development and use of a taxonomy to carry out a systematic review of the literature on methods described to effect distal movement of maxillary molars. J Orthod. 2002;29(3):211–6; discussion 195–6. https://doi.org/10.1093/ortho/29.3.211.

9. Fudalej P, Antoszewska J. Are orthodontic distalizers reinforced with the temporary skeletal anchorage devices effective? Am J Orthod Dentofacial Orthop: official publication of the American Association of Orthodontists, its constituent societies, and the American Board of Orthodontics. 2011;139(6):722–9. https://doi.org/10.1016/j.ajodo.2011.01.019.

10. Bondemark L, Karlsson I. Extraoral vs intraoral appliance for distal movement of maxillary first molars: a randomized controlled trial. Angle Orthod. 2005;75(5):699–706.

11. Patel MP, Janson G, Henriques JF, de Almeida RR, de Freitas MR, Pinzan A, et al. Comparative distalization effects of Jones jig and pendulum appliances. Am J Orthod Dentofac Orthop. 2009;135(3):336–42. https://doi.org/10.1016/j.ajodo.2007.01.035.

12. Paul L, O'Brien K, Mandall N. Upper removable appliance or Jones jig for distalizing first molars? A randomized clinical trial. Orthod Craniofacial Res. 2002;5(4):238–42.

13. Burhan AS. Combined treatment with headgear and the frog appliance for maxillary molar distalization: a randomized controlled trial. Korean J Orthod. 2013;43(2):101–9. https://doi.org/10.4041/kjod.2013.43.2.101.

14. Soheilifar S, Mohebi S, Ameli N. Maxillary molar distalization using conventional versus skeletal anchorage devices: a systematic review and meta-analysis. Int Orthod. 2019;17(3):415–24. https://doi.org/10.1016/j.ortho.2019.06.002.

15. Bayome M, Park JH, Bay C, Kook YA. Distalization of maxillary molars using temporary skeletal anchorage devices: a systematic review and meta-analysis. Orthod Craniofac Res. 2021;24(Suppl 1):103–12. https://doi.org/10.1111/ocr.12470.

16. Cornelis MA, De Clerck HJ. Maxillary molar distalization with miniplates assessed on digital models: a prospective clinical trial. Am J Orthod Dentofac Orthop. 2007;132(3):373–7. https://doi.org/10.1016/j.ajodo.2007.04.031.

17. Oberti G, Villegas C, Ealo M, Palacio JC, Baccetti T. Maxillary molar distalization with the dual-force distalizer supported by mini-implants: a clinical study. Am J Orthod Dentofac Orthop. 2009;135(3):282.e1–5; discussion -3. https://doi.org/10.1016/j.ajodo.2008.11.018.

18. Al-Thomali Y, Basha S, Mohamed RN. Pendulum and modified pendulum appliances for maxillary molar distalization in class II malocclusion - a systematic review. Acta Odontol Scand. 2017;75(6):394–401. https://doi.org/10.1080/00016357.2017.1324636.

19. Mohamed RN, Basha S, Al-Thomali Y. Maxillary molar distalization with miniscrew-supported appliances in class II malocclusion: a systematic review. Angle Orthod. 2018;88(4):494–502. https://doi.org/10.2319/091717-624.1.

20. Bechtold TE, Kim JW, Choi TH, Park YC, Lee KJ. Distalization pattern of the maxillary arch depending on the number of orthodontic miniscrews. Angle Orthod. 2013;83(2):266–73. https://doi.org/10.2319/032212-123.1.

21. Kircelli BH, Pektas ZO, Kircelli C. Maxillary molar distalization with a bone-anchored pendulum appliance. Angle Orthod. 2006;76(4):650–9. https://doi.org/10.1043/0003-3219(2006)076[0650:MMDWAB]2.0.CO;2.

22. Ravera S, Castroflorio T, Garino F, Daher S, Cugliari G, Deregibus A. Maxillary molar distalization with aligners in adult patients: a multicenter retrospective study. Prog Orthod. 2016;17:12. https://doi.org/10.1186/s40510-016-0126-0.

23. Bellini-Pereira SA, Pupulim DC, Aliaga-Del Castillo A, Henriques JFC, Janson G. Time of maxillary molar distalization with non-compliance intraoral distalizing appliances: a meta-analysis. Eur J Orthod. 2019;41(6):652–60. https://doi.org/10.1093/ejo/cjz030.

24. Godt A, Kalwitzki M, Goz G. Retrospective analysis of casts to assess cervical headgear treatment in the presence of vertical growth pattern. J Orofac Orthop. 2005;66(3):230–40. https://doi.org/10.1007/s00056-005-0433-4.

25. Godt A, Kalwitzki M, Göz G. Retrospective analysis of casts to assess cervical headgear treatment in the presence of vertical growth pattern. J Orofac Orthop / Fortschritte der Kieferorthopädie. 2005;66(3):230–40. https://doi.org/10.1007/s00056-005-0433-4.

26. Flores-Mir C, McGrath L, Heo G, Major PW. Efficiency of molar distalization associated with second and third molar eruption stage. Angle Orthod. 2013;83(4):735–42. https://doi.org/10.2319/081612-658.1.

27. Karlsson I, Bondemark L. Intraoral maxillary molar distalization. Angle Orthod. 2006; 76(6):923–9. https://doi.org/10.2319/110805-390.
28. Kinzinger GS, Fritz UB, Sander FG, Diedrich PR. Efficiency of a pendulum appliance for molar distalization related to second and third molar eruption stage. Am Orthod Dentofacial Orthop: official publication of the American Association of Orthodontists, its constituent societies, and the American Board of Orthodontics. 2004;125(1):8–23. https://doi.org/10.1016/j.ajodo.2003.02.002.
29. Flores-Mir C, McGrath LM, Heo G, Major PW. Efficiency of molar distalization with the XBow appliance related to second molar eruption stage. Eur J Orthod. 2013;35(6):745–51. https://doi.org/10.1093/ejo/cjs090.
30. Acar AG, Gürsoy S, Dinçer M. Molar distalization with a pendulum appliance K-loop combination. Eur J Orthod. 2010;32(4):459–65. https://doi.org/10.1093/ejo/cjp136.
31. de Oliveira JN Jr, de Almeida RR, Rodrigues de Almeida M, de Oliveira JN. Dentoskeletal changes induced by the Jasper jumper and cervical headgear appliances followed by fixed orthodontic treatment. Am J Orthod Dentofac Orthop. 2007;132(1):54–62. https://doi.org/10.1016/j.ajodo.2005.07.028.
32. Toy E, Enacar A. The effects of the pendulum distalising appliance and cervical headgear on the dentofacial structures. Aust Orthod J. 2011;27(1):10–6.
33. Sun W, Xia K, Huang X, Cen X, Liu Q, Liu J. Knowledge of orthodontic tooth movement through the maxillary sinus: a systematic review. BMC Oral Health. 2018;18(1):91. https://doi.org/10.1186/s12903-018-0551-1.

3

Growth Modification Treatment in Class II Malocclusion

Contents

© The Author(s), under exclusive license to Springer Nature Switzerland AG 2023   43
S. Mheissen, H. Khan, *Orthodontic Evidence*,
https://doi.org/10.1007/978-3-031-24422-3_3

Abbreviations

CCTs	Controlled clinical trials
CVMs	Cervical vertebra maturation stages
div	Division
F	Female
FA	Forsus appliance alone
FFA	Fixed functional appliances
FMP	Forsus appliance with skeletal miniplate anchorage
FR-2	Fränkel-2
FT	Full time
HG	Headgear
HWM	Hand writs method
M	Male
MB	Modified Bionator
MIsHA	Miniscrews supported Herbst appliance
mo	Month
NSTB	non-Southend clasps TB
OB	Overbite
OJ	Overjet

PT   Part time
RFA   Removable functional appliances
SCTB   Southend clasp TB
TB   Twin block
TFBC   Twin Force Bite Corrector
TMJ   Temporomandibular joint

Introduction

Class II malocclusion is a prevalent problem in orthodontics involving 23–26% of Caucasians in mixed dentition [1]. Class II malocclusion has molars mostly in Class II relationships, while the incisor relationship can be either Class II division 1 or division 2. Class II division 1 is more common than class II division 2 as in the United Kingdom, one-quarter of children at 12 years of age have prominent maxillary incisors [2]. The etiology of Class II malocclusion is multifactorial, with both genetic and environmental factors involved. The malocclusion can have a dental or skeletal origin, or it can be a combination of both [3, 4]. There are many philosophies for Class II treatment; growth modification at the early stage (two phases) versus growth modification at a late stage (one phase), camouflage in permanent dentition, and orthognathic surgery [4–6].

Growth modification is an established procedure in orthodontics to modify jaw growth. This is done when the patient is still growing. The theory behind growth modification is that when the bone is exposed to a functional stimulus, it has the capacity to remodel. This functional stimulus is provided by using bite jumping or anterior mandibular advancement appliances in cases of retrognathic mandible or headgears that restrict the growth of the maxilla in case of prognathic maxilla. The proposed benefit of Class II growth modification is that it improves the patient profile by correcting the skeletal and dental relationships of the patient. Theoretically, it would also increase the self-esteem of the patient, provide him with a stable occlusion and decrease the chances of traumatic injuries to the teeth. According to a systematic review [7], children with an overjet larger than 3 mm have approximately twice the chances of trauma to anterior teeth than children with an overjet smaller than 3 mm, with higher chances of trauma for boys than girls.

There are different methods to achieve the growth modification for skeletal Class II malocclusion:

1. *Orthopedic appliances*, in theory, directly modify jaw growth. These appliances include mostly headgear (HG).
2. *Functional appliances* affect either the mandible position or the muscular environment of the oral cavity to enhance the mandibular growth and restrict the maxillary growth. These appliances include:
   - Fixed functional appliances (FFA) such as Herbst, Sabbagh Universal Spring(SUS), or Jasper Jumper.
   - Removable functional appliances (RFA) like Activator, Twinblock, or Frankel appliance [8, 9].

Growth Modification Prospect

Clinical Question 1: Is Class II Growth Modification Effective?

Evidence

Systematic Reviews and Meta-Analyses
Batista/2018 [10]

In this Cochrane review, seven included trials compared late functional treatment with no treatment and found that the overjet decreased in the fixed functional treatment group by 5.46 mm (MD; −5.46, 95% CI: −6.63 to −4.28; 2 trials, 61 participants) and 4.62 mm (MD; −4.62, 95% CI −5.33 to −3.92; 3 trials, 122 participants) in the removable functional group, respectively, when compared with no treatment group. ANB angle decreased in the removable functional appliance group by 2.37° (MD; −2.37°, 95% CI −3.01 to −1.74; 2 trials, 99 participants) when compared with no treatment group. While the ANB decreased by 0.53° (MD; −0.53°, 95% CI −1.27 to −0.22; 3 trials, 89 participants) with fixed functional appliances versus the control group. The quality of evidence for the findings was low in this review.

Ehsani/2015 [11]

This review investigated the short-term effects of twin block (TB) appliance. The authors included 10 papers; 6 were prospective controlled clinical trials (CCTs), and 4 were retrospective studies. The review found that there was a statistically significant decrease in SNA angle (MD;−0.7°, 95% CI: −1.2 to −0.2, 5 trials) using the TB appliance. An increase in SNB angle (MD; 1.2°, 95% CI: 0.9–1.4, 3 trials) favoring the TB appliance group was also reported, along with an increase in mandibular body length Go-Gn (MD; 2.95 mm, 95% CI: 1.9–4.0, 3 trials). However, the increase in facial height (2.1 ± 0.47 mm, 3 trials) during treatment might reduce the impact of positive changes on the mandible. The dental changes were retroclination of upper incisors (MD; −9.2°, 95% CI: −9.9 to −8.5, 3 trials) and proclination of the lower incisors (MD;3.9°, 95% CI: 1.4–6.3, 3 trials). The risk of bias in most studies was assessed as medium to low, as retrospective studies were included in this review, thus decreasing the level of evidence.

Evidence Summary

Looking at the evidence collectively, the best available evidence supports that the functional treatment is effective in correcting the Class II malocclusion with both skeletal and dental changes when compared with non-treated controls. The skeletal changes are; a reduction in ANB angle by 2.37° and 0.53° in removable (RFA) and fixed functional appliance (FFA) groups, respectively [10]. There was a decrease in SNA angle by 0.7°, an increase in SNB angle by 1.2°, and an increase in mandibular body length Go-Gn by 2.9 due to functional treatment [11]. The dental changes were retroclination of upper incisors by 9.2° and proclination of the lower incisors by 3.9°. The overall reduction of the OJ was 5.46 mm and 4.62 mm in fixed and removable functional appliance groups, respectively.

Evidence Interpretation

Class II growth modification is an effective method to modify jaw growth in growing patients with mild to moderate Class II malocclusion. Functional appliances can effectively reduce overjet by almost 5 mm. Also, functional treatment may reduce the ANB by 2° due to restraining the growth of the maxilla by less than 1° and enhancing the mandible growth by more than 1°.

For young patients with an OJ between 7 and 9 mm, growth modification appliances, ideally removable, should be given to bring the OJ to normal limits. Ideally, cases with proclined upper incisors (Class II division 1) and retroclined lower incisors would have more favorable effects with growth modification treatment. In growing patients with moderate and severe Class II skeletal relationships, functional appliances can still be used, but full skeletal correction cannot be achieved in most cases. The benefit of functional treatment in those patients is that after growth modification, a case of definite surgery might be treated by orthodontic or surgical camouflage, or at least, the future surgical morbidity would be reduced.

Viewpoint

The well-conducted systematic reviews for RCTs represent the highest evidence in the research. As such, Batista et al. review [10] was a well-conducted review published by Cochrane. Interestingly, most of the included studies were at high risk of bias and the author judged that the overall quality of the evidence as low.

Ehsani review [11] was a well-conducted review. However, there were some limitations in this review; there was no information on the inter-rater reliability, which may lead to bias in conducting the review. The authors used a modified tool for risk of bias assessment and reported that the tool is subjective and not validated. There was no information about the risk of bias between studies or grading the level of the evidence. Including retrospective studies, lack of randomization and blinding, and insufficient description of the included studies reduce the overall quality of the evidence. Furthermore, the authors used a random effect model in the forest plot without a clear definition for the statistical heterogeneity measures.

Growth in Class II Patients

Clinical Question 2: What Is the Fate of Patients with Class Malocclusion if Growth Modification Is not Done?

Evidence

Randomized Controlled Trials
Tulloch/1997 [12]
In this randomized controlled trial (RCT), the authors recruited 180 Class II patients with OJ of more than 7 mm. They randomly assigned 166 Class II patients to three groups; 61 patients with OJ of 8.4 mm in the control group, 52 patients with OJ of 8.3 mm in the modified bionator (MB) group, and 52 patients with OJ of 8.3 mm in

HG group. The authors found that the non-treated control group showed minor changes without treatment, as there was no OJ change on average (0.0.9 ± 0.98), but the range of changes was very wide (OJ increased in 50% and decreased in 50% of the control group). Most patients in the treatment groups showed a reduction in ANB, which also happened in many patients in the control group (overall changes: −0.17 ± 0.73). Interestingly, some of the patients in HG group showed an increase in SNA and 20% of patients in the functional group showed mandible growth less than the control group.

Tulloch/1997 [13]

This study is a published paper for the same trial [12]. The author noted that 30% of untreated patients (control) had a favorable growth.

Tulloch/1998 [14]

This study is a published paper for the same trial with different outcomes. The authors reported that 4% of the control group showed favorable growth, and 15% showed unfavorable growth. Also, 75% of the treatment group showed favorable growth.

Evidence Summary

Looking into the evidence collectively, the best available evidence suggests that favorable growth happened in 4–30% of untreated patients. Fifty percent of untreated patients showed OJ improvement, while 50% did not. The functional treatment reduced ANB and OJ, which also happened in many untreated patients.

Evidence Interpretation

It is difficult to predict the future degree of Class II malocclusion in untreated patients due to the unpredictable nature of growth. Favorable growth does happen in untreated patients but there is a wide range of it, and the present evidence is weak. As Class II growth modification is an effective method and is associated with skeletal changes, the clinician should not wait for the chance of favorable growth to happen and should start the treatment when the patient is near his/her pubertal growth spurt. In case if there is favorable growth, it would enhance the treatment effects.

Viewpoint

Tulloch studies [12–14] were well-conducted RCTs, but the allocation concealment was not clear and there was some difference in reporting of the trial many times, which may increase the selected reported outcome bias. The loss to follow-up issue was treated with ITT analysis. For applicability, the mean of ANB Angle was 6.2°with a wide range (0.4°–12.2°) which may be a problem for the internal validity. The mean overjet was 8.4 mm with a wide range (range 7–15 mm) as well.

As these RCTs provide very low evidence, we have very little confidence in their findings, and the true effect of the treatment is likely to be substantially different from this trial's findings.

Success Rate

Clinical Question 3: What Is the Success Rate of Growth Modification Appliances in Class II Malocclusion?

Evidence

Randomized Controlled Trials
Tulloch/1997 [12]

As discussed before, this trial analyzed 166 Class II patients who were either treated using MB or HG, or did not have any treatment as a control group. The researchers found that most patients in treatment groups showed a reduction in ANB. Interestingly, some of the patients in HG group showed an increase in SNA, while 20% of patients in the functional group showed mandible growth less than the control group.

Tulloch/1997 [13]

This trial was discussed before. The author reported that a high percentage (nearly 80%) of treated patients, either with a functional appliance or with HG, had a favorable change in skeletal jaws relationship. However, the authors found that there was no linear relationship between the skeletal response and the severity of the skeletal discrepancy, the growth pattern, and the cooperation of the patients.

Tulloch/1998 [14]

This study has been discussed before. The authors reported that 75% of the treatment group showed favorable growth.

Retrospective Study
Casutt/2007 [15]

The authors collected data of 222 Class II patients from two centers (Giessen and Berne). The patients were treated in three functional treatment groups: 92 patients were treated using the Andresen activator, 72 patients were treated by Herren activator, and 58 patients were treated using Van Beek activator. The average patients' age was 10 and 11.2 years in the two centers. The authors defined success as the net improvement in the sagittal molar relationship of at least half cusp. They found that the success rate was 64% in Giessen center and 66% in Berne center. The functional treatment led to ideal occlusion in 27% of patients and marked improvement in 38% of the patients. The total improvement in the molar relationship has a large inter-individual variation with a range of 0–1.5 cusp widths. Interestingly, there was no improvement at all in the sagittal molar relationship for 5 patients (4%) in Giessen and 7(8%) in Berne. The treatment time was statistically longer by 0.6 years in the successful group than in the failure group. The level of patient cooperation was a significant predictor of the successful treatment; 75% were classified as cooperating well in the success group versus 29% in the failure group ($P < 0.001$).

Evidence Summary

Looking at the evidence collectively, the best available evidence suggests that the success rate of the functional treatment range from 64% to 66% using different functional appliances. Only in 27% of the patient's ideal occlusion was achieved after functional treatment. Favorable growth happened in 75–80% of treated patients by Bionator or HG appliances. Furthermore, 20% of treated patients by Bionator showed less mandibular growth than the untreated control. Some of the treated patients by HG showed an increase in SNA angle.

Evidence Interpretation

The success rate of growth modification is above 60% with most of the patients showing favorable sagittal growth. Favorable growth by this treatment is seen in a wide range of skeletal patterns.

In clinical practice, good cooperation is necessary for successful growth modification, but it does not guarantee favorable results in all cases. The clinician should inform his/her patients and parents that there is a failure in functional treatment in Class II patients by approximately 35%, and good cooperation does not guarantee the favorable outcome.

Viewpoint

Casutt study [15] was from a retrospective design that may lack some patients' records, and it is more prone to selection bias. The success rate in the functional treatment has many confounding factors such as the design of the appliance, the experience of the clinician, and the cooperation and growth stage of the patients. As the researchers could not control or adjust these confounders, this may reduce the confidence in the findings. As such, new evidence may substantially change the success rate of the functional treatment.

Treatment Timing

Clinical Question 4: What Is the Best Time for Growth Modification (Early vs. Late) in Class II Patients?

Evidence

Systematic Reviews and Meta-Analyses
Batista/2018 [10]

This Cochrane systematic review for randomized clinical trials looked for the best time for Class II growth modification. Three included trials compared early treatment in two phases (7–11 years) versus late treatment in one phase (12–16 years) by functional appliances and found that there is no difference between groups in final OJ (MD; 0.21, 95% CI −0.10 to 0.51, $P = 0.18$; 343 participants, low-quality evidence) or ANB (MD; −0.02, 95% CI −0.47 to 0.43; 347 participants, moderate

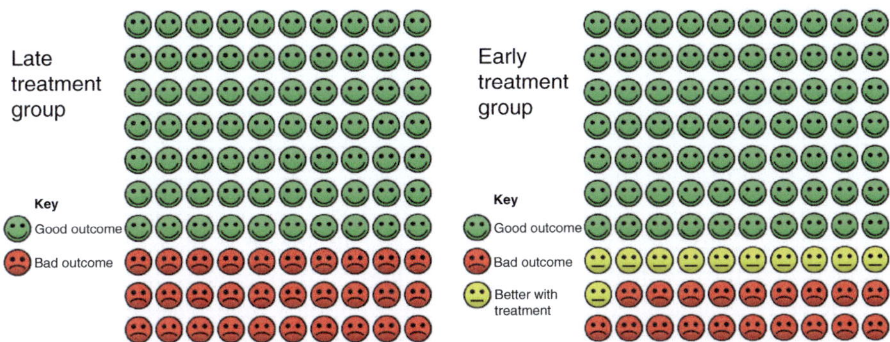

Fig. 3.1 In the late treatment group, 30% of Class II patients had Incisors' trauma, while only 19% in the early treatment group have a new trauma. The red emojis represent the patients who got trauma in the late vs. early treatment group

quality evidence). These studies also concluded with moderate quality evidence that the early treatment with functional appliances had reduced the incidence of incisal trauma (OR; 0.56, 95% CI 0.33–0.95; 332 participants) in comparison with late treatment. So, early treatment has 44% less chance of trauma than late treatment. Incidence of new trauma in the early group was 19% and in the late group was 30% and this difference was clinically significant (Fig. 3.1). Two included studies compared early treatment versus late treatment using HG and found that at the end of treatment there was no difference between groups in OJ (MD; −0.22, 95% CI −0.56 to 0.12; 238 participants, low-quality evidence) and ANB (MD; −0.27, 95% CI −0.80 to 0.26; 231 participants). Also, the early treatment using HG has reduced the incidence of incisal trauma (OR; 0.45, 95% CI 0.25–0.80; 237 participants, low quality) in comparison with the late treatment. Early treatment has no significant difference in self-concept score (MD −3.63, 95% CI −7.66 to 0.40, P value = 0.08; one study, 135 participants).

Perinetti/2015 [16]

This meta-analysis included 11 studies investigating the effectiveness of functional treatment in the pre-pubertal and pubertal growth phases. Researchers found that the skeletal change after removable functional treatment is more effective in the pubertal period. The annual increase in the mandible length was 0.95 mm (96%CI: 0.38–1.51, p = 0.001, 5 trials) and 2.91 mm (95%CI: 2.04–3.79, p < 0.001, 6 trials) in the pre-pubertal and pubertal group, respectively. The annual increase in the mandibular ramus height was 0 mm (95%CI: −0.52 to 0.53, p = 0.99, 3 trials) and 2.18 mm (95%CI: 1.51–2.86, p < 0.001, 4 trials) in the pre-pubertal and pubertal group, respectively. ANB was decreased by 0.73 mm (MD; −0.73, 95%CI: −0.95 to −0.50, p < 0.001, 3 trials) in the pre-pubertal period, and decreased by 2.14 mm (MD; −2.14, 95%CI: −3.09 to −1.18, p < 0.001, 3 trials) in the pubertal period. The evidence was of low quality except for the total mandible and ramus length in the pubertal period, where it was moderate.

Randomized Controlled Trials
O'Brein/2009 [17]

A large multicenter trial evaluated the effects of early versus late treatment with TB in 174 Class II division 1 patients aged 8–10 years. Of them, 89 patients (41 girls, 48 boys) were allocated to the early treatment group and 85 patients (39 girls, 46 boys) to the late treatment group. This study concluded that the final ANB angle was 4.0° ± 2 and 3.8° ± 2.2 for early and late treatment groups, respectively. The overall treatment was statistically longer in the early treatment group than in the late treatment group. Also, the cost of treatment was also greater for the early treatment group because of the additional time. The dental trauma incidence was 8% and 14% for early and late treatment groups, respectively, with no statistical difference.

Tulloch/2004 [18]

This RCT recruited 175 adolescent Class II patients in the mixed dentition stage with OJ ≥7 mm and randomized them into three groups: the combination headgear group, the modified Bionator group, and the observation group. The phase one treatment was followed by a fixed appliance at the permanent dentition stage, and the late treatment group was only treated using a fixed appliance at the permanent dentition stage. At the end of the treatment, the final ANB angle was (3.79° ± 2.12), (4° ± 1.91), and (4.36° ± 2.06) for Bionator, headgear, and late treatment groups, respectively, without statistically significant difference. The final OJ was 3.72 mm, 3.48 mm, and 3.99 mm for Bionator, headgear, and late treatment groups, respectively, without statistically significant difference.

O'Brein/2003 [19]

This large multicenter trial evaluated the psychosocial effects of early treatment with Twin-block (TB) in 89 patients with Class II division 1 versus untreated 78 Class II patients. The study concluded that the self-concepts were higher in TB group and negative social experiences were lower in TB group in comparison with a non-treated group at phase one. The total Piers-Harris score increased by 4.95 in the early treatment group versus 1.52 in the untreated control.

O'Brein/2009 [20]

This study aimed to assess whether early treatment using TB improves the facial attractiveness of Class II patients. It was found that the profile of early treated patients was statistically more attractive than those who did not receive treatment. The attractiveness was correlated with less OJ, less jaw discrepancy, less facial convexity, and a slightly more acute labiomental angle.

Tulloch/1997 [12]

This study has been discussed before. The researchers found that the early treatment reduced the severity of the Class II discrepancy either with the functional appliance or with HG, and the difference was only in the mechanism. The reduction in OJ was statistically different between the three groups: -2.66 ± 1.8, -1.5 ± 1.36, and $-0.0.9 \pm 0.98$ in MB, HG, and control groups, respectively. The researchers found that gender does not have any impact on the treatment outcome.

Tulloch/1998 [14]
This study has been discussed before. There was a statistically significant reduction in ANB angle in early treated groups in the first phase of treatment, while the late treatment group showed more ANB reduction in the second phase with small differences between late and early treatment at the end of treatment.

Evidence Summary
Looking at the evidence collectively, the best available evidence supports that there is no difference between early (7–11 years of age) and late (12–16 years of age) treatment for Class II malocclusion in regard to OJ and ANB using functional appliances or HG. However, the early treatment enhances the self-esteem of the child and reduces the chances of incisal trauma, which mean the early treatment does not confer treatment advantage except for incisal trauma reduction and transitory changes in self-esteem. On the other hand, early treatment may have some disadvantages; increased cost, length of treatment, and attendance.

Evidence Interpretation
It is mostly recommended to start the treatment near the initiation of the pubertal growth spurt. However, if the patient has low self-esteem or negative social experiences, and there are more chances for trauma due to special sports, bullying, or excessive overjet, early treatment is favored. While if the patient has good self-esteem, there is no negative social experience, and the probability of dental trauma is low, late treatment is favored and will also decrease the cost, number of visits, loss to follow-up, and the overall treatment duration.

Viewpoint
The two systematic reviews represent the highest evidence in research. Perinetti review [16] is a well-conducted review. However, most of the included studies have a significant risk of bias, particularly the non-randomized studies. Pooling Frankel with other appliances such as TB in forest plot can lead to clinical heterogeneity. The methodological heterogeneity and the risk of bias may lead to imprecision in this evidence.

O'Brein trials [17, 19, 20] were a well-conducted multicenter trials with a large sample size. These trials were done in real-life settings in England. However, the orthodontist should take some points into his account; the dropout was higher in the early treatment group (14 patients) versus one patient in the late treatment group for the functional stage, and this may bias the results, but the authors treat this problem by using intention to treat analysis. The initial malocclusion was not described in detail, which may be a confounding factor in this study as more spaces or crowding can affect the outcomes, as well as, the anterior teeth inclination. For applicability, the overjet was 10.77 ± 2.5 mm, and the buccal segment's blocks of the TB were 7 mm with advancement of 7–8 mm and the inclined planes were at about 70° to the occlusal plane.

Most of the RCTs included in the reviews were graded as low to moderate evidence, therefore the actual effect for the late versus the early functional treatment is likely to be similar to the current effect.

Cervical Vertebra Maturation and Growth Modification

Clinical Question 5: Can Cervical Vertebra Maturation Stages be Considered a Reliable Method to Predict the Pubertal Growth Spurt?

Evidence

Systematic Reviews
Szemraj/2018 [21]
This review included 10 studies that investigated the correlation between the cervical vertebral maturation stages (CVMs) and the hand writs method (HWM). The authors found that the correlation between the two methods was high and ranged from 0.62 to 0.98. Also, they concluded that, based on eight included studies, the CVMs could be used instead of HWM. While the CVMs were an additional method in two trials.

Santiago/2012 [22]
This review included 23 trials; six studies were from moderate to high quality and 17 studies were of low-quality studies in terms of methodological quality. The authors excluded the low-quality studies from their results. They found that some studies suggested a good correlation between the two methods with a considerable level of reproducibility. The authors judged the evidence as low with limited studies.

Evidence Summary
The best available evidence suggests that there is a good correlation between CVM and HWM. There is an absence of evidence regarding the reliability of CVM in predicting the growth velocity.

Evidence Interpretation
There is an absence of conclusive evidence regarding the reliability of CVM. So, while evaluating growth spurt, CVM should be used as an adjunctive method than solely relying on it.

Viewpoint
Szemraj review [21] was a low-quality review as the authors did not follow robust standards. The search was limited to only one database. There was no clear description of the data extraction, risk of bias assessment, or the data syntheses. The aforementioned issues may increase the bias in this review.

Santiago review [22] was a good review. However, the limitation in reporting and not following rigorous guidelines may reduce the quality of the systematic review. There was a lack of methodological details for the included studies. Selecting some studies for reporting may lead to a selection bias.

Dental Versus Skeletal Effects

Clinical Question 6: What Are the Effects of Functional Appliances on Facial Structures? Are These Effects Skeletal, Dental, or Both?

Evidence

Systematic Reviews and Meta-Analyses
Batista/2018 [10]
This Cochrane systematic review has been discussed before. Seven included studies compared late treatment with functional appliances versus no treatment. The final OJ reduced by 5.46 mm (MD; −5.46, 95% CI −6.63 to −4.28; 2 trials, 61 participants), and 4.62 (MD; − 4.62, 95% CI −5.33 to −3.92; 3 trials, 122 participants) in fixed and removable functional appliances, respectively, when compared with no treatment group. The ANB reduction was 2.37° (MD; −2.37°, 95% CI −3.01 to −1.74; 2 trials, 99 participants) in the functional group when compared to the no treatment group. The evidence for these findings was low.

Ehsani/2015 [11]
As discussed earlier, this review included 10 trials investigating the short-term effects of TB appliance. The effects of TB were a statistically significant reduction of SNA angle (MD; −0.7°, 95% CI: −1.2 to −0.2, 5 trials) and a statistically significant increase in SNB angle (MD; 1.2°, 95% CI: 0.9–1.4, 3 trials) along with an increase in mandibular body length Go-Gn (MD; 2.95 mm, 95% CI: 1.9–4.0, 3 trials). The dental changes were retroclination of upper incisors (MD; −9.2°, 95% CI: −9.9 to −8.5, 3 trials) and proclination of the lower incisors (MD; 3.9°, 95% CI: 1.4–6.3, 3 trials).

Randomized Controlled Trial
O'Brein/2003 [23]
This large multicenter trial evaluated the effectiveness of early treatment for Class II division I malocclusion with Twin-block appliance. The reduction of overjet was 6.93 mm with a skeletal change of 1.88 mm (27%) and dental change of 5.05 mm (73%). The skeletal reduction (27%) was a result of growth modification of both jaws to a similar degree; 13% (0.88 mm) maxillary restriction and 14% (1 mm) mandibular advancement. The dental reduction in overjet (73%) was due to severe retroclination for the upper incisors 44% (3.03 mm) and proclination of the lower incisors 29% (2.03 mm).

The molar correction was a combination of 41% (1.88 mm) skeletal change and 59% (2.71 mm) dental change. The skeletal molar relationship correction was a result of growth modification of both jaws 19%, 22% for maxillary and mandibular bases, respectively. The dental molar correction was 26% and 33% for maxillary and mandibular molars, respectively.

Evidence Summary

The best available evidence supports that the functional treatment in Class II patients affects the growth of both maxilla and mandible and results in more dental than skeletal changes. Less than half of the OJ reduction is from the ANB improvement, which is contributed more by mandibular growth [10, 11]. In one RCT [23] the dental and skeletal changes were 73:27. Interestingly, the dental changes were mainly upper incisors retroclination ($-9.2°$) then lower incisors proclination ($3.9°$) [11]. The upper and lower incisors changes were 60:40 in one RCT [23].

Evidence Interpretation

Functional treatment reduces the skeletal discrepancies by both skeletal and dental effects, with major contributions coming from the dental effects (almost 70%). As functional treatment results in retroclination of maxillary and proclination of mandibular incisor so pretreatment incisor inclinations, gingival biotype, nasolabial and labiomental angle must be taken into consideration during the planning for the functional treatment.

Viewpoint

The aforementioned evidence was discussed previously.

Effects on TMJ

Clinical Question 7: What Is the Effect of the Functional Treatment on the Temporomandibular Joint?

Evidence

Systematic Review and Meta-Analysis
Kyburz/2019 [24]

This study included 11 papers for 8 trials that investigated the influence of functional treatment on TMJ in Class II patients compared to non-treated patients. The review found that the functional treatment was associated with a condylar width increase by 1.1 mm (95% CI: 0.1–2.2; 2 trials; very low evidence), anterior joint space decrease by 0.7 mm (MD; −0.7, 95% CI: − 0.5 to −0.9; 2 trials; very low evidence), posterior joint space increase by 1.0 mm (95% CI: 0.9–1.2; 2 trials; very low evidence), superior joint space increase by 0.7 mm (95% CI: 0.5–1.0 mm; 2 trials; very low evidence), and vertical displacement of the glenoid fossa by 0.4 mm(95% CI: 0.1 to 0.7; 2 trials; very low evidence). All the findings in the present review have a very low level of evidence.

Systematic Review
Ivorra-Carbonell/2016 [25]
This systematic review included 21 studies investigating the effects of Class II functional treatment on TMJ. Some of the included studies reported that there was an anterior movement of the condyle with adaptive changes in the glenoid fossa. Other studies demonstrated that these changes were not significant and have a short-term effect. One included study [26] investigated Herbst appliance outcomes and found that there was an anterior-inferior displacement of the glenoid fossa and posterior superior condylar growth, especially in hyperdivergent patients. The included studies reported no deleterious effects of Class II functional treatment on TMJ.

Retrospective Study
Pancherz/2004 [26]
This long-term trial investigated the effects of Herbst appliance on TMJ in Class II patients. The authors divided 68 patients aged 10–16 years (average 12.4 years) into three groups according to the facial type; 13 hyperdivergent patients ((ML/NSL $\geq 37°$)), 17 hypodivergent patients (ML/NSL $\leq 26°$), and 38 normodivergent patients (ML/NSL = $26.5°–36.5°$). The average treatment duration was 7 months (5–12 months), and the measuring of the TMJ parameters were done after finishing the treatment and after 5 years. The authors found that there is no significant difference between the three groups. The fossa was displaced in the anterior and inferior direction during the treatment and displaced posteriorly after the treatment. Also, the condyle growth was in a posterior and superior direction.

Evidence Summary
The best existing evidence indicates that the functional treatment for Class II malocclusion is associated with short-term positional and skeletal effects on the temporomandibular joint. During functional treatment, there is an anterior and inferior displacement of the condyle, increased condyle width, and vertical displacement of the glenoid fossa. However, there are no harmful effects of functional treatment on TMJ.

Evidence Interpretation
Functional treatment has an adaptive effect on the temporomandibular joint and the glenoid fossa, but these effects are mostly in the short term.

Viewpoint
Kyburz review [24] was a well-conducted systematic review. However, most included studies were from very low-quality studies due to a high risk of bias, non-randomized design, and methodological issues, which result in heterogeneity and inconsistency between studies. Also, the limited samples may lead to imprecision.

Ivorra-Carbonell review [25] included another systematic review with different designs of studies which may represent confusion in the inclusion criteria. Furthermore, the inclusion of different types of studies may reduce the quality of the evidence. The authors used the reporting tools to assess the included studies without interest in the internal validity.

Pancherz study [26] was a cephalometric study for the long term. Without randomization, the selection bias and the confounding factors may affect the outcome.

As such, we are uncertain about the estimate, and further high-quality trials may substantially provide a different estimate of the Class II functional treatment effect on the TMJ.

Effects on Mandibular Growth

Clinical Question 8: What Is the Influence of Functional Treatment on Mandibular Growth?

Evidence

Systematic Reviews and Meta-Analyses
Perillo/2011 [27]
The authors included nine trials, investigating the effect of Fränkel-2 (FR-2) appliance on mandibular growth by comparing functional treatment using FR-2 versus no treatment in growing patients. Meta-analysis demonstrated that FR-2 increased the mandibular body length by 0.4 mm/year (95%CI: 0.18–0.62; 9 trials), mandibular ramus height by 0.65 mm/year (95%CI, 0.24–1.06; 9 trials), and the total mandibular length by 1.07 mm/year (95%CI, 0.68–1.5; 9 trials). The quality of the included studies was low to medium.

Perinetti/2015 [16]
This meta-analysis included 12 articles with 8 pre-pubertal and 7 pubertal groups to assess the skeletal and dentoalveolar change after removable functional treatment. The authors revealed that the annual increase in the total mandible length was 0.95 mm (95%CI: 0.38–1.51) in the pre-pubertal group and 2.91 mm (95%CI: 2.04–3.79) in the pubertal group. The annual increase in the mandibular ramus height was 0 mm (95%CI: −0.52 to 0.53) in the pre-pubertal group and 2.18 mm (95%CI: 1.51–2.86) in the pubertal group. The quality of the evidence was low for the pre-pubertal studies and moderate for the pubertal studies. The annualized increase in the mandibular base was 1.01 mm/year (95%CI: 0.21–1.8) and 1.63 mm/year (95%CI: 0.98–2.28) in pre-pubertal and pubertal groups, respectively.

Systematic Review
Cozza/2006 [28]
In this review, the authors included 22 trials; 4 RCTs, 2 prospective CCTs, and 16 retrospective CCTs investigating the mandibular changes using different Class II functional appliances. The quality was low in three studies, medium in 13 studies, and medium to high in 6 studies with only 8 studies performing a suitable statistical analysis. The researchers concluded that the elongation of the mandible after functional treatment was 0.16 mm/month. Two-thirds of the included studies reported a

clinically significant elongation in total mandibular length as a result of overall active treatment with functional appliances.

A greater mandibular elongation was reported using Herbst appliance (0.28 mm/mo) in four trials. Likewise, the mandibular elongation was 0.23 mm/mo using TB appliance in 7 trials. Only Tümer and Gültan study reported a clinical and statistical increase in ANB angle by 2.2° [29].

Evidence Summary

The available evidence suggests an increase in the mandible's total length, ranging from 1.07 mm/year to 3.12mm/year (0.26 mm/month). The increase in mandibular ramus height ranged from 0.65 to 2.18 mm/year, while mandibular body length increase ranged from 0.4 to 1.63 mm/year. The mandibular growth was greater in the pubertal than the pre-pubertal period.

Evidence Interpretation

Functional treatment increases the total mandibular length, especially in the pubertal period. This increase involves both the mandibular body and ramus height. As most of the results are only statistically significant and the values were calculated per year, the clinician should keep in mind that there would be some amount of the mandible growth which might not be clinically significant during the treatment period, even in the pubertal period.

Viewpoint

Included studies in Perilla's meta-analysis [27] have a high clinical and statistical heterogeneity resulting from differences between studies like patients' age, treatment duration, and measurements. Also, the included studies were at low to medium quality due to methodological limitations; no reported method error, and lack of blinding in measurement. This may reduce the certainty of the evidence.

Cozza review [28] has a restriction on the search date and language. Most of the included trials were from retrospective design and were of low to moderate quality due to methodological limitations and lack of blinding in the measurements that may reduce the quality of the evidence. Furthermore, the authors were unable to perform a meta-analysis.

Effects on Maxillary Growth

Clinical Question 9: What Are Headgear Effects And Do Functional Appliances Have a Headgear Effects?

Evidence

Systematic Reviews and Meta-Analyses
Batista/2018 [10]

Two studies in this Cochrane systematic review compared HG in the early treatment group with the observation group. They found that the effect of HG was statistically significant in overjet reduction (MD: −1.07 mm, 95% CI: −1.63 mm to −0.51 mm) and in ANB reduction by −0.72° (95% CI: −1.18° to −0.27°).

Antonarakis/2007 [30]

This systematic review included 9 studies to evaluate the short-term effects of functional appliances such as TB and activator, and the effect of orthopedic appliances like HG on Class II malocclusion. To restrain maxillary growth, three included trials found that TB statistically decreased SNA by 1.03° (MD; −1.03°, 95% CI: −1.94 to −0.13) when compared to a non-treated control group, while the activator appliance decreased the SNA angle by 0.31(MD; −0.31, 95% CI: −0.65 to −0.04). On the other hand, extraoral appliances (high/cervical HG) statistically decreased SNA by 1.01° (MD; −1.01°, 95% CI: −1.34 to −0.69) when compared to the non-treated control group in two trials. Functional appliances mainly act on the mandible and the extraoral appliances mainly act on the maxilla apart from TB, which affects both the jaws.

Randomized Controlled Trial
Tulloch/1997 [12]

This RCT, which was included in Antonarakis review [30], randomly assigned 180 Class II patients into three groups: control group, modified Bionator (MB)group, and headgear (HG) group. The researchers found that the main effect of HG was maxillary restriction as SNA was statistically decreased by 0.91° ± 1.11 in the HG group while increased in the functional and control groups by 0.11° ± 1.26 and 0.26 ± 1.17, respectively. The main effect of the MB functional appliance was a forward position of the mandible with an increase in its length when compared with the control and HG groups; SNB increased by 1.07° ± 0.91 in the MB group, 0.15 ± 0.88 in the HG group, and 0.43 ± 0.9 in the control group. The reduction in OJ was statistically different between the three groups; −2.66 ± 1.8, −1.5 ± 1.36, and − 0.0.9 ± 0.98 in MB, HG, and control groups, respectively.

The researchers found that gender does not have any impact on the treatment outcome.

Evidence Summary

The best available evidence suggests that the extraoral traction appliances restrain the maxilla by 1.01° reduction in SNA angle. In contrast, the Twin-block appliance seems to restrain the maxilla by 1.03° in SNA angle, while the activator has less effect on the maxillary growth. As such, the main effect of functional appliances is on the mandible, while the main and only effect of headgear is on the maxilla.

Evidence Interpretation

Functional appliances seem to have small headgear effects as they restrain the growth of the maxilla. So functional appliances stimulate the growth of the mandible and restrain the growth of the maxilla. In Class II patients, if the problem is only maxillary excess, headgear can be preferred, while if the problem is a mandibular deficiency or both maxillary excess and mandibular deficiency, TB may be a better option in the light of the available evidence, as it affects both jaws. The present evidence interpretation of TB should be taken with caution as it is very low. Some clinicians also combine TB with HG to get more maxillary restraining effects but at present there is no evidence for this.

Viewpoint

Antonarakis [30] review had some shortcomings; there was no duplication in the selection of included studies or extraction of the data, and the authors did not assess the quality of the studies. So, evidence interpretation regarding the use of TB should be taken with caution. Furthermore, new high-quality research is needed, which may substantially provide a different estimate of the functional/orthopedic treatment effect on the maxilla and mandible.

Effect on the Vertical Pattern

Clinical Question 10: What Are the Effects of Functional Appliances on Vertical Growth?

Evidence

Systematic Reviews and Meta-Analyses
Ehsani/2015 [11]

In this systematic review and meta-analysis, short-term effects of twin block were reviewed. This systematic review has a conflict between studies about the main effect of functional treatment on vertical growth. Three included studies reported an increase in the vertical dimension (MD; 2.1 mm, 95%CI: 1.2–3.1) in the TB group when compared to non-treated controls. Another included study [31] added occlusal rests on the bite blocks to control the vertical dimensions by preventing the eruption of molars in high-angle cases and they revealed that they controlled the vertical dimension by this technique. One included study [32] found that the TB did not restrict the vertical eruption of posterior teeth, and they interpreted that it was not pure extrusion but distal tipping of the molars and extrusion of the mesial cusp. The systematic review concluded that the vertical dimension can be changed in patients who can benefit from it.

Perinetti/2015 [16]

This review has been discussed previously. The reviewers investigated the effect of different functional appliances such as TB, FR2, and Bionator on jaw growth. The researchers found that the annual increase in the facial divergence was not statistically significant (MD; $0.27°$, 95%CI: -0.25 to 0.79, $p = 0.31$, 4 trials) in pre-pubertal group, while this increase was statistically but not clinically significant (MD; $0.8°$, 95%CI: $0.34–1.26$, $p < 0.001$, 5 trials) in the pubertal group.

Evidence Summary

The best available evidence suggests that there is a small increase of nearly 2 mm in the vertical dimension [11] when TB was used, while it was 0.8° in the facial divergence by using different removable appliances in pubertal period.

Evidence Interpretation

Functional treatment slightly increases the vertical dimension. So removable functional appliances may have a benefit in low-angle cases where they can add some improvement in the vertical dimension of the patient. The vertical dimension can be improved in low-angle cases in TB by selective grinding of the upper block. Usually, not more than 1 mm of the upper block is trimmed in a 4-week visit. In high-angle cases, there can be slight deterioration of the vertical dimension by a functional appliance. In twin block, this can be prevented by placing occlusal rest on the lower molars in a twin block appliance.

The present evidence interpretation should be taken with caution due to the low-level evidence provided by the studies.

Viewpoint

As previously discussed, Perillo's meta-analysis [27] has high clinical and statistical heterogeneity. Ehsani et al. review [11] has conflicting findings regarding the vertical dimensional changes, includes retrospective studies in the review, and has a low to medium risk of bias in most of the included studies. Further research is necessary on the effect of functional appliances on the vertical dimension, which may substantially provide a different estimate of this effect.

Functional Treatment and Soft Tissue

Clinical Question 11: What Are the Effects of the Functional Appliances on Soft Tissue?

Evidence

Systematic Reviews
Ehsani/2015 [11]
In this review, two included trials assessed the short-term effects of TB on soft tissues. The two included studies [33, 34] did not find statistically significant changes in the upper lip position. Also, there was no significant change in facial convexity, but the authors [34] detected forward movement of soft tissue B point (2.9 mm) and lower lip (2.9 mm). They also noticed an increase in lower facial height soft tissue (2.7 mm) and lower lip length (3.2 mm). Likewise, the other included study [33] found statistically significant differences for most of the mandibular soft tissue

landmarks, including a forward movement of soft tissue pogonion and increase of both nasolabial and labiomental angles.

Flores-Mir/2006 [35]

This systematic review included 11 studies evaluating soft tissue changes in Class II patients treated using either bionator or activator. For the activator, the results were contradictory in the position of the upper lip, where three studies reported upper lip retrusion (−1.1 to −3 mm) while the other two trials did not find any change in the upper lip. There was no change in the lower lip or soft tissue menton.

For Bionator, the results of facial angles were conflicted. One study [36] reported an increase in the facial convexity (2.7°), another trial [34] mentioned a decrease in the facial convexity (−2.2°), while another study [37] did not report any change. Also, one study [36] reported a large increase in labiomental angle (17°), while another study [34] mentioned no changes. Interestingly, no studies reported significant nasolabial angle change. Two studies reported upper lip retrusion (−0.89 to −1.4 mm) versus no change in one study [34]. Also, two studies reported lower lip protrusion (2.2–4.9 mm) versus no change in others. Most of the soft tissue changes reported in this review have questionable clinical significance.

Evidence Summary

Based on the best available evidence, the effects of functional treatment on the soft tissues, using an activator or bionator, are conflicting. So, we cannot conclude a good summary about this topic. However, the nose tip and labionasial angle are not affected by functional treatment. Upper lip retrusion was reported in activator (−1.1 to −3 mm) and bionator (−0.89 to −1.4 mm) groups with different values between studies. Lower lip protrusion was reported in bionator group with a wide range (2.2–4.9 mm). There were statistically significant changes in the mandibular soft tissue landmarks with no clear changes in the facial convexity.

Evidence Interpretation

The effects of the functional treatment on soft tissues are not clear, and many factors play a role. Small changes in upper and lower lip positions can be anticipated after functional treatment.

Viewpoint

Flores-Mir review [35] was a well-conducted review. The included studies were low to moderate quality due to the lack of randomization and blinding. The head position and the used reference structures to quantify soft tissue changes may play a vital role in the precision of the measurements. Interestingly, conventional lateral cephalometric analyses may not be suitable for a comprehensive evaluation of 3D changes. As such, further robust RCTs are needed to draw a crucial conclusion regarding the effect of the functional treatment on the soft tissues.

Fixed Versus Removable Functional Appliances

Clinical Question 12: What Should be the Appliance of Choice for Functional Treatment: Fixed or Removable?

Evidence

Systematic Reviews and Meta-Analyses
Batista/2018 [10]

This Cochrane systematic review has included three trials compared removable versus fixed functional appliances in adolescent Class II patients. This review found that the fixed functional appliance is better than the removable appliance in reducing the OJ (MD; 0.74, 95% CI: 0.15–1.33, $P = 0.01$), and the removable appliance is better than the fixed appliance in reducing ANB (MD; $-1.04°$, 95% CI: -1.60 to -0.49, $P < 0.001$). The quality of evidence for these findings was low.

Systematic Reviews
Pacha/2015 [38]

This systematic review included 4 trials; two trials compared Twin-block (TB) versus fixed rigid appliance (Herbst), and two trials compared fixed hybrid appliances; Forsus and Twin Force Bite Corrector (TFBC) versus Activator. The authors found a significant overjet reduction by 5 mm using the Herbst appliance versus 4.5 mm when TB was used. The soft tissue improvement was 2 ± 2.8 in the convexity angle in the Herbst group versus 0.75 ± 2.3 in the TB group. The treatment time was significantly shorter in the Herbst group (5.8 months, 95% CI: 5.1–6.5) than TB group (11.2 months, 95%CI: 9.5–12.9) with a higher cost for the fixed functional appliances. There was a significant increase in mandible length by 1.3 mm using Forsus appliance, 3.7 mm using TFBC, and 3.7–6.6 mm using Activator appliance, with a lower incisors proclination in all groups.

Cozza/2006 [28]

As discussed before, this systematic review concluded that the average elongation of the mandible after functional treatment was 0.16 mm/month, and this was greater in Herbst appliance at 0.28 mm/mo than twin block at 0.23 mm/mo.

Randomized Control Trials
O'Brein/2003 [39]

This trial randomly assigned 215 Class II division 1 patients into two groups; 110 patients (62 F: 48 M) with an average age of 12.41 years in the TB group and 105 patients (55 F:50 M) with an average age of 12.74 years in Herbst appliance group. The authors found that 37 patients (33.6%) in TB group and 18 patients (12.9%) in Herbst group did not complete the functional phase and this was statistically significant ($p = 0.01$). As such, using TB decreased the chance of completing the functional appliance treatment phase by 2.4 times when compared with the Herbst appliance. The authors found that the functional phase period was significantly longer in the TB group, 11.22 months when compared with Herbst group 5.81 months

($p = 0.0005$), but there was no statistically significant difference in the total treatment time between groups. TB increases the duration of treatment by 1.5–2.2 months, but the overall treatment time was equal. At the end of treatment, there was no difference in terms of skeletal or dental effects between the two appliances. The overjet reduction was 6.24 mm (MD; −6.24 mm, 95%CI: −5.47 to −7) and 5.8 mm (MD; −5.8, 95%CI: −6.42 to −5.18) in TB and Herbst groups, respectively. The mandible length increased by 3.46 mm (95%CI: 2.45–4.47) and 3.36 mm (95%CI: 2.51–4.21) in TB and Herbst groups, respectively.

Baysal/2014 [40]

This trial randomly assigned 60 patients; 20 each, to compare TB versus Herbst with the control group. There was more overjet correction by Herbst (5.08 mm) than TB (4.86 mm). The overjet correction was combination of 29% skeletal and 70.9% dental in Herbst group, while it was 70% skeletal and 30% dental in TB group. Molar correction was more skeletal in TB group (71.5%) than in Herbst appliance group (36.7%). In TB group, more mandibular skeletal changes were observed. TB mainly corrected the Class II malocclusion with mandibular advancement, while Herbst appliance did the Class II correction mainly by retroclination of upper incisors and proclination of lower incisors. There was a 13% dropout in Herbst appliance and 16% in TB.

Evidence Summary

The available evidence suggests that there is little difference between fixed functional (FFA) and removable appliances in the reduction of OJ with evidence favoring FFA. For reducing skeletal discrepancies such as ANB or mandible length increase, the evidence favors removable appliances. Moreover, these evidences reported less treatment duration with a higher cost and higher chance of completing the treatment using FFA.

Evidence Interpretation

The choice of fixed or removable functional appliance depends upon the expertise of the clinician and patient-related factors. If patient compliance is a concern, and the patient is in the last of the growth spurt with obvious proclination of upper incisors and retroclination of lower incisors FFA is a favorite option. But if the patient is cooperative, there is ample growth remaining and more skeletal effects are desired while the cost is a concern, a removable functional appliance should be the appliance of choice.

Viewpoint

The included studies, in Batista review [10] and Pacha's review [38], were from low quality. The risk of bias and the heterogeneity between the included studies may reduce the evidence in Pacha review [41].

O'Brein study [39] was a well-conducted RCT with a large sample size. The authors performed ITT analysis to treat the missing data. However, there was attrition bias due to the high dropout of 37% in the TB group, which may be more than in the real-life settings. This may be due to the differences between the study centers and the design of the TB as the thickness of the appliance was 7 mm in this study.

Baysal [40] RCT has no clear description for allocation concealment and blinding of accessors. The loss to follow up was 3 and 4 from Herbst and TB groups, respectively, without treating this issue with ITT analysis which increases the risk of attrition bias. For the applicability, the initial ANB was 6° ± 1.17° and the mean OJ was 8.5 ± 2.3 mm. Also, the clinician should consider the results of this study under the following instructions; the bite registration was an edge to edge in Herbst appliance, and 70% of the maximum protrusive path with 2–4 mm beyond freeway space in TB.

Skeletal Anchorage and Fixed Functional Appliances

Clinical Question 13: Can Skeletal Anchorage Devices Improve the Outcome of Functional Treatment by Fixed Functional Appliances?

Evidence

Systematic Review and Meta-Analysis
Elkordy/2016 [42]

This review compared the dentoskeletal effects of FFA with or without skeletal anchorage devices (miniplates and miniscrews). The reviewers included five studies in their meta-analysis. After treatment, the mandibular length was greater in FFA with skeletal anchorage than conventional appliances but not statistically significant (SMD; 1.98, 95%: −0.11 to 1.19, $p = 0.06$, 3 trials). SNB angle change was insignificant and slightly greater in the FFA group with skeletal anchorage (SMD; 1.2°,95%CI: −0.37 to 2.77, $p = 0.14$, 3 trials). Also, ANB angle had no statistically significant difference between the two groups (SMD; 0.7, 95% CI −1.55 to 0.14). Skeletal anchorage with FFA had no statistically significant decrease in SNA angle (SMD; −0.23, 95% CI −0.70 to 0.25, $p = 0.35$). The review reported significant differences between lower and upper incisors inclination between the two groups. FFA with skeletal anchorage reduced the inclination of lower and upper incisors during treatment; (SMD; −1.43, 95% CI: −2.59 to −0.27) and (SMD; −1.04, 95% CI: −1.57 to −0.51), respectively.

Randomized Clinical Trial
Elkordy/2019 [43]

In this RCT, 48 patients were randomized into three equal groups to compare Forsus appliance alone (FA), Forsus appliance with skeletal miniplate anchorage (FMP), and a control group. Mandibular length showed a significant increase in the FMP group only 4.05 ± 0.78 mm versus 0.86 ± 0.79 mm in the FA group and 1.11 ± 0.74 mm in the control group. The FMP group showed a retroclination of lower incisors (−1.49 ± 4.70), while the FA group showed significant proclination of the lower incisors (9.17 ± 2.42). The failure rate of miniplates was 13.3%. Only in FMP group, the ANB change (−1.62° ± 1.37) and the vertical dimension change (MP/SN; 2.06 ± 1.44) were statistically significant.

Controlled Clinical Study
Manni/2019 [44]

This was a prospective controlled study, recruited 26 Class II patients; 13 patients to Herbst Appliance (HA) group, and 13 patients to miniscrews supported Herbst appliance (MIsHA) group. The mean treatment time was 10.0 ± 0.8 months in MIsHA group and 10.8 ± 2.1 months in the HA group. Skeletal effects were statistically higher in MIsHA group than HA group. The increase in SNB angle was statistically higher in MIsHA group (2.9°) when compared with HA group (1.1°). The ANB decrease was statistically greater in MIsHA group (−3.3 mm) than HA group (−1.3 mm). There was a statistically significant difference in the vertical dimension (SN-GoGn) between the groups; it increased slightly in MIsHA group (0.5°) and decreased in HA group (−2.2°, $p = 0.007$). There was no statistically significant difference in SNA changes (−0.7 and − 1 in MIsHA group and HA group, respectively, $p = 0.62$). The lower incisors showed protrusion and proclination in both groups with no statistically significant difference between groups (Li-GoGn: 1.6 and 3.7 in MIsHA and HA groups, respectively, $p = 0.40$).

Evidence Summary

Looking into the available evidence, the skeletal anchorage devices may enhance the sagittal skeletal effects of functional appliances. These devices also increased the vertical dimensions while decreasing the lower incisors proclination, but these effects do not have a large effect size.

Evidence Interpretation

Skeletal anchorage devices improve the outcome of functional treatment with more sagittal effects and decreased lower incisors proclination than conventional appliances. So, these devices would be useful in Class II patients with a hypodivergent face and proclined lower incisor (if no proclination of lower incisors is desired) and there is a need for greater skeletal change.

Viewpoint

Elkordy systematic review [42] was well conducted. The included studies were assessed as low to very low-quality studies, which may reduce the quality of the evidence. Interestingly, the forest plots were confusing that lead to a difficulty in reading the results. Elkordy [43] RCT misreported the consort diagram about the dropout of the patients. The measurement of the two groups was at different follow up times which might raise bias in the study.

Manni study [44] was a pilot study. There was a lack of randomization, allocation concealment, and blinding in this trial that left the study at serious risk of bias. Interestingly, the number of girls was extremely larger in the conventional treatment group (10 females: 3 males with a mean age of 12.2 years). By this age they might have passed their growth spurt period which can decrease the skeletal effects. The comparison group was mostly treated retrospectively. The blinding was an issue in this study as the principal author was the same operator. So, the findings of this study should be interpreted carefully. Further researches are needed to be certain about the real effect of the skeletal anchorage devices in Class II functional treatment.

Twin Block Versus Other Functional Appliances

Clinical Question 14: Which Removable Appliance Should be Favored for the Functional Treatment?

Evidence

Systematic Review and Meta-Analysis
Batista/2018 [10]
A Cochrane systematic review included six trials that compared TB with other functional appliances. Four RCTs found that there is no statistically significant difference in terms of the OJ (MD: 0.08 mm, 95% CI −0.60 to 0.76). Three RCTs concluded that the TB performed a statistically significant reduction in ANB (MD: −0.56°, 95% CI −0.96 to −0.16) in comparison with other functional appliances.

Randomized Controlled Trial
Campbell/2019 [45]
This study randomly assigned 60 Class II division 1 patients into two parallel groups 30 each; Frankel 2 (FR2) group with mean patients age of 12.6 ± 1.4 years and OJ of 10.8 ± 1.3 mm, and a modified twin block (MTB) group with an average age of 13.1 ± 1 years and OJ of 10.3 ± 1.3 mm. Forty-two participants completed the study (FR2: 20, MTB: 22), with a high number of dropouts in the two groups. There was no statistically significant difference in the treatment time (FR2: 376 days, MTB: 340 days; $P = 0.41$, MD:36 days, 95% CI: [−44, 95]), appliance breakage (FR2: 0.3; MTB: 0.4; $P = 0.67$), child OHRQoL, or Piers-Harris scores.

Evidence Summary
Looking at the evidence collectively, TB may have greater skeletal effects than other appliances like FR2 or Monoblock. There is no difference in regard to the treatment time and the appliance breakage between FR2 and TB. However, the FR2 cost was double the MTB cost in Campbell et al. study [45].

Evidence Interpretation
TB seems to be a better and more cost-effective removable functional appliance (RFA) than other commonly used appliances. As the present evidence is low so other factors such as the clinician's experience with functional appliances, the patient's cooperation and characteristics, and the resources should be considered during the selection of the RFA.

Viewpoint

In Batista's review [10], the quality of the included studies was low. In Campbell trial [45], the dropout of patients was 30% which is a concern as it is high, but the authors used ITT to treat this problem. However, the compliance issue and missing outcome data should be borne in mind and the results should be interpreted with caution.

Incremental Versus Maximum Bite Advancement

Clinical Question 15: Which Is Better, the Incremental or the Maximum Bite Advancement in the Functional Treatment?

Evidence

Randomized Controlled Trial
Banks/2004 [46]

This study treated 189 Class II patients with TB, by allocating 94 patients with an average age of 12.6 years (12.30–12.87) to the maximum bite advancement group and 95 patients with an average age of 12.62 years (12.41–12.83) to the incremental advancement group. The maximum advancement was constructed in an edge-to-edge position, while the incremental group had an initial advancement of 2 mm and 2 mm further advancement after 6 weeks in the clinic by incorporating an advancement screw in the Twin-block. The researchers found that there is no difference between incremental or maximum advancement regarding the outcomes of treatment. The success rate of maximum advancement Twin-block was 70%, while in the incremental advancement Twin-block it was 81%. Interestingly, they revealed that patients younger than 12.3 years are 3 times more likely to complete the treatment than patients older than 12.3 years. Also, they found that the operator has an effect on the treatment completion.

Evidence Summary

The available evidence suggests that the method of advancement does not have an impact on the functional treatment outcome. On the other hand, the success rate of completing the treatment was higher in the incremental advancement group than the maximum advancement group by 11%.

Evidence Interpretation

In functional treatment, incremental and maximum bite advancement can produce the same outcomes. With incremental advancement, TB has a slightly more success rate than single advancement TB, and it is usually taken as more acceptable by the patient. Incremental advancement either in removable or fixed functional appliances is usually a more expensive option than a single advancement appliance. For small overjet, a single advancement appliance can be used. For a large overjet, incremental advancement is preferred.

Viewpoint

The loss to follow up in Banks study [46] were 20–30%, which represents a high number of dropouts, but the authors treated this lost data using ITT. Interestingly, the treatment was considered as discontinued after 3 failed appointments, 10% or less overjet reduction over 6 months, or excessive appliance breakages or loss at the operator's discretion. The discontinuation has three different cut-off points that may widen the success rate/completion definition and mislead the results.

Stability of Class II Fixed Functional Appliance Therapy

Clinical Question 16: Does the Functional Treatment Relapse?

Evidence

Systematic Review and Meta-Analysis
Bock/2016 [47]

This review aimed to investigate the changes after at least 1 year of functional treatment of Class II cases. The study included 20 articles; 19 trials detected treatment using Herbst appliance, and one study evaluated twin force bite corrector (TFBC). The average post-treatment period ranged from 12 to 382 months (median = 36 months). The meta-analysis revealed that the average relapse in the retention period was 0.2° out of 1.5° (12.5%) in ANB, as the reduction in ANB during functional treatment was 1.5°. The overjet relapse was 1.8 mm out of 6.5 mm OJ reduction during treatment, while the overbite relapse was 1.2 mm out of 2.9 mm OB reduction during treatment. The wits appraisal relapse was 0.5 mm and the molar relation relapse was 1.2 mm (21.8%) as the molar relation correction was 5.1 mm. For the soft tissue, the convexity angle decreased by 3.2° during the treatment, and the relapse was 0.1° in the retention phase. The evidence level was low.

Randomized Controlled Trial
Dolce [48]

This randomized controlled trial comprised three groups: Bionator, headgear and bite plane, and a observation group with no growth modification treatment. The first phase involved the growth modification stage. The second phase was orthodontic treatment for the three groups by fixed orthodontic appliances. ANB angle significantly decreased in the first two groups in the first phase. By the end of treatment, the ANB angle was similar in the three groups.

Evidence Summary

The available evidence found that there is relapse after the functional treatment of Class II patients. The functional treatment relapse was reported as (12.5%); 0.2° out of 1.5° correction of the ANB during the functional treatment. Also, it was 27.7% in OJ; which is 1.8 mm relapse from 6.5 mm reduction in the OJ during the treatment. The relapse of overbite was (41%); 1.2 mm from 2.9 mm overbite reduction during the treatment in Class II division I cases, and the relapse was (25%); 1 mm from OB reduction of 4 mm during the treatment in Class II division II cases.

Evidence Interpretation

There is always some relapse in post-functional phase or the retention phase. Patients should be communicated about this relapse at the start of treatment and end of treatment, and signed consent should be taken. Overcorrection of molar relations and overjet should be aimed during the functional phase. It is a well-established practice to make the incisor relations edge to edge as an end-functional phase treatment goal to accommodate relapse in Class II growth modification.

Viewpoint

Bock review [47] was a good review with no clear following for rigorous guidelines. The included studies were low-quality evidence with a moderate risk of bias and further research may change the estimate of relapse after functional treatment. A related point to notice is the wide range of post-treatment follow up that may increase the clinical heterogeneity between studies and affect the findings.

Dolce study [48] was a well-conducted trial with a large sample size. However, there are some limitations in this study; there was no information regarding allocation concealment or blinding, which may increase the risk of bias. Interestingly, the dropout was higher in Bionator group 11.5% than HG group 7%, so differential dropout should be considered as there are differences in the appliance design or the instructions and that may increase the risk of bias due to deviations from the intended interventions.

Class II Elastic and Functional Appliance

Clinical Question 17: Are Class II Elastic Effective in Treating Class II Malocclusion in Growing Children?

Evidence

Systematic Review
Janson/2013 [49]

The authors included 11 articles investigating Class II elastics usage with different forces (1–4 oz., mean force 2.6 oz. (73.7 g)) in treating Class II patients. Interestingly, only one included study mentioned the mean active treatment (8.5 months) using Class II elastics. In correcting the OJ, Class II elastics resulted in 4% skeletal effect, while Herbst produced 51% of skeletal changes in the short term. In regard to the molar relationship, Class II elastics produced only 10% of skeletal effects while Herbst achieved 66% of it.

According to this review, the Class II elastics proclined the lower incisors and reduced the OJ by 5.8 mm, and this effect was 71.1% of dental and 18.9% of skeletal changes. The overbite reduction was 3 mm and the correction of molars' relationship was 3 mm with 63% due to dental and 37% due to skeletal effects. The mandibular growth increased 1.1 mm more than maxillary growth, and the facial height increased 5 mm. The elastics increased the upper and lower lip thicknesses by 0.7 and 1.2 mm, respectively, and decreased Holdaway soft tissue angle by 1.48°.

Randomized Clinical Trial
Aras/2017 [50]

In this study, the author allocated 34 Class II subdivision patients into two groups; Forsus appliance treatment group (mean age 14.19 ± 1.02 years), and elastics treatment group (mean age 13.75 ± 1.16 years, elastic ¼ inch/6 Oz). They found that the treatment time in Forsus group was 4.53 ± 0.91 months and 6.85 ± 1.08 months in the elastic group. The upper incisors retroclination and extrusion was statistically greater in the elastic group. The lower incisors protrusion had no significant difference between groups. There was lower incisors' intrusion in Forsus group and extrusion in the elastics group. The improvement in molar relationship and OJ was greater in the Forsus group. The Class I molar relationship was seen in 12 (85%) and 10 (71%) patients in Forsus and elastics groups, respectively.

Evidence Summary

Class II elastic seems to be effective in treating Class II malocclusion with some limitations. The daily full-time wear of Class II elastics can correct 5.8 mm of the OJ and 3 mm of molar relationship with a 5 mm increase in the height of the face and increases in the lip thickness. Functional appliance like Herbst can produce more skeletal changes than elastics, while most effects of elastics are dentoalveolar. The best available evidence supports that the FFA, such as Forsus and Herbst, are more effective in Class II treatment than Class II elastics.

Evidence Interpretation

Class II elastics can treat Class II malocclusion, but are not as effective as fixed functional appliances, as most effects of Class II elastics are dentoalveolar. Class II elastics can be used if there is no residual growth, the facial height is decreased, and the patient can wear the elastics 24 hours per day for an average of 8 months.

As the present evidence is very low, the findings interpretation should be taken with caution.

Viewpoint

Janson review [49] has a lot of shortcomings; there is a lack of following to robust guidelines in conducting and reporting. There is no risk of bias assessment between or within the individual studies, and there is no reporting for the quality or the design of the included studies that may reduce the quality of the evidence.

Aras trial [50] was a good study. There is some limitation in this study. The authors did not conceal the group allocation with no information about the blinding. The authors deleted some data, two from elastics and one from the Forsus group, from the final analysis without treating the missing data by a statistical analysis.

Also, they calculated the power of the study for midline coincidence correction and the study aimed to figure out the effectiveness of both treatment modalities. However, using intermaxillary Class II mechanics have dental effects on both arches, so if the authors comprised patients only with lower midline shift, how they will manage the effects on the upper arch?. For applicability, the clinician should consider the patients' cooperation when using the elastics, as 2/17 patients in this trial did not show cooperation.

WEAR Time of Removable Functional Appliances

Clinical Question 18: Is There Any Difference Between Part-Time Versus Full-Time Wearing of Twin Block on the Treatment Results?

Evidence

Randomized Clinical Trial
Parekh/2019 [51]
This trial comprised 62 Class II patients aged between 10 and 14 years. The investigators randomly allocated the patients into two parallel groups; full-time TB wearing group (FT, 22 hours daily) and part-time wearing group (PT, 12 hours daily). The authors measured the wearing time using a temperature-sensitive TheraMon microsensor. They found that there was no statistically significant difference between the two groups regarding the reduction of OJ. The OJ reduction was 7 ± 2.92 mm in the PT group and 6.5 ± 2.62 mm in the FT group. Also, there was no statistically significant difference between groups in terms of skeletal changes; ANB angle decreased by $1.51°$ in PT group and $1.25°$ in FT group ($P = 0.83$, 95% CI: 0.68–0.849). Interestingly, the mean wear durations were 8.78 ± 3.77 hours per day in the PT group and 12.38 ± 5.89 hours per day in the FT group.

Evidence Summary
The mean wear duration of twin block was (8.78–12.38 per day). There was a more loss to follow up in the full-time wear group. Informing the patients that the wear time is a full day can increase the duration by only 3 hours per day as compared to part-time wear group. Interestingly, there was no statistically significant difference in skeletal or dental outcomes between full- or part-time wear of TB.

Evidence Interpretation
It is worth mentioning that orthodontic patients do not wear the appliance for full time. Part-time wear has the same effects as full-time wear; however, full-time wear has a greater failure to complete rate. The patient can be asked to wear the appliance part time to get better compliance without compromising the outcome.

As the compliance rate in both groups was low, so the present interpretation should be taken with caution.

Viewpoint

Parekh trial [51] was a well-conducted RCT. The main shortcomings were; confounding factors related to more girls in FT group as the girls may be more compliance than boys, more Asian British origin patients in PT group than FT group (71% vs 51.6%), the attrition bias, and underpowering the study where the acquired sample size was 56 patients (28 per group) and the loss to follow up was 6 patients in FT group and 1 patient in PT group. Interestingly, the authors adjusted for the Covariates; age, sex, overbite, and lower anterior face height, with a similar result. Furthermore, the actual comparison was made between two part-time wear groups with 3 hours difference.

Twin Block Design

Clinical Question 19: Does Adding Southend Clasps in Twin Block Affect the Treatment Results?

Evidence

Randomized Clinical Trial
Trenouth/2012 [52]

This study randomly allocated two parallel groups for functional treatment using TB with or without Southend clasps on upper and lower incisors. The trial enrolled 52 patients and analyzed 41 who continued the study. The findings showed that the dental changes have a statistically significant difference between the two groups. The upper incisors retroclination was less in the Southend clasp TB (SCTB) (6.1° ± 6) than in the non-Southend clasps TB group (NSTB) (12° ± 6.6). Lower incisors were proclined by (3° ± 3.6) for the SCTB and (6.9° ± 4.5) for the NSTB, which was statistically significant $p = 0.005$. However, the skeletal changes were statistically higher in the Southend clasps TB group. The reduction in ANB was statistically higher in the Southend clasp TB group (−3.5° ± 1.1) than in the non-Southend TB group (−2.6° ± 0.7, $p = 0.004$). The increase of SNB has no statistically significant difference between the two groups (3.2° and 2.4° for the Southend and non-Southend clasp group, respectively).

Evidence Summary

The best available evidence suggests that placing Southend clasps on the lower and upper incisors can improve the skeletal outcome of the treatment by Twin-block, and also can decrease the dental effect of this treatment.

Evidence Interpretation

Adding Southend clasps to TB appliance minimizes the dental effects and yields more skeletal effects with no reported harm. As these are findings of a single RCT with a limited sample that may represent low or very low evidence.

Viewpoint

This was a well-conducted trial [52]. The rate of loss to follow up was 21% of patients who did not complete the study, which lead to the attrition bias. The authors' inclusion criteria defined the age range as 9–30 years which is a very wide range and suggests a typo error; however, they included patients were from age range of 12.6 to 17.2 years. Though, it is hard to get skeletal effects after 15 years of age, the mean age was 15 years in this study. This raise up a question regarding the female growth and skeletal effects at this age.

Clinical Question 20: Which Is Better, Using Torquing Spurs with Headgear or a Labial Bow in the Twin Block Design?

Evidence

Randomized Controlled Trial
Yaqoob/2012 [53]

This trial randomly allocated 64 patients for functional treatment using TB either with or without a labial bow in the upper part of TB. Due to the loss to follow up, the authors analyzed 60 patients' records. Interestingly, although the upper incisors' inclination was less by 2.4° without a labial bow, but it was not statistically significant. The author did not find any statistically significant difference between the two groups regarding the amount of skeletal change, anterior facial height, or the rate of OJ reduction. The ANB angle decreased by 2.83° ±2.12 and 3.07° ±1.51, with and without a labial bow, respectively, with no statistically significant difference between both of them.

Clinical Trial
Parkin/2001 [54]

This clinical trial allocated 36 patients for functional treatment by TB with a labial bow and 27 patients for functional treatment using TB with torquing spurs on the upper centrals with a combination of headgear. The main findings suggested that the torquing spurs decreased the upper incisors retroclination and the headgear increased the vertical and sagittal control on the maxilla. In regard to SNA angle, the pre- and post-treatment changes had a significant difference between the traditional TB group (MD; -0.1°) and the HG with TB group (MD; -1.4°). The upper incisors angle has a statistically significant difference between the TB group (MD; -11°) and the torquing spurs HG TB group (MD; -6.9°) after the treatment.

Evidence Summary

The available evidence suggests that the design of TB appliances can affect the treatment outcomes. Interestingly, the labial bow has no effect on the treatment outcomes. The modified TB by adding torquing spurs on the upper centrals with HG combination can decrease the upper incisors retroclination and reinforce maxilla restrain.

Evidence Interpretation

Torquing spurs may reduce the upper incisors retroclination and thus give a room for more skeletal changes, while the use of HG reinforces maxillary restraining effects of twin block. The use of a labial bow is not effective in controlling incisor inclination.

When making a decision regarding the choice of appliance component to control upper incisors position, the Southend clasp seems to be effective in controlling the incisors torque with more skeletal effects according to the available evidence.

Viewpoint

Yaqoob study [53] was a well-conducted trial. The attrition was 4/64, and the authors did not use a proper test to deal with the dropouts (such as m-ITT or ITT). However, the authors calculated the sample size to get 5 degrees differences in the upper incisors' inclination, which may be large to detect.

In Parkin study [54], there was no randomization, allocation concealment, or blinding, and this addresses the study at a high risk of bias. Also, torque spurs were used in combination with headgear, so it is hard to investigate the true effects of torquing spurs. The authors did not calculate the sample size so the power of this study is questionable. The aforementioned points conclude that the quality of this trial is very low.

Clinical Question 21: Does Using Lower Incisors' Acrylic Capping Influence Their Proclination?

Evidence

Retrospective Study
Van der Plas/2017 [55]
This study calculated records of 56 Class II patients treated with TB; 29 patients were treated with TB appliances with acrylic capping on the lower incisors, and 27 patients were treated with TB appliances with ball-ended clasps in the lower incisors. The results showed that there is no statistically significant effect of the appliance design (with or without acrylic capping) on the lower incisors proclination. The lower incisors proclined up to 3° with acrylic capping and 2° with ball end clasp.

Evidence Summary

This evidence suggests that the acrylic capping in the Twin-block design does not influence the lower incisors' proclination. Adding acrylic capping on the lower incisors does not statistically prevent or decrease the lower incisors' proclination compared to ball-ended clasps.

Evidence Interpretation

The acrylic capping in TB design does not have any impact on the lower incisors' proclination. Trenouth et al. trial [52] also reported that almost similar amount of lower incisor proclination using Southend clasps, and the fact that it was a prospective randomized trial with higher quality than the Van der Plas et al. [55] study. So, a Southend clasp should be preferred for control of lower incisor inclination.

Viewpoint

This design [55] of study suffers from selection bias and confounding factors that mean the study is susceptible to a high risk of bias. The true effect is likely to be substantially different from this study estimate, and the study quality is very low.

Authors' Recommendations

- Class II growth modification is an effective method with a good success rate in growing children. It acts by restricting maxillary growth and augmenting mandibular growth.
- Removable functional appliances are more effective in terms of skeletal outcomes and cost, but have lower success rates than fixed functional appliances. In most cases, a Twin-block appliance with Southend clasps on upper and lower incisors is the best choice. The authors prefer a Herbst appliance in fixed functional appliances as it is a time-tested appliance with proven benefits.
- Functional appliances are effective in most cases of Class II growth modification. But in cases of moderate to severe maxillary prognathism, an orthopedic appliance like headgear can be combined with functional appliances for better skeletal outcomes.
- The removable functional appliance can be given part time, but if patient compliance is good, he can be advised to wear the appliance as much as he can.
- Late treatment (12–16 years) is more beneficial for the patient and the clinical practice than early treatment (7–11 years). Early treatment should only be done if the patient has psychological problems and wants to decrease the chances of incisor trauma chances.
- Class II growth modification should ideally be done before the start of the pubertal growth spurt. Multiple methods such as CVM, the patient's height, and secondary sexual characteristics should be used to assess the patient's pubertal peak spurt.
- Skeletal anchorage can be used to improve the effectiveness of functional appliances. This technique is so far novel and not very well taken by children/parents as it is invasive.
- Class II elastics can be used for Class II malocclusion correction but their effects are mainly dental, and they increase vertical dimensions of the face.
- Growth modification has no effects on TMJ in the long term.

References

1. Alhammadi MS, Halboub E, Fayed MS, Labib A, El-Saaidi C. Global distribution of malocclusion traits: a systematic review. Dental press. J Orthod. 2018;23(6):40:e1–e10. https://doi.org/10.1590/2177-6709.23.6.40.e1-10.onl.
2. Batista KB, Thiruvenkatachari B, Harrison JE, O'Brien KD. Orthodontic treatment for prominent upper front teeth (class II malocclusion) in children and adolescents. Cochrane Database Syst Rev. 2018;3(3):CD003452.
3. Bondemark L, Kurol J, Bernhold M. Repelling magnets versus superelastic nickel-titanium coils in simultaneous distal movement of maxillary first and second molars. Angle Orthod. 1994;64(3):189–98. https://doi.org/10.1043/0003-3219(1994)064<0189:rmvsnc>2.0.co;2.
4. Bondemark L, Kurol J. Distalization of maxillary first and second molars simultaneously with repelling magnets. Eur J Orthod. 1992;14(4):264–72.
5. Samson GS, Hechtkopf MJ. Supervision of class II discrepancies. Pediatric Dentisitry. 1988;10(4):331–5.
6. Bondi M. Lower body mesialization, upper distalization or combined therapy of the distal bite with horizontal growth. Mondo Ortod. 1979;4(1):24–38.
7. Nguyen QV, Bezemer PD, Habets L, Prahl-Andersen B. A systematic review of the relationship between overjet size and traumatic dental injuries. Eur J Orthod. 1999;21(5):503–15. https://doi.org/10.1093/ejo/21.5.503.
8. Logn JR, Casamassimo PS. Corrective methods for Class II patients. Pediatr Dent. 1988;10(4):342–4. PMID: 3272961.
9. Vaid NR, Doshi VM, Vandekar MJ. Class II treatment with functional appliances: a meta-analysis of short-term treatment effects. Semin Orthod. 2014;20(4):324–38. https://doi.org/10.1053/j.sodo.2014.09.008.
10. Batista KB, Thiruvenkatachari B, Harrison JE, O'Brien KD. Orthodontic treatment for prominent upper front teeth (class II malocclusion) in children and adolescents. Cochrane Database Syst Rev. 2018;3:Cd003452. https://doi.org/10.1002/14651858.CD003452.pub4.
11. Ehsani S, Nebbe B, Normando D, Laġravere MO, Flores-Mir C. Short-term treatment effects produced by the twin-block appliance: a systematic review and meta-analysis. Eur J Orthod. 2015;37(2):170–6. https://doi.org/10.1093/ejo/cju030.
12. Tulloch JFC, Phillips C, Proffit WR. The effect of early intervention on skeletal pattern in Class H malocclusion: a randomized clinical trial. Am J Orthod Dentofacial Orthop. 1997;111(4):391–400.
13. Tulloch JFC, Phillips C, Proffit WR. Influences on the outcome of early treatment for class H malocclusion. Am J Orthod Dentofacial Orthop. 1997;111(5):533–42.
14. Tulloch JFC, Phillips C, Proffit WR. Benefit of early class II treatment: Progress report of a two-phase randomized clinical trial. Am J Orthod Dentofac Orthop. 1998;113(1):62–72.
15. Casutt C, Pancherz H, Gawora M, Ruf S. Success rate and efficiency of activator treatment. Eur J Orthod. 2007;29(6):614–21. https://doi.org/10.1093/ejo/cjm066.
16. Perinetti G, Primozic J, Franchi L, Contardo L. Treatment effects of removable functional appliances in pre-pubertal and pubertal class II patients: a systematic review and meta-analysis of controlled studies. PLoS One. 2015;10(10):e0141198. https://doi.org/10.1371/journal.pone.0141198.
17. O'Brien K, Wright J, Conboy F, Appelbe P, Davies L, Connolly I, et al. Early treatment for class II division 1 malocclusion with the twin-block appliance: a multi-center, randomized, controlled trial. Am J Orthod Dentofacial Orthop: official publication of the American Association of Orthodontists, its constituent societies, and the American Board of Orthodontics. 2009;135(5):573–9. https://doi.org/10.1016/j.ajodo.2007.10.042.
18. Tulloch JFC, Proffit WR, Phillips C. Outcomes in a 2-phase randomized clinical trial of early class II treatment. Am J Orthod Dentofac Orthop. 2004;125(6):657–67. https://doi.org/10.1016/j.ajodo.2004.02.008.

19. O'Brien K, Wright J, Conboy F, Chadwick S, Connolly I, Cook P, et al. Effectiveness of early orthodontic treatment with the twin-block appliance: a multicenter, randomized, controlled trial. Part 2: psychosocial effects. Am J Orthod Dentofac Orthop. 2003;124(5):488–94. https://doi.org/10.1016/j.ajodo.2003.06.001.

20. O'Brien Kevin TM, Wright J, Conboy F, Appelbe P, Birnie D, Chadwick S, Connolly I, Hammond M, Harradine N, Lewis D, Littlewood S, McDade C, Mitchell L, Murray A, O'Neill J, Sandler J, Read M, Robinson S, Shaw I, Turbill E. Early treatment for class II malocclusion and perceived improvements in facial profile. Am J Orthod Dentofacial Orthop. 2009;135(5):580–5. https://doi.org/10.1016/j.ajodo.2008.02.020.

21. Szemraj A, Wojtaszek-Slominska A, Racka-Pilszak B. Is the cervical vertebral maturation (CVM) method effective enough to replace the hand-wrist maturation (HWM) method in determining skeletal maturation?-a systematic review. Eur J Radiol. 2018;102:125–8. https://doi.org/10.1016/j.ejrad.2018.03.012.

22. Santiago RC, de Miranda Costa LF, Vitral RW, Fraga MR, Bolognese AM, Maia LC. Cervical vertebral maturation as a biologic indicator of skeletal maturity. Angle Orthod. 2012;82(6):1123–31. https://doi.org/10.2319/103111-673.1.

23. O'Brien K, Wright J, Conboy F, Sanjie Y, Mandall N, Chadwick S, et al. Effectiveness of early orthodontic treatment with the twin-block appliance: a multicenter, randomized, controlled trial. Part 1: dental and skeletal effects. Am J Orthod Dentofac Orthop. 2003;124(3):234–43. https://doi.org/10.1016/s0889-5406(03)00352-4.

24. Kyburz KS, Eliades T, Papageorgiou SN. What effect does functional appliance treatment have on the temporomandibular joint? A systematic review with meta-analysis. Prog Orthod. 2019;20(1):32. https://doi.org/10.1186/s40510-019-0286-9.

25. Ivorra-Carbonell L, Montiel-Company JM, Almerich-Silla JM, Paredes-Gallardo V, Bellot-Arcis C. Impact of functional mandibular advancement appliances on the temporomandibular joint - a systematic review. Med Oral Patol Oral Cir Bucal. 2016;21(5):e565–72. https://doi.org/10.4317/medoral.21180.

26. Pancherz H, Michailidou C. Temporomandibular joint growth changes in hyperdivergent and hypodivergent Herbst subjects A long-term roentgenographic cephalometric study. Am J Orthod Dentofacial Orthop: official publication of the American Association of Orthodontists, its constituent societies, and the American Board of Orthodontics 2004;126(2):153–61; quiz 254–5. https://doi.org/10.1016/j.ajodo.2003.07.015.

27. Perillo L, Cannavale R, Ferro F, Franchi L, Masucci C, Chiodini P, et al. Meta-analysis of skeletal mandibular changes during Frankel appliance treatment. Eur J Orthod. 2011;33(1):84–92. https://doi.org/10.1093/ejo/cjq033.

28. Cozza P, Baccetti T, Franchi L, De Toffol L, McNamara JA Jr. Mandibular changes produced by functional appliances in class II malocclusion: a systematic review. Am J Orthod Dentofac Orthop. 2006;129(5):599 e1-12:discussion e1-6. https://doi.org/10.1016/j.ajodo.2005.11.010.

29. Tümer N, Gültan AS. Comparison of the effects of monoblock and twin-block appliances on the skeletal and dentoalveolar structures. Am J Orthod Dentofac Orthop. 1999;116(4):460–8. https://doi.org/10.1016/S0889-5406(99)70233-7.

30. Antonarakis GS, Kiliaridis S. Short-term anteroposterior treatment effects of functional appliances and extraoral traction on class II malocclusion. A meta-analysis. Angle Orthod. 2007;77(5):907–14. https://doi.org/10.2319/061706-244.

31. Illing HM, Morris DO, Lee RT. A prospective evaluation of Bass, Bionator and Twin Block appliances. Part I--The hard tissues. Eur J Orthod. 1998;20(5):501–16. https://doi.org/10.1093/ejo/20.5.501.

32. Lund DI, Sandler PJ. The effects of twin blocks: a prospective controlled study. Am J Orthod Dentofac Orthop. 1998;113(1):104–10. https://doi.org/10.1016/s0889-5406(98)70282-3.

33. Varlik SK, Gültan A, Tümer N. Comparison of the effects of twin block and activator treatment on the soft tissue profile. Eur J Orthod. 2008;30(2):128–34. https://doi.org/10.1093/ejo/cjm121.

34. Morris DO, Illing HM, Lee RT. A prospective evaluation of Bass, Bionator and Twin Block appliances. Part II--The soft tissues. Eur J Orthod. 1998;20(6):663–84.

35. Flores-Mir C, Major PW. A systematic review of cephalometric facial soft tissue changes with the activator and Bionator appliances in class II division 1 subjects. Eur J Orthod. 2006;28(6):586–93. https://doi.org/10.1093/ejo/cjl034. Epub 2006 Nov 9
36. Lange DW, Kalra V, Broadbent BH Jr, Powers M, Nelson S. Changes in soft tissue profile following treatment with the bionator. Angle Orthod. 1995;65(6):423–30. https://doi.org/10.1043/0003-3219(1995)065<0423:Cistpf>2.0.Co;2.
37. Maltagliati L, Henriques JF, Janson G, Almeida RR, Freitas MR. Influence of orthopedic treatment on hard and soft facial structures of individuals presenting with class II, division 1 malocclusion: a comparative study. J Appl Oral Sci. 2004;12(2):164–70. https://doi.org/10.1590/s1678-77572004000200016.
38. Pacha MM, Fleming PS, Johal A. A comparison of the efficacy of fixed versus removable functional appliances in children with class II malocclusion: a systematic review. Eur J Orthod. 2016;38(6):621–30. https://doi.org/10.1093/ejo/cjv086.
39. O'Brien K, Wright J, Conboy F, Sanjie Y, Mandall N, Chadwick S, et al. Effectiveness of treatment for class II malocclusion with the Herbst or twin-block appliances: a randomized, controlled trial. Am J Orthod Dentofac Orthop. 2003;124(2):128–37. https://doi.org/10.1016/s0889-5406(03)00345-7.
40. Baysal A, Uysal T. Dentoskeletal effects of twin block and Herbst appliances in patients with class II division 1 mandibular retrognathy. Eur J Orthod. 2014;36(2):164–72. https://doi.org/10.1093/ejo/cjt013.
41. Madurantakam P. Fixed or removable function appliances for class II malocclusions. Evid Based Dent. 2016;17(2):52–3. https://doi.org/10.1038/sj.ebd.6401171.
42. Elkordy SA, Aboelnaga AA, Fayed MM, AboulFotouh MH, Abouelezz AM. Can the use of skeletal anchors in conjunction with fixed functional appliances promote skeletal changes? A systematic review and meta-analysis. Eur J Orthod. 2016;38(5):532–45. https://doi.org/10.1093/ejo/cjv081.
43. Elkordy SA, Abouelezz AM, Fayed MMS, Aboulfotouh MH, Mostafa YA. Evaluation of the miniplate-anchored Forsus fatigue resistant device in skeletal class II growing subjects: a randomized controlled trial. Angle Orthod. 2019;89(3):391–403. https://doi.org/10.2319/062018-468.1.
44. Manni A, Migliorati M, Calzolari C, Silvestrini-Biavati A. Herbst appliance anchored to miniscrews in the upper and lower arches vs standard Herbst: a pilot study. Am J Orthod Dentofacial Orthop: official publication of the American Association of Orthodontists, its constituent societies, and the American Board of Orthodontics. 2019;156(5):617–25. https://doi.org/10.1016/j.ajodo.2018.11.015.
45. Campbell C, Millett D, Kelly N, Cooke M, Cronin M. Frankel 2 appliance versus the modified twin block appliance for phase 1 treatment of class II division 1 malocclusion in children and adolescents: a randomized clinical trial. Angle Orthod. 2019;90(2):202–8. https://doi.org/10.2319/042419-290.1.
46. Banks P, Wright J, O'Brien K. Incremental versus maximum bite advancement during twin-block therapy: a randomized controlled clinical trial. Am J Orthod Dentofac Orthop. 2004;126(5):583–8. https://doi.org/10.1016/j.ajodo.2004.03.024.
47. Bock NC, von Bremen J, Ruf S. Stability of Class II fixed functional appliance therapy--a systematic review and meta-analysis. Eur J Orthod. 2016;38(2):129–39. https://doi.org/10.1093/ejo/cjv009.
48. Dolce C, McGorray SP, Brazeau L, King GJ, Wheeler TT. Timing of class II treatment: skeletal changes comparing 1-phase and 2-phase treatment. Am J Orthod Dentofacial Orthop: official publication of the American Association of Orthodontists, its constituent societies, and the American Board of Orthodontics. 2007;132(4):481–9. https://doi.org/10.1016/j.ajodo.2005.08.046.
49. Janson G, Sathler R, Fernandes TM, Branco NC, Freitas MR. Correction of class II malocclusion with class II elastics: a systematic review. Am J Orthod Dentofacial Orthop: official publication of the American Association of Orthodontists, its constituent societies, and the American Board of Orthodontics. 2013;143(3):383–92. https://doi.org/10.1016/j.ajodo.2012.10.015.

50. Aras I, Pasaoglu A. Class II subdivision treatment with the Forsus fatigue resistant device vs intermaxillary elastics. Angle Orthod. 2017;87(3):371–6. https://doi.org/10.2319/070216-518.1.
51. Parekh J, Counihan K, Fleming PS, Pandis N, Sharma PK. Effectiveness of part-time vs full-time wear protocols of twin-block appliance on dental and skeletal changes: a randomized controlled trial. Am J Orthod Dentofacial Orthop: official publication of the American Association of Orthodontists, its constituent societies, and the American Board of Orthodontics. 2019;155(2):165–72. https://doi.org/10.1016/j.ajodo.2018.07.016.
52. Trenouth MJ, Desmond S. A randomized clinical trial of two alternative designs of twin-block appliance. J Orthod. 2012;39(1):17–24. https://doi.org/10.1179/14653121226788.
53. Yaqoob O, Dibiase AT, Fleming PS, Cobourne MT. Use of the Clark twin block functional appliance with and without an upper labial bow: a randomized controlled trial. Angle Orthod. 2012;82(2):363–9. https://doi.org/10.2319/041411-268.1.
54. Parkin NA, McKeown HF, Sandler PJ. Comparison of 2 modifications of the twin-block appliance in matched class II samples. Am J Orthod Dentofacial Orthop: official publication of the American Association of Orthodontists, its constituent societies, and the American Board of Orthodontics. 2001;119(6):572–7. https://doi.org/10.1067/mod.2001.113790.
55. van der Plas MC, Janssen KI, Pandis N, Livas C. Twin block appliance with acrylic capping does not have a significant inhibitory effect on lower incisor proclination. Angle Orthod. 2017;87(4):513–8. https://doi.org/10.2319/102916-779.1.

Growth Modification Treatment in Class III of Malocclusion

4

Contents

© The Author(s), under exclusive license to Springer Nature Switzerland AG 2023

S. Mheissen, H. Khan, *Orthodontic Evidence*,

https://doi.org/10.1007/978-3-031-24422-3_4

Abbreviations

ALt-RAMEC	Alternating rapid maxillary expansion and constriction
BAIMT	Bone-anchored intermaxillary traction
CC	Chin cup
CCHFG	Chin cup with high applied force and acrylic bite plane
CCLFG	Chin cup with low applied force and acrylic bite plane
CG	Controls group
CrI	Credibility intervals
FM	Facemask
FM/RME	Facemask with rapid maxillary expansion
FM-BARME	Bone-anchored rapid maxillary expansion
FM-MTAD	Facemask with a maxillary temporary anchorage device
FR3	Frankel-III
MFM	Modified face mask
MJJ	Modified Jasper Jumper
mo	Month
NMA	Network meta-analysis
RTB	Reverse twin block
Y	Year

Introduction

Class III malocclusion has the lowest prevalence among Angle's malocclusions. The global prevalence of Class III malocclusion ranges from 1 to 20%, with the highest prevalence reported in Mongoloids [1]. In this type of malocclusion, the molars or incisor relationship can be in Class III, with associated negative overjet in most cases. The etiology of Class III malocclusion is multifactorial, with genetic and environmental factors involved [2, 3]. The malocclusion can have a dental or skeletal origin, or it can be a combination of both.

The age of the patient plays a vital role in the treatment of Class III malocclusion. In young patients, ideally before the age of 10 years, growth modification is the treatment of choice [4]. It is mostly undertaken in cases with mild to moderate malocclusion. In permanent dentition, camouflage treatment can be done only if the problem is mild. For Class III camouflage treatment in growing patients, the extraction should be avoided in patients with a family history of Class III, because the pattern of camouflage extraction is opposite to the surgical decompensation. So, if the camouflage fails due to further mandibular growth, it should not limit the scope of future surgery. Patients with moderate to severe Class III malocclusion are mostly treated with orthognathic surgery once the mandibular growth has ceased.

Growth modification for Class III malocclusion is based on the same principle as Class II growth modification. Both functional and orthopedic appliances are effective for growth modification, at least in the short term [5]. In the literature, many different appliances have been suggested to treat this malocclusion, with most of them trying to direct the growth in a favorable way. The growth modification of Class III malocclusion can be undertaken using:

Orthopedic appliance: Most of these appliances use an extraoral force to stimulate the maxillary growth; such as the facemask, or to restrain/redirect the mandibular growth as in the case of chin cup.

Myofunctional appliance: These are intraoral appliances and can be tooth-borne such as reverse twin block, or tissue borne such as Frankel-III regulator.

Most recently temporary skeletal anchorage devices (TSADs) such as mini-implants and miniplates have been used to provide direct Class III traction using either intermaxillary elastics or support the Class III orthopedic appliances.

Class III Growth Modification Effectiveness

Clinical Question 1: Is Class III Growth Modification Effective?

Evidence

Systematic Reviews and Meta-Analyses
Woon/2017 [5]

This systematic review included 15 studies; three trials compared Class III patients treated using facemask (FM) with non-treated controls. Meta-analysis for the three trials showed statistically significant skeletal and dental changes in the short term. ANB increased in facemask group by 3.90° (95% CI: 3.54–4.25; $P < 0.0001$), and the overjet increased by 2.5 mm (95% CI: 1.21–3.79; $P = 0.0001$, one trial). The overall quality of evidence for these findings was low.

Zhang/2015 [6]

This review included 12 papers investigating the treatment of Class III malocclusion using the facemask. The authors pooled four studies in meta-analysis, and compared treatment using facemask versus non-treated patients. They found that there was a statistically significant increase in the SNA angle (MD; 1.78°, 95% CI: 1.57–1.99, $P < 0.00001$) favoring the treated group. Similarly, a statistically significant increase was found in ANB angle (MD; 3.64°, 95% CI: 3.10–4.19, $P < 0.00001$), favoring FM treated group when compared to untreated controls. Also, the authors found a statistically significant decrease in SNB angle (MD; −1.75°, 95% CI: −2.28 to −1.23, $P < 0.00001$).

Four trials in meta-analysis compared the facemask along with rapid maxillary expansion (FM/RME) versus non-treated controls. The researchers found statistically significant differences between FM/RME and non-treated controls regarding the skeletal changes. The treated group showed a statistically significant increase in SNA (MD; 1.39°, 95% CI: 0.85 to 1.94, $P < 0.00001$) than controls. The SNB angle decreased statistically in FM/RME group (MD; −2.54°, 95% CI: −3.08 to −2.01,

$P < 0.00001$) than controls. Furthermore, there was a statistically significant difference in ANB angle (MD; 3.25°, 95% CI: 2.06–4.44, $P < 0.00001$) favoring the treatment group.

Watkinson/2013 [7]

This Cochrane systematic review included seven RCTs with 339 Class III patients under 16 years of age. The reviewers investigated the effectiveness of orthopedic appliances in treating Class III malocclusion. They found that the FM showed statistically significant effects regarding the overjet correction (MD; 4.10 mm, 95%CI: 3.04–5.16; $P < 0.0001$) when compared with non-treated patients. Likewise, there was a statistically significant difference in ANB angle favoring facemask (MD; 3.93°, 95% CI: 3.46–4.39, $P < 0.0001$) over non-treated controls. Interestingly, one primary study reported adverse effects of FM, showing temporomandibular joint (TMJ) signs and symptoms, but there was a very low prevalence of these effects.

Two included studies compared the chin cup versus no treatment and found a statistically significant difference in ANB (MD; 1.96°, 95%CI: 1.58–2.34, $P < 0.0001$). While one included study found a statistically significant difference between Tandem traction bow appliance and non-treated controls in regard to overjet (MD; 3.30 mm, 95% CI: 2.46–4.14, $P < 0.0001$, one trial), and ANB (MD; 1.70°, 95% CI: 1.09–2.31, $P < 0.0001$, one trial) favoring Tandem traction bow appliance.

Randomized Controlled Trial
Mandall/2010 [8]

The authors conducted a multicenter RCT with 15 months of follow up to investigate the effectiveness of Class III early treatment (7–9 years old) using FM/RME. They allocated 35 patients out of 73 to the FM/RME group and 38 to the non-treated controls group (CG). In the FM/RME group, they used a bonded acrylic expansion device. The extraoral force was gradually increased every 2 weeks from 3/8;8 oz. to 5/16;16 oz. until the applied force reached 400 g per side. The active treatment time was 8.6 ± 3.5 months. The researchers found statistically significant differences between groups regarding the skeletal and dental changes. SNA angle increased by 1.4° ± 2.1 in the FM/RME group versus 0.3° ± 2 in the CG, which was statistically significant ($p = 0.018$). There was a statistically significant difference between both groups regarding SNB angle changes ($p < 0.001$); SNB statistically decreased by −0.7° ± 1.5 in FM/RME group, while it increased in the CG by 0.8° ± 1.4. Likewise, ANB mean difference between groups was statistically significant (2.6°, $p < 0.001$) favoring the FM/RME group. The increase in maxillary-mandibular angle was small but statistically significant. For the dental changes, there was a statistically significant difference between groups in regards to retroclination of lower incisors (−4.9° ± 4.1 for FM/RME versus −1.2° ± 4.3 for CG). The overjet increased 4.4 ± 2.7 mm in FM/RME group versus 0.3 ± 1.6 mm in CG, and this was a statically significant difference between groups ($p < 0.001$). The success rate of FM/RME was 70%, with the patient attaining positive overjet.

Mandall/2012 [9]
This is the continuation of the previous RCT with 3 years of follow-up. The authors analyzed 63 records after 3 years, with 10 patients lost to follow-up. The mean age was 12.1 and 12.3 years for FM/RME and CG, respectively. They found that the skeletal differences were statistically significant between groups in ANB improvement (1.5° ± 2 in FM/RME group and 0.1° ± 1.9 in CG, $p = 0.001$). The FM appliance maintained more advancement at A point (FM/RME 2.3° ± 2.1 versus CG 1.6° ± 2.6, $p = 0.14$) and more retrusion at B point (FM/RME 0.8° ± 1.5 versus CG 1.5° ± 2.3, $p = 0.26$), but these effects were not statistically significant on their own. A statistically significant backward and downward maxillary rotation were found between groups 4.1° ± 4.1 in FM/RME group and 4.3° ±2.8 in CG. The difference between groups regarding the lower facial height and the mandibular angle change was not statistically significant.

Evidence Summary

The best available evidence indicates that FM is an effective orthopedic treatment for early age Class III patients. There were statistically significant effects induced by FM treatment on the skeletal changes for both jaws in different studies. The SNA increase ranged from 1.39° to 1.78°, while the SNB decrease was between 0.7° and 2.54°. The highest SNB change (2.54°) was reported in the meta-analysis of Zhang [6] though the overall change for SNB in the systematic reviews was less than the SNA change. The ANB improvement ranged from 2.6° to 3.93° using FM. Chin cup and Tandem traction bow appliance also improved ANB angle.

Dental changes included lower incisors retroclination by 4.9° in FM/RME versus 1.2° in CG with an overjet increase of 4.4 mm in the FM group and 0.3 mm in CG. In the long term of 3 years of follow-up, the early orthopedic treatment started before 10 years of age achieved a statistically significant improvement in ANB angle (MD; 1.5°) and positive overjet in 70% of patients with no harmful effects (TMJ) in the long term.

Evidence Interpretation

Class III growth modification is an effective treatment in growing children that is associated with maxillary protraction and restriction of mandibular growth. Ideally, it is recommended in children less than 10 years of age. More skeletal effects are seen in the maxilla than in the mandible with the facemask appliance. So, the ideal cases for growth modification are one with maxillary retrognathism. Consent must be taken from the patients as the treatment is successful in only 70% of the patients with the treatment duration ranging from 6 to 12 months.

Viewpoint

Woon study [5] was a well-conducted review. The included studies were graded as low to moderate quality evidence. The included trials have variations in the age range of the patients. Two studies were assessed with some concerns according to the risk of bias tool. However, there was a substantial statistical heterogeneity without adjusting the meta-analysis using a random model to account the between studies' variability.

Zhang review [6] have the following limitations: There was a restriction on the search language. The authors did not provide information about data screening and inclusion. They assessed the quality of the included studies as fair to good and those studies were from case-control design. As such, these reduce the overall quality of the evidence.

Watkinson review[7] was a well-conducted Cochrane review. The quality of the evidence varied between low to very low quality according to the small number of participants, the heterogeneity, and the risk of bias.

Mandall study [8, 9] was a well-conducted study with a low attrition bias. Although this study was done in real-world settings, the authors excluded high hyperdivergent cases (NL-ML >35°) and cases with TMJ signs or symptoms. In contrast, the forward displaced mandible cases were included that increases the probability of treating mild Class III cases. Interestingly, the points mentioned above limit the applicability of the trial to Caucasian children, average and hypodivergent faces, and patients with no history of TMJ problems.

Further research with a long-term follows up may change our certainty as the true effects of Class III growth modification may be different from the recent estimate.

Treatment Timing

Clinical Question 2: What Is the Best Time for Orthopedic Treatment of Class III Malocclusion?

Evidence

Systematic Reviews and Meta-Analyses
Zhang/2015 [6]

In this review, the authors pooled four studies in meta-analysis to compare the early versus the late Class III treatment. The early treatment comprised participants with an age range of 7–10 years and having early mixed dentition, whereas the late treatment group comprised participants with an age range of 11–14 years in their late mixed dentition or early permanent dentition.

The review found that the FM treatment yielded greater effects in the early treatment group than the late treatment group. The SNA change was greater in the early treatment group than the late treatment group, but insignificant (MD; 1.09, 95% CI: −0.70 to 2.88, $P = 0.23$, 3 trials). The SNB change was statistically greater in the early than the late treatment group (MD; −1.42, 95% CI: −1.95 to −0.90, $P < 0.00001$, 3 trials). Likewise, the ANB change was greater in early age treatment than late treatment group, but not statistically significant (MD; 1.72, 95% CI: −0.76 to 4.19, $P = 0.17$, 3 trials).

Kim/1999 [4]

In this systematic review, the treatment time was classified into two categories: early treatment for patients younger than 10 years of age, and late treatment for patients older than 10 years of age. The authors included six studies investigating the effectiveness of early Class III treatment using FM, versus seven studies assessing the late treatment effects of the facemask. The researchers found that the skeletal effects were larger in the younger group than the older group. The pre and post-treatment skeletal changes in younger participants (4–10 years) were 2.2° ± 2.1 in SNA angle, −1.6° ± 1.7 in SNB angle, and 3.8°±2.7 in ANB. In the older age group (10–15), these changes were 1.6° ± 1.6 in SNA, −1.2° ± 1.4 in SNB, and 2.8°±1.8 in ANB. The differences between the early and the late treatment were 0.6° in SNA, −0.5° in SNB, and 1° in ANB, favoring early treatment. As such, skeletal changes were greater if treatment was done before 10 years of age.

Retrospective Studies
Baccetti/1998 [10]
The authors selected 46 Class III patients from 105 patients for facemask treatment, and divided them into two groups: An early treatment group having 23 patients with a mean age of 6 years and 9 mo ± 1 year, and the late treatment group having 23 patients with a mean age of 10 years and 3 mo ± 1 year. The mean treatment time was 11 ± 4 months using FM and bonded maxillary expander with an incremental force of 3/8-inch 8Oz, ½ inch 14Oz, and finally 5/16 inch 14Oz. The investigators found that the skeletal changes favored the early treatment group (Co-A: 4.91 ± 2.36 mm, Co-Gn: 1.8 ± 2.04 mm) over the late treatment group (Co-A: 3.12 ± 1.96 mm, Co-Gn: 3.26 ± 2.68 mm) but this was statistically insignificant.

Yavuz/2009 [11]
This study divided 28 females into two groups: the adolescent group comprised 15 females with a mean age of 11.8 y ± 0.8 (Fishman; SMI 1–3), and the young adults' group in which 13 females with a mean age of 14.02 y ± 0.63 (Fishman; SMI 10–11) were included. The treatment duration was 6.89 ± 1.53 months for adolescents and 8 ± 1.65 months for adults. The researchers found that the SNA changes were statistically significant in the adolescent group (2.31° ± 1.29) and the young adults' group (0.78° ± 0.67), with a higher effect size in the adolescents' group. The comparison between the two groups revealed that the difference in ANB changes was statistically significant between the two groups favoring the adolescents' group (3.65° ± 1.56) over the young adults' group (2.25° ± 1.20). The dental changes were greater in the adolescent group than young adults' group, but not statistically significant; UI/SN: 5.13° ± 4.32 and 2.69° ± 2.43 for adolescents and young adults, respectively. Similarly, the changes in the lower incisors were −4.17° ± 3.34 and − 3.95° ± 4.85 for adolescents and young adults, respectively. Furthermore, the vertical increase was similar between groups and not statistically significant; MP/SN: 1.87° ± 1.86 and 1.33° ± 1.79 in adolescents and adults, respectively.

Evidence Summary
The best available evidence supports that the early orthopedic treatment provides more skeletal changes than the late orthopedic treatment. In one systematic review[6], a statistically significant difference was found in SNB (MD; −1.42°, 95% CI: −1.95 to −0.90, $P < 0.00001$), but not in SNA (MD; 1.09°, 95% CI: −0.70 to 2.88, $P = 0.23$) and ANB (MD; 1.72°, 95% CI: −0.76 to 4.19, $P = 0.17$). Another

review [12], reported a minor difference between early and late treatment and that was 0.6° in SNA, −0.5° in SNB, and 1° in ANB. One trial[10] reported more favorable skeletal linear changes in the early age group (Co-A: 4.91 mm, Co-Gn: 1.8 mm) than the late group (Co-A: 3.12 mm, Co-Gn: 3.26 mm). Though these differences were not statistically significant regarding SNA and ANB between older and younger groups, the differences have a large effect. On the other hand, a statistically significant difference was found in SNB angle between both groups.

Evidence Interpretation

The best time for undertaking Class III growth modification is before 10 years of age. But if the patient presented at the age range between 10 and 14 years, the treatment should not be denied, but the patient must be cautioned that the chances of success might be less, and there might be limited skeletal and more dental effects due to the treatment.

Viewpoint

Kim et al. review [12] provided good information about FM treatment. Unfortunately, there was a lack of following a well-structured guidelines with no clear description for the included studies and their quality, that may reduce the quality of this evidence.

Baccetti [10] and Yavuz studies [11] lack sample size calculation, randomization, allocation concealment, and blinding. In Baccetti et al. [10] study, there were retrospective control records from another institution, and the authors did not correct the cephalometric enlargement for liner measurements which may lead to some concerns in the pre- and post-treatment linear measurements. Also, the authors only included European-American ethnicity which may increase the selection bias and limit the generalizability of the results. The error of the method ranged from 0.13 to 0.81 mm for the linear measurements and from 0.19° to 0.93° for the angular measurements, which may increase the uncertainty in the measurements. In Yavuz [11] study, the authors only included females with OJ and ANB less than zero, so the applicability is restricted to the sample characteristics. The sample size was small, and the researchers did not provide the differences between groups at the baseline.

Dental Versus Skeletal Effects

Clinical Question 3: What Are the Skeletal and Dental Effects of Class III Orthopedic Treatment?

Evidence

Systematic Reviews and Meta-analyses
Jäger/2001 [13]

In this systematic review and meta-analysis, the reviewers included 12 trials to investigate the skeletal and dental effects of maxillary protraction using FM. The meta-analysis demonstrated that the main effect of FM therapy was an increase in SNA angle up to 1.4° ± 0.2 with a statistically significant anterior maxillary rotation

(NL-NSL 0.9° ± 0.2). Additionally, the ANB angle increased by 2.6° ± 0.3, and the SNB angle reduced by −1.3° ± 0.2 with a posterior rotation of the mandible. FM increased the lower facial height (LAFH) by 1.6 ± 0.3 mm. FM has also a significant effect on the dentoalveolar components; the protrusion of the upper incisors was 1.5° ± 0.6, and the retrusion of the lower incisors was −3.7° ± 0.7°.

Woon/2017 [5]
This review included 15 articles: 9 were RCTs, and 6 were CCTs. The age of patients varied from 7.3 to 11.75 years in the included studies. As discussed before, more ANB and overjet changes were noted in the FM group when compared to CG; after FM traction, ANB increased by 3.90° (95% CI: 3.54–4.25; $P < 0.001$), and the overjet increased by 2.5 mm (95% CI: 1.21–3.79; $P = 0.001$, one trial).

Tandem traction bow appliance also has a good result in terms of skeletal and dental measures when compared to untreated controls. After the treatment, ANB angle was statistically greater in tandem appliance group (MD; 1.7°, 95% CI: 1.54–1.86; $P < 0.001$) with more statistically significant correction in the overjet (MD; 3.30 mm, 95% Cl: 3.08–3.52; $P < 0.001$).

Evidence Summary
The best available evidence suggests that growth modification using FM provides both skeletal and dental changes. For the skeletal changes, there was a statistically significant difference between the FM group and the untreated CG; ANB (MD; 2.6°–3.90°), SNA (MD; 1.4° ± 0.2), NL-NSL (MD;0.9° ± 0.2), SNB (MD; −1.3° ± 0.2), and LAFH (MD; 1.6 ± 0.3 mm) favoring FM group. Furthermore, a statistically significant difference was found between the FM group and CG in terms of dental changes. After the treatment, the FM group has more protrusion in upper incisors (MD; 1.5° ± 0.6), and more retrusion in lower incisors (MD; −3.7° ± 0.7) than CG. As a result, the overjet significantly increased in the FM group (MD; 2.5 mm, $p = 0.0001$) when compared to CG.

Evidence Interpretation
Growth modification in Class III cases results in both skeletal and dental changes. There was a significant improvement in ANB, but this was associated with undesirable incisors' inclination. Furthermore, Class III growth modification increases the facial vertical proportions by downward and backward rotation of the mandible. Keeping these treatment changes in mind, the ideal cases for Class III growth modification are ones with a deficient maxilla with normal or low vertical proportions. As the posterior rotation of the mandible causes a decrease of the overbite, cases with increased overbite are favored more for FM treatment than decreased overbite or openbite cases. As such, the undesirable effects of growth modification should be kept in mind during treatment planning of skeletal open bites and cases with dentoalveolar compensation.

Viewpoint
In Jäger [13] review, the search was not comprehensive, and the authors searched only the Medline database which may miss some related studies and increase the potential publication bias. There was no reporting for the risk of bias assessment,

the quality of the included studies, the data extraction, and the screening or full-text reading. As such, Jäger [13] review is a very low-quality systematic review.

Woon review [5] was a well-conducted systematic review, and the included studies were graded as low to moderate quality evidence.

The aforementioned evidence suggests a little confidence in the effect estimate of the Class III growth modification, and further research may change the real effect of this treatment.

Facemask Versus Chin Cup

Clinical Question 4: What Should be the Appliance of Choice for Early Orthopedic Treatment: Facemask or Chin Cup?

Evidence

Systematic Reviews and Meta-Analyses
Rongo/2017 [14]

This systematic review and meta-analysis included 21 studies; 7 RCT, 8 CCT, and 6 retrospective studies. Out of those studies, 15 FM studies and 3 chin cup (CC) studies were pooled in the meta-analysis. The age in the FM group ranged from 5.6 ± 1.0 years to 12.5 ± 0.7 years, and in the CC ranged from 4.8 ± 1.4 years to 11.5 ± 1.1 years. The treatment duration varied between 5.6 and 6 months. The authors found that there was a statistically significant skeletal improvement in the FM and CC groups after treatment; ANB (SMD;2.59 in CC versus 3.65 in FM), SNA (SMD; 0.59 in CC versus 2.09 in FM), and SNB (SMD; -2.23 and -1.49 in CC and FM, respectively), but the authors were unable to compare the groups directly. Likewise, the dental changes were statistically significant. Upper incisors inclination was (SMD; 0.87 in CC and 0.62 in FM groups), and the lower incisors inclination was (SMD; -2.14 in CC and -0.27 in FM groups). Moreover, FM and CC increased the mandibular divergence and caused a mandibular clockwise rotation (SMD; 1.66 and 1.03 in CC and FM, respectively).

Watkinson/2013 [7]

This Cochrane systematic review included seven RCTs. The reviewer authors inspected the effectiveness of orthopedic appliances in treating Class III malocclusion. They found that the FM showed statistically significant effects in regard to overjet (MD; 4.10 mm, 95%CI: 3.04–5.16; $P < 0.001$) and ANB (MD; 3.93°, 95% CI: 3.46–4.39; $P < 0.001$) when compared with non-treated patients. Two studies compared chin cup (CC) versus no treatment and found a statistically significant increase in ANB (MD; 1.96°, 95%CI: 1.58–2.34, $P < 0.0001$, two trials) favoring the CC group. Likewise, a significant increase was found in the CC group regarding Wits appraisal (MD; 4.94 mm, 95% CI: 4.45–5.42, $P < 0.0001$, two trials). The evidence was of low quality.

Randomized Controlled Trial
Abdelnaby/2010 [15]

This clinical trial comprised 50 patients with skeletal Class III (ANB <1°). The patients were randomly assigned into three groups; 20 patients in the occipital pull chin cup with high applied force and acrylic bite plane CCHFG (600 g per side group), 20 patients in the chin cup with low applied force and acrylic bite plane CCLFG (300 g per side group), and 10 patients in the control group. The mean age was 9.6, 10.1, and 9.2 years in CCHFG, CCLFG, and control groups, respectively. The wearing time was 14 hours per day, and the data were collected after 1 year. The researchers found that there was a statistically significant difference between groups in regard to ANB (2.5° ± 0.51, 2.40° ± 0.50, and 0.50° ± 0.52 in CCHFG, CCLFG, and CG, respectively), SNB (−2.20° ± 0.41, −2.00 ± 0.79, −0.30° ± 0.48 in CCHFG, CCLFG, and CG, respectively), SN-MP(1.50° ± 0.51, 1.40° ± 0.50, 0.50° ± 0.52 in CCHFG, CCLFG, and CG, respectively), Na-Me increase (4.20 ± 1.93, 4.70 ± 2.05, 1.40 ± 0.69 in CCHFG, CCLFG, and CG, respectively). On the other hand, no statistically significant difference was found between the three groups regarding SNA (0.3° ± 0.47, 0.4° ± 0.50, 0.2° ± 0.42 in CCHFG, CCLFG, and CG, respectively). However, the intergroup dental changes were statistically different regarding the lower incisors angle (LI-MP; −3.90° ± 2.22, −2.80° ± 1.10, −0.20° ± 0.63 in CCHFG, CCLFG, and CG, respectively), but not for the upper incisor angle with the SN plane. Interestingly, no significant difference was found between the two treatment groups except the ramus height reduction; the reduction was statistically higher in the high force group than in the low force group; Ar-Go; −0.95 ± 0.67 in CCHFG vs. -0.10 ± 0.64 in CCLFG.

Evidence Summary

The orthopedic appliances are effective in early Class III treatment. FM has a higher skeletal effect than CC in terms of ANB (MD; 3.93° and SMD; 3.65 in FM vs. 2.59 in CC). FM has a greater effect on maxilla than the CC appliance; SNA (SMD; 2.09 in FM vs. 0.59 in CC). FM has lesser effects on the mandible than CC; SNB (SMD; −2.23 and −1.49 in CC and FM, respectively). Greater lower incisors retroclination was found in the CC than the FM group (SMD; −2.14 in CC and −0.0.27 in FM). Also, there was a more vertical increase in the CC group when compared with non-treated controls (SN-MP; 1.50°–1.40° in CC group vs. 0.50° in the control group) and with FM (SMD; 1.66 and 1.03 in CC and FM, respectively), Na-Me (4.20–4.70 in CC group vs. 1.40 in the control group). A high force chin cup (600 g/side) has a greater effect size than the low-force chin cup, but this was not statistically significant in most of the parameters.

Evidence Interpretation

In Class III growth modification, if there is maxillary deficiency and greater correction of ANB is required, FM should be the appliance of choice. FM also produces a less vertical increase than CC, which usually is a desirable effect in Class III treatment. The indications for the chin cup are limited and can be used if only the mandible is prognathic, the patient has short anterior face height, and lower incisors are proclined with no signs or symptoms of TMJ.

Viewpoint

Rongo [14] review was a well-conducted review with some limitations; the included studies were graded as very low to moderate quality studies. The pooled studies in the meta-analysis were heterogeneous in the methods (RCT, CCT, and retrospective studies), and clinical applicability with substantial statistical variability between studies.

Abdelnaby study [15] was a well-conducted RCT with some limitations; there was no sample size calculation, and the authors did not report enough details for the randomization process with a lack of proper allocation concealment. The blinding of the operators was not possible as the intervention needs force measurement with no information regarding the blinding of the assessors or data collectors. For the generalizability or the external validity, the study recruited Class III patients with a mild sagittal skeletal discrepancy (initial ANB; 0.1° to −0.8°) and average vertical growth (SN-MP; 34–35). Further research may have a significant impact on our confidence in the estimate of the effect of those appliances.

Facemask Versus Functional Appliances

Clinical Question 5: Which Is Better for Class III Treatment, Facemask, or Functional Appliances?

Evidence

Systematic Review and Meta-Analysis
Yang/2014 [16]

This systematic review and meta-analysis included seven cohort studies. Of the included studies, five trials investigated the short-term effects of Frankel-III (FR3) appliance versus non-treated control group, and two studies investigated the long-term effects of FR3 appliance versus non-treated controls. The meta-analysis showed that there was no significant effect of FR3 on the SNA angle in the short term (MD; 0.43°, 95% CI: −0.52° to 1.39°, $P = 0.37$) or the long term (MD; 0.37°, 95% CI: −0.29° to 1.03°, $P = 0.28$) when compared with CG. SNB angle showed a statistically significant difference between FR3 and CG in the short (MD; −1.62°; 95% CI: −2.62° to −0.62°, $P < 0.01$) and long terms (MD; −1.50°, 95% CI: −2.12° to −0.88°, $P < 0.001$). The meta-analysis showed a statistically significant difference between FR3 and CG regarding ANB angle changes in the short term (MD; 1.84°, 95% CI: 0.96°–2.71°, $P < 0.001$) but not in the long term (MD; 0.07°, 95% CI; −3.17° to 3.30°, $P = 0.97$). Also, there was a difference in overjet between groups in the short term (MD; 3.47 mm; 95% CI, 2.93–4.01 mm, $P < 0.001$) and the long term (MD; 4.56 mm; 95% CI, 3.78–5.35 mm, $P < 0.001$) favoring FR3 group.

Controlled Clinical Trial
Kılıçoğlu/2017 [17]

This clinical trial enrolled 46 Class III patients into three groups; 13 patients in the untreated control group, 17 patients in FM group, and 16 patients in a modified Jasper Jumper group (MJJ), which was fixed between the upper canine and the lower molar. The patients' age ranged from 8 to 11 years. The authors found a statistically significant improvement in both treated groups versus no improvement in the control group. The overjet correction in the MJJ group was statistically higher than CG (4.78 ± 1.96 mm and 0.15 ± 0.37 in MJJ and CG, respectively), with 51.4% skeletal and 48.6% dental changes. Also, the overjet correction in the FM group was statistically greater than CG (5.32 ± 0.54 mm and 0.15 ± 0.37 mm in FM and CG, respectively), but this was due to 70.6% skeletal and 29.4% dental changes. In regard to Class III molar correction, a greater statistically significant correction was noted in the MJJ group when compared with CG (MD; 4.77 ± 1.00 mm, 49.9% skeletal, and 50.1% dental changes). Similar findings were reported for the FM group versus CG (MD; 4.87 ± 1.80 mm, $P = 0.001$, 75% skeletal, and 25% dental). The main dental effects were upper incisor protrusion in the MMJ group (MD; 1.77 ± 0.80 mm in UI, and − 0.48 ± 1.48 mm in LI) and lower incisor retrusion in the FM group (MD; +0.05 ± 0.70 mm in UI, and − 1.47 ± 0.85 mm in LI).

Retrospective Studies
Seehra/2012 [18]

This retrospective cohort study collected records from a previous clinical trial and consecutively treated cases. The sample consisted of 9 facemask patients, 13 reverse twin block (RTB) patients, and 10 untreated control patients. The mean age was 8.5 ± 0.5 years in the control group, 8.8 ± 0.56 years in the FM group, and 9.9 ± 0.99 years in the RTB group. The treatment duration was 9.23 months for RTB, 9.46 months for FM, and 17.1 observation months in the control group. The findings revealed that greater SNA changes were noted in the FM group (2.1° ± 0.9) when compared to the RTB group (1.2° ± 0.7) and the control group (−0.3 ± 0.8). Similarly, a more considerable ANB change was noted in the FM group (3.8° ± 1.3) than RTB (1.0° ± 1.3) group and the control (−0.5 ± 1.1). There was a statistically significant reduction in SNB in both treated groups (−1.7° ± 2 in the FM group versus −2.1° ± 1.2 in the RTB group) when compared to the control group (0.7 ± 0.8). The dental changes were different between the groups. The upper incisors inclination significantly increased in both treated groups (4.0° ± 2.4 in the FM group vs. 9.0° ± 3.1 in the RTB group and 0.3 ± 1.9 in the control group), and the lower incisors inclination statistically decreased in the three groups (−2.2° ± 2.1 in FM group vs. -5.3° ± 2.2 in RTB group and − 1.5° ± 3 in the control group). Furthermore, the lower anterior facial height increased in both treatment groups with a more increase in the FM group (1.4 ± 1.6 mm in the FM group vs. 0.7 ± 0.8 mm in the RTB group and 0.3 ± 0.5), but this increase was not statistically significant.

Fareen/2017 [19]

This study comprised 95 Class III Malay children treated in a previous RCT; 49 patients were treated using RTB, and 46 patients were treated using FM. The authors divided them into two subgroups; the early mixed dentition group (8–9 years), and the late mixed dentition group (10–11 years). The authors analyzed the records using Ricketts analysis by computer software. They found that there were significant skeletal and dental changes in the FM group, especially in the late mixed dentition group. In the RTB group, facial taper and lower lip to E-plane values significantly reduced after the treatment, while maxillary convexity and U1 to A-Pog values significantly increased after the treatment.

Evidence Summary

Looking at the evidence collectively, the best available evidence suggests that FR3 does not move the maxilla forward, but restricts the mandibular growth SNB (MD; $-1.62°$ in the short term to $-1.5°$ in the long term), with a good improvement in overjet (MD; 3.47 mm in the short term and 4.56 mm in the long term), and ANB in the short term (MD; $1.84°$). The overjet correction using FM was greater than MJJ ($5.32 ± 0.54$ mm vs.$4.78 ± 1.96$ mm) and more skeletal in nature (70.6% vs. 51.4%).

Furthermore, the evidence suggests that the facemask has more skeletal effects on the maxilla (SNA;$2.1°$) than RTB (SNA;$1.2°$), and more effects on ANB ($3.8°$ vs $1°$ in FM and RTB, respectively). There was a greater anterior facial height increase in the FM group by 1.4 mm vs. 0.7 mm in the RTB group. Regarding the dental effects, the RTB group showed a greater upper incisor proclination and lower incisor retroclination than FM ($4.0°$ UI and $- 2.2°$ LI in the FM group vs. $9.0°$ UI and $- 5.3°$ LI in the RTB group), The skeletal effects of FM in terms of ANB angle were greater than FR3.

Evidence Interpretation

Facemask treatment is more predictable and produces greater skeletal effects in terms of ANB than treatment using FR3, MJJ, or RTB. As such FM should be favored over functional appliances for Class III growth modification. FM being an extraoral appliance might have some limitations for compliance in some patients. In patients who are reluctant to have the FM appliance, functional appliances can be used, but only if the skeletal discrepancy is mild.

Viewpoint

Yang [16] review is a well-conducted review with a comprehensive search. The authors have undertaken the screening by two reviewer authors that may reduce the bias. The included studies were assessed as low to high-quality evidence. The included studies were cohort studies which have lower evidence than randomized trials and more prone to bias and confounding factors.

Kılıçoğlu study [17] has some limitations; the lack of randomization, allocation concealment, and blinding, which increase the risk of bias and put the study at a high risk of bias. For the external validity, the authors recruited skeletal Class III patients with maxillary retrognathism (SNA < 79°) with a horizontal growth pattern (S-N/Go-Me: 30–32°), so the clinician should keep this in mind when they employ this evidence. Interestingly, the patient's selection was based on the criteria that the patient can bite edge to edge anteriorly, which means there is a mild skeletal discrepancy in these cases, and might be the skeletal discrepancy is associated with centric occlusion-centric relation shift.

Seehra study [18] was a retrospective study, and this type of study is more prone to selection bias. The authors have undertaken a statistical regression analysis to detect the gender and treatment duration effects on the outcomes as confounding factors. The researchers included anterior crossbite on three to four incisors in ICP and edge to edge relation in RCP in the RTB group. Also, ANB was −1.8° in RTB and −2.4° in the FM group, which means there is a difference between groups in the baseline and there is no matching between them. However, the researchers excluded the repeated history of broken appliances and failed appointments, and this does not happen in the real life, so it will increase the bias and minimize the applicability of the results. For the statistical power, they did a calculation for the power and that was good, but they used 2.58° ± 3 ANB change in the calculation between the two groups without a reference.

In Fareen study [19], the authors reported that it is a cross-sectional study while they collected records from finished RCT and this means it is a retrospective study. They calculated the power of the study using an unclear effect size, and they supposed that the dropout is 30%, which is not possible in a retrospective study. Also, the inclusion criteria were limited to overjet of 0 mm, so the clinician should not apply the results of this study to patients with overjet less than 0 mm.

Optimal Orthopedic Force

Clinical Question 6: What Are the Ideal Force Magnitude, Duration, and Direction When Using a Facemask in Early Class III Treatment?

Evidence

Systematic Review
Yepes/2014[20]
This systematic review included 14 studies: 2 were clinical trials, and 12 were cohort studies. The authors aimed to assess the optimal FM force for maxillary protraction. They found a variation in force magnitude (180–800 g per side); two studies used low force which was less than 300 g/side, 9 studies used a medium force of 300–400 g/side, and three studies used a high force of more than 500 g/side, with no favored force magnitude. The daily wear duration varied from 10 hours to 24 hours per day, with an average of 12–16 hours per day for 9–12 months as total treatment duration. Likewise, the force vector direction varied between 15° and 30° below the occlusal plane or paralleled either to the occlusal or Frankfurt plane. The review provided a contradictory conclusion regarding the right force magnitude, force duration, and direction of the force.

Randomized Controlled Trial
Keles/2002 [21]
This pilot study randomized 20 Class III patients into two groups: 9 patients (5 females, 4 males) with a mean age of 8.58 years (7.3–10.8 years) in the FM group and 11 patients (6 males and 5 females) with a mean age of 8.51 years (7.8–10.9 years) in the modified facemask group (MFM). In the FM group, the force direction angle

was 30° to the occlusal plane. In the MFM group, the force was parallel to the Frankfurt plane in an anterior direction. The authors soldered tubes in the molar region to receive an adjustable face bow, and they bent the outer bows in the upward direction of 30°. The researchers applied a protraction force of 500 g/side and used the same type of acrylic expanders in each group. The duration of appliance wear was 16 hours per day. The data were collected after 6 months. The authors found that there was no significant difference between groups regarding SNA angle changes. SNA increased by 3.11° ± 1.05 in the FM group and 3.09° ± 1.7 in the MFM group. Interestingly, the counterclockwise rotation of the maxilla occurred only in the FM group, SN-PP also decreased only in the FM group by (−2.44° ± 2.35) while it did not change significantly in the MFM group (0.27 ± 0.65). The occlusal plane angles SN-OP did not change significantly in the FM group (−1 ± 2.12) but increased by (8.91° ± 4.59) degrees in the MFM group.

Evidence Summary

The systematic review for this question suggests that there is no enough evidence to decide the optimal force magnitude, direction, or duration for FM treatment in early Class III malocclusion. However, there was a wide variation; the force magnitude ranged from 180 g to 800 g per side, and the direction was parallel to the occlusal plane or 15°–30° below it. Only one RCT [21] reported a greater vertical facial increase and counterclockwise maxillary rotation in the FM group than MFM. The range of daily use of FM ranged from 16 to 24 per day due to clinician preferences with no information regarding the actual use by patients. The total treatment duration ranged from 9 to 12 months.

Evidence Interpretation

There is an absence of evidence regarding facemask force magnitude, force vector direction, or treatment duration. Usually, 300–500 gram/side protraction force is given with the help of extraoral elastics. The direction of force usually affects the facial vertical proportions and the overbite. A 15–30° downward directed force may lead to counterclockwise rotation of the maxilla and a decrease in the overbite. This is ideal in a case where the clinician encounter increased overbite at the start of treatment. If the overbite was decreased at the start of treatment the direction of the force should be directed upward or parallel to the occlusal plane. This will theoretically lead to a clockwise rotation of the maxilla and may increase the overbite. Though not evidence based, it is usually suggested that if the clinician does not want to change the existing overbite, the direction of force should be parallel to the occlusal plane. The duration of FM wear should be from 12 to 16 hours. As Class III growth modification is done in young children, it is usually advisable that the appliance should not be worn during school and playing time to avoid any bullying or injury to the child.

Viewpoint

Yepes review [20] was a well-conducted review with a restriction on the search language, which may miss some relevant studies. The included studies were graded as very low-quality clinical trials to high-quality cohort studies that lead to very low evidence when taking into account the study design, the heterogeneity, and the inconsistency between studies.

To our knowledge, Keles [21] RCT was a pilot study with some limitations: There was no sample size calculation that means the study does not represent good evidence with the low number of patients. There was a difference in the baseline characteristics of patients suggesting selection bias, as the SNA angle was −0.44 in the FM group and −1.55 in the MFM group, and SN-OP was 19.44 in the FM group and 22.18 in the MFM group. Also, there was no clear description of the blinding that suggesting no blinding with a high risk of bias. There was a difference in the level of force application between groups which the authors did not take into their account as a confounding factor. For external validity, it is not possible to generalize the finding of this study due to the aforementioned limitations. Furthermore, the confidence in the effect is low, and high-quality research may substantially change the estimate.

ALt-RAMEC/FM Versus RME/FM

Clinical Question 7: Should Expansion be Done with a Facemask, and What Is the Best Expansion Protocol?

Evidence

Systematic Review and Meta-Analysis
Almuzian/2018 [22]

This systematic review included five trials to compare the effectiveness of the FM and alternating rapid maxillary expansion and constriction (ALt-RAMEC) with the FM and the conventional RME. The mean age of patients was 10.11 to 12.1 years in the ALt-RAMEC group and 9.81–11.94 years in the RME group. The ALt-RAMEC protocol was 0.4-1 mm/day expansion or constriction rate (1-week expansion and 1-week constriction) for 4–7 weeks. The reviewers found that the statistical difference was more considerable in the ALt-RAMEC group. The change in overjet was 7.13 ± 2.09 mm in the ALt-RAMEC group and 4.97 ± 2.07 mm in the RME group ($P < 0.0003$). The change in SNA was statistically higher in the Alt-RAMEC group than in the RME group (MD; 1.16°, 95%CI: 0.65–1.66, $P < 0.00001$, 4 trials, 117 participants). The ANB change was higher in the ALt-RAMEC group (MD; 0.66°, 95%CI: 0.08–1.25, $P = 0.03$, 4 trials). However, the change in SNB was smaller in the ALt-RAMEC group (MD; 0.67°, 95%CI: 0.32–1.02, $P = 0.0002$, 4 trials). The change in the MP-SN angle was insignificant between the two groups (MD; −0.21, 95%CI: −1.73 to 1.30, $p = 0.78$, 4 trials). Furthermore, the dental changes had insignificant differences between groups for mandibular incisors (MD; 0.38, 95%CI: −0.76 to 1.52, $p = 0.51$, 3 trials) and maxillary incisors (MD; 0.02, 95%CI: −1.56 to1.60, $p = 0.98$, 2 trials). The evidence was moderate for the skeletal effects and low for the dental effects.

Randomized Controlled Trials
Liu/2015 [23]

This trial, was included in the previous review [22], recruited 44 Chinese patients with skeletal Class III (midface deficiency) and randomly allocated them into two parallel groups; FM-ALt-RAMEC (mean age 10.11 years), and FM with conventional RME (mean age 9.81 years). The expansion was initiated by 1 mm per day in both groups. The ALt-RAMEC was done for 7 weeks in a sequence giving a week for each phase. The instruction for wearing time of facemask was 14 hours per day but the researchers found that the actual wearing time by patients was 11.5 hours. The protraction time was statistically longer in the RME group (10.84 ± 2.76 months) than the ALt-RAMEC group (9.06 ± 2.55 months). The advancement of the maxilla was statistically larger in the ALt-RAMEC group; SNA changes were 2.67° in the ALt-RAMEC group vs. 1.93° in the RME group (MD; 0.73, 95% CI: 0.07–1.4; $P = 0.03$). The counterclockwise rotation of the palatal plane was statistically greater in the ALt-RAMEC group than the RME group (MD; 0.9°, 95% CI: 0.08–1.73; $P = 0.03$). Similarly, there was a statistically significant difference between groups regarding the mandible; the decrease in SNB was statistically smaller in the ALt-RAMEC group than RME group (MD; −0.87°, 95% CI: −1.52 to −0.21, $P = 0.01$). The downward rotation of the mandible was 2° in the ALt-RAMEC group and 3.32° in the RME group (MD; 1.32, 95% CI: 0.24–2.4, $P = 0.017$). However, the dental changes had no statistically significant difference between groups.

Vaughn/2005 [24]

The researchers randomly assigned 46 Class III patients with an age range of 5–10 years into three groups. Fifteen patients in the FM-RME group, 14 patients in FM with a passive intraoral appliance group, and 17 patients in the non-treated control group. After 12 months of observation of the control group, they reassigned this group of patients to the two experimental groups. Six patients were randomly assigned to the first group, and eight patients were randomly assigned to the second group. The expansion in the first group was done by 0.5 mm/day for 7 days. The researchers applied FM with 300–500 g of force, 15°–30° downward to the occlusal plane with full-day wearing time. They found that there is no statistically significant difference between the first two groups in terms of the SNA angle (3.02° and 2.78° for the expansion and non-expansion groups, respectively). ANB angle changes were 3.87° and 3.99° in the expansion and non-expansion groups, respectively, and this difference was statistically insignificant. Also, SNB angle changes were −0.86° and −1.23° for the expansion and non-expansion groups, respectively.

Importantly, the first two groups had statistically significant skeletal changes when compared with the control group.

Evidence Summary

Looking into the evidence collectively, the best available evidence suggests that the ALt-RAMEC/FM protocol is better than the FM-RME protocol. There was a statistically significant difference in skeletal changes between the groups; ANB

(MD;0.66°, $P = 0.03$) and SNA (MD;1.16°, $P < 0.00001$) in favor of the ALt-RAMEC protocol, and SNB (MD; 0.67°, $P = 0.0002$) in support of FM-RME group. There was a greater downward rotation of the mandible in the RME/FM group (MD; 1.32, 95% CI; 0.24–2.4, $P = 0.017$). On the other hand, there was no statistically significant difference between groups in terms of dental changes.

The treatment duration was slightly lesser in the ALt-RAMEC group, with 11.5 hours of daily wearing of the facemask appliance. Considering Vaughn [24] RCT, which found similar effects of FM-RME and FM alone, it can be said that ALt-RAMEC/FM have more skeletal change than FM alone.

Evidence Interpretation

The ALt-RAMEC/FM protocol is preferable over the FM-RME and FM alone if the patient's age is more than 10 years. In these cases, with no maxillary constriction, the ALT-RAMEC protocol can be used. But in cases with maxillary constriction, the ALt-RAMEC protocol can be used for 7 weeks to loosen the suture, and then the required amount of expansion should be achieved.

If the patient age is less than 10 years conventional expansion should be done in cases with maxillary constriction and in the case without maxillary constriction only FM treatment is sufficient.

Viewpoint

Almuzian review [22] was a well-conducted review. The authors followed the high standards for conducting and reporting. However, they made a typo mistake in reporting SNB changes in the results section. The included studies were graded as low to moderate evidence in their review.

Liu study [23] was a well-conducted RCT. The authors reported a good sample size calculation and increased the sample size by 40%. They did sample randomization with balanced groups. There was no blinding for the patients and the operators, and they discussed that in the limitation section. For the applicability, the range of patients' age was wide (8–12 years), the average ANB was −3° with mainly maxillary retrusion, and the ethnicity was Chinese. The authors mentioned that the patient's education is important to wear the appliance, and 11.5/14 hours is the average wearing time. However, the authors treated missingness using per-protocol analysis, which excludes the missing data, and ideally, the intention to treat analysis should have been used as it is more conservative.

Vaughn [24] RCT was a well-conducted trial. However, there are always some limitations in each study, and the clinician should be aware of those limitations during the interpretation of the findings. The age range was very wide, from 5 to 10 years without a clear description of the baseline characteristics of the malocclusion or the cephalometric variables that suggest a problem in the randomization and increase the selection bias. Also, the authors did not exclude cases with pseudo or dental Class III, which is considered a confounding factor. Three of the reassigned patients from the control group to the experimental group failed to finish the treatment, and this may affect the outcome. The blinding for the operators or patients was not possible, but the tracing of the cephalometric radiograph was claimed to be done blindly, although it is easy to recognize the expander in the first group. Re-assigning the control group to treatment groups increases the concern in the measurement method. Statistically, using a t-test for three groups and more than a cutoff point increases the type I error. Finally, the confidence in the finding of this study is low according to the aforementioned issues. So, with low confidence, there is no significant difference in treating mild Class III cases using facemask with or without expansion.

Skeletal Anchorage and Orthopedic Appliances

Clinical Question 8: Which Is Better for Treating Class III Patients: Conventional Facemask or Skeletal Anchored Appliances?

Evidence

Systematic Review and Meta-Analysis
Rodriguez de Guzman-Barrera/2017 [25]

This systematic review included nine studies; eight studies were from case control design, and one was a controlled clinical study. The authors pooled seven studies in the meta-analysis. Two of the included studies used mini-screws, while seven studies used miniplates for the skeletal anchorage. The skeletal anchorage devices were used as bone-anchored rapid maxillary expansion (FM-BARME), facemask with maxillary temporary anchorage devices (FM-MTAD), or bone-anchored intermaxillary traction (BAIMT). The skeletal anchorage devices showed significant changes in all variables when compared to the non-treated control group. TSADs statistically increased the overjet (MD; 6.52 mm, 95% CI: 6.17–6.88, $P < 0.001, 4$ trials), and the ANB angle by 6.07° (95% CI: 5.56–6.58, $p < 0.001$, 3 trials) when compared to the control group. Similarly, the SNA increase was statistically significant (MD; 2.70°, 95% CI 2.16–3.24, $p < 0.001$, 3 trials), and the decrease in SNB was statistically significant (MD; −3.07, 95% CI −3.52 to −2.62, $p < 0.001$) when compared to the control group. Interestingly, there was no statistically significant difference between skeletal anchorage groups (TSADs) and conventional FM-RME regarding overjet (MD; −0.03 mm, 95%CI; −0.7 to 0.64, $p = 0.9$, 2 trials), ANB (MD; 0.29°, 95%CI; −0.28 to 0.87, $p = 0.31$, 3 trials), or SNB (MD; 0.06°, 95%CI; −0.32 to 0.44, $p = 0.76$, 3 trials). In contrast, there was a statistically significant difference between TSADs and FM-RME regarding SNA (MD; 0.60°, 95%CI; 0.13–1.07, $p = 0.01$, 3 trials) and Wits appraisal (MD; 1.28 mm, 95%CI; 0.28–2.28, $p = 0.01$, 2 trials) favoring skeletal anchorage devices.

Controlled Clinical Trial
Aglarcı/2015 [26]

This controlled clinical trial comprised 50 Class III patients: 25 patients were treated using a facemask with a bite plate and 25 patients were treated using mini plates with a force of 200 g provided by Class III elastics. The average age of patients was

11.21 ± 1.32 years in the FM group and 11.75 ± 1.23 years in the skeletal anchorage devices (TSADs) group. The treatment duration was 0.53 ± 0.10 years in the FM group and 0.76 ± 0.09 years in the TSADs group. The researchers revealed that the effect of the treatment was similar between the two groups. There was no statistically significant difference between the groups in regard to the skeletal changes; SNA (1.34° ± 0.91 in FM group, and 1.63° ± 1.3 in TSADs group, $p = 0.37$), SNB ($-1.16°$ ± 1.3 in FM group, and $-$ 1.54° ± 1.6 in TSADs group, $p = 0.35$), ANB (MD; 2.50° ± 1.32 in FM group, and 3.08° ± 1.56 in TSADs group, $p = 0.17$), and SN/Go-Gn (MD; 1.30° ± 2.11 in FM group, and 1.66° ± 187 in TSADs group, $p = 0.53$). On the other hand, the dental changes were different between the groups. Upper incisors change was statistically higher in the FM group; U1/NA (4.89° ± 3.47 in FM group, and 2.06° ± 4.23 in TSADs group, $p = 0.013$). Also, lower incisor changes were statistically different between the groups LI/NB (MD; $-2.25°$ ± 2.9in FM group, and 2.69° ± 3.03 in TSADs group, $p < 0.001$).

Evidence Summary

Looking into the evidence collectively, the best available evidence suggests that there is no statistically significant difference between skeletal anchorage and conventional anchorage with a facemask in treating Class III patients in regard to SNB, ANB, overjet, and mandible rotation. However, there was a statistically significant difference in regard to SNA (MD; 0.60°), and Wits appraisal (MD; 1.28 mm) favoring the skeletal anchorage devices group. Similarly, a trial [26] indicated a significant difference between skeletal anchorage and conventional anchorage in terms of dental effects; U1/NA (MD; 4.89° in FM group, and 2.06° in SA group, $p = 0.013$), and L1/NB (MD; $-2.25°$ in FM group, and 2.69° in TSADs group, $p < 0.001$) favoring TSADs.

Evidence Interpretation

In cases with skeletal Class III growth modification, if there are already dentoalveolar compensations for Class III, skeletal anchorage is a preferred technique over conventional appliances. Skeletal anchorage is more beneficial if there is maxillary retrognathia in a Class III pattern. The skeletal anchorage has a vital role in cases where maxillary dentition provides no support or poor support for the application of extraoral forces.

When the lower incisors are proclined and/or upper incisors are retroclined, conventional facemask treatment may be an effective and less invasive choice.

Other factors that can dictate between TSADs and conventional FM treatment are the compliance of the patient, the age of the patient, the medical condition, and the affordability. Many patients prefer to wear an intraoral appliance rather than an extraoral one. In patients with mixed dentition or early permanent dentition, the position of tooth buds or their path of eruption may interfere with skeletal anchorage devices, and FM treatment might be the only choice. Some patients may not like the idea of an invasive procedure, or their medical condition is a contraindication for an invasive procedure as involved in the placement and removal of the mini plates/screws. Moreover, TSADs are more expensive than FM, and patients in many instances might not be able to afford this mode of treatment.

Viewpoint

Rodriguez de Guzman-Barrera review [25] was a well-conducted review. The authors assessed the included studies as having a moderate quality according to the Newcastle-Ottawa Scale. The case control design may downgrade the quality of the evidence due to inherent shortcomings in the design. The authors made an erratum in the selection criteria paragraph by including systematic review and meta-analyses in their review.

Aglarcı trial [26] was a good clinical trial. However, there were some limitations; The authors mentioned that the treatment was allocated according to patients' treatment preferences, not by randomization and they did not report anything about the blinding which may increase the bias. The loss to follow-up was 9 patients; 4 patients per group for cooperation reasons and one in the TSADs group due to failure of the mini plates, but the authors did not use an optimal analysis for the missing data, which may increase the bias. For the applicability, the authors included patients with ANB° between (0° and −4°) and SN/Go-Gn (less than 40°) that means mild to moderate Class III cases with a normal divergent face.

The Best Orthopedic Protocol

Clinical Question 9: What Is the Best Early Orthopedic Treatment Protocol?

Evidence

Systematic Review and Network Meta-Analysis
Wu/2019 [27]

This systematic review included 25 studies: 6 RCTs and 19 CCTs. The reviewers pooled six interventions in network meta-analysis (NMA): FM-Alt-RAMEC for 88 patients, bone-anchored intermaxillary traction (BAIMT) for 58 patients, bone-anchored rapid maxillary expansion (FM-BARME) for 53 patients, facemask with a maxillary temporary anchorage device (FM-MTAD) for 96 patients, FM-RME 467 patients, and controls 203 patients. According to the methodology, the authors separated RCTs from CCTs in the NMA.

Network Meta-Analysis/RCTs

In comparison with FM-RME, SNA changes were greater in BAIMT group (MD: 2.3°,95% CrI; −0.1.4 to 5.6), FM-MTAD group (MD: 0.97°,95% CrI; −1.8 to 3.4) and FM-Alt-RAMEC group (MD: 0.80°, 95% CrI; −0.98 to 2.6). SNB changes were less in FM-Alt-RAMEC group (MD: 0.71°,95% CrI; −0.91 to 2.3) and BAIMT group (MD: 1.6°, 95% CrI; −1.3 to 4.9) when it compared with FM-RME group. ANB changes did not have statistically significant differences between FM-MTAD and other groups (versus FM-RME: MD 0.017°; versus BAIMT: MD −0.07°; versus FM-Alt-REMEC: MD 0.02°).

NMA/CCTs

In comparison with FM-RME, SNA changes were greater in FM-Alt-RAMEC group (MD: 1.3°), BAIMT group (MD: 1.2°), FM-MTAD group (MD: 1.0°), and FM-BARME group (MD: 1.0°).

Also, SNB showed less mandibular retrusion in BAIMT group (MD: 0.96°), FM-MTAD group (MD: 0.29°), and FM-BARME group (MD: 0.38°) in comparison with FM-RME group.

ANB changes were greater in FM-Alt-RAMEC group (MD: 1.5°), FM-MTAD group (MD: 0.85°) when compared with FM-RME group. In regard to overjet, the FM-Alt-RAMEC group showed more improvement (MD: 2.2 mm) than the FM-RME group, while the OJ improvement in FM-MTAD group (MD: 0.2 mm) was similar to the FM-RME group. However, the vertical changes showed significant differences between BAIMT group and the control group (BAIMT group versus FM-RME: MD = −2.2°; control group versus FM-RME: MD = −2.3°), while the FM-MTAD group and the FM-RME group were similar (MD: −0.16°) in regard to SN-Go/Gn. The FM-Alt-RAMEC group and the FM-RME group (MD: 0.04°) have the same increase in the SN-Go/Gn angle.

The dental effects showed statistically significant changes between groups. The BAIMT group showed more control on the lower incisors angle in all the treatment groups (versus control group: MD: 1.5°), while the FM-MTAD group (MD: −5.5°), FM-Alt-RAMEC group (MD: −5.1°), and FM-RME group (MD: −5.1°) showed greater lingual inclination than the control group. In comparison with the control group, upper incisors showed less proclination in the BAIMT group (MD: 0.86°), FM-MTAD group (MD: −0.81°), and FM-BARME group (MD: −0.66°).

Evidence Summary

The best available evidence suggests that the most effective interventions in increasing SNA are: BAIMT (MD: 1.2° and 2.3° in CCTs and RCTs, respectively), FM-BARME (MD: 1.0°), FM-MTAD (MD: 1.0° and 0.97°in CCTs and RCTs, respectively) and FM-Alt-RAMEC (MD:1.3°and 0.8° in CCTs and RCTs, respectively) when they compared with conventional FM-RME. In contrast, the following interventions showed less mandibular retrusion; BAIMT (MD: 0.96°, 1.6° in CCTs and RCTs, respectively), FM-Alt-RAMEC (MD: 0.71°), FM-BARME (MD: 0.38°), FM-MTAD (MD: 0.29°) than FM-RME. ANB was greater in FM-Alt-RAMEC group (MD: 1.5°), FM-MTAD group (MD: 0.85°) when compared with FM-RME group.

FM-Alt-RAMEC showed more improvement in the overjet (MD: 2.2 mm) than FM-RME, while MTAD showed similar changes to FM-RME. BAIMT significantly decreased the vertical dimension (MD −2.2°) more than FM-RME, while FM-Alt-RAMEC had a similar effect to FM-RME on the vertical dimension.

For the dental effects, BAIMT showed control on the lower incisors versus the control group (MD: 1.5°), FM-MTAD showed the most retroclined lower incisors (MD: −5.5°), while Alt-RAMEC and FM-RME decreased the inclination (MD: −5.1°) when they are compared with controls. Upper incisors inclination was (MD: −0.81°) in FM-MTAD, (MD: −0.66°) in FM-BARME, and (MD: 0.86°) in FM-BAIMT group.

Evidence Interpretation

The aforementioned protocols are effective in treating Class III cases; however, most of the sagittal skeletal differences between these protocols were neither statistically nor clinically significant due to the confidence/credibility intervals. As such, treatment decisions should be based on the clinician's skills, patients' preferences and characteristics, and the available sources.

Treatment with FM-Alt-RAMEC or FM-MTAD is the most effective in ANB improvement, but the clinician should keep in mind that FM-Alt-RAMEC is less invasive, so it would always be the first choice for most patients. However, FM-MTAD can be used when the anchor teeth provide poor support for FM-Alt-RAMEC.

FM-Alt-RAMEC provides greater overjet correction than other treatment modalities. But FM-Alt-RAMEC is associated with greater vertical and dental changes as compared to BAIMT, so FM-Alt-RAMEC can be used in low or average angle cases where no dentoalveolar compensation is present for the Class III skeletal pattern.

In Class III patients with increased vertical dimension and with normal or decreased lower incisors angle, BAIMT is a preferred option if the patient is ready to undergo an invasive procedure. BAIMT offers less dental and vertical changes during treatment.

Viewpoint

Wu et al. [27] review was a well-conducted review with a very informative network meta-analysis. The included studies varied between low and moderate quality. The authors did a meta-regression to figure out the effect of age, force magnitude, and initial ANB on the heterogeneity between studies, and they found that there is no effect of these variables in their study. Other limitations were the small sample sizes, no power calculation, results in the short term, and the wide credibility interval (CrI) in the included studies, which may reduce the quality of the evidence.

Orthopedic Treatment AND Orthognathic Surgery

Clinical Question 10: Does Early Class III Treatment Using the Facemask Reduce Orthognathic Surgery Needs?

Evidence

Randomized Controlled Trial
Mandall/2016 [28]

This multicenter (8 UK hospitals) 2-arm parallel randomized controlled trial recruited 73 Class III patients aged 7–9 years. The authors treated 35 patients using FM versus 38 patients without treatment and followed them for 6 years. After 6 years of follow-up, the researchers found that 36% of the treatment group and 66% of the control group needed orthognathic surgery ($P = 0.027$), and the early treatment decreased the odds of orthognathic surgery need by 3.3 (odds ratio = 3.34 95% CI 1.21 to 9.24) (Fig. 4.1).

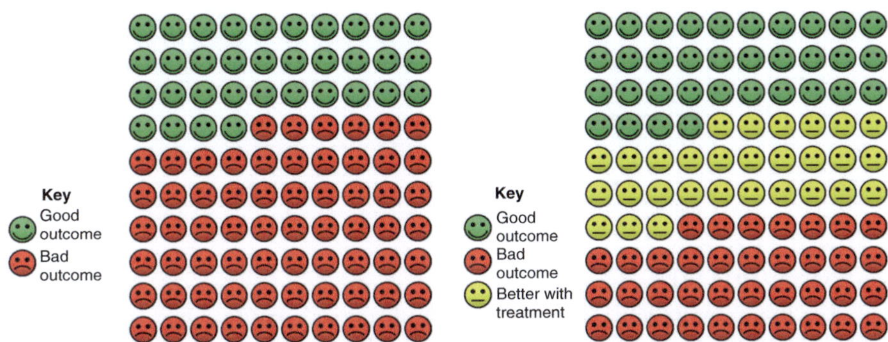

Fig. 4.1 Cates Plot depicts the need for surgery in the untreated control group and in the facemask group, with a 30% drawn in yellow in treatment groups does not need surgery after treatment by FM

Evidence Summary

The available evidence suggests that the odds of needing surgery are 3.3 times more in non-treated Class III patients versus treated patients using a facemask. In other words, untreated Class III patients are 2.3 more likely to have surgery than early treated patients.

Evidence Interpretation

Early treatment of the Class III patients decreases the need of orthognathic surgery in the treated patients as compared to the controls. The clinician should undertake this form of treatment whenever possible in the best interest of the patients.

Viewpoint

This [28] is a worthy multicenter randomized controlled trial. The authors could not calculate the sample size for the need of surgery, but they calculated it for Peer Assessment Rating (PAR) improvement between groups. They performed stratified randomization by gender. The average ANB angle was lesser in the control group by 0.5°, which may suggest including the more severe cases in the control group. The loss to follow up was 21% of the sample; however, the researchers used per-protocol analysis (PP), which is less optimal than Intention to Treat (ITT) analysis in case of missing data.

Adverse Effects

Clinical Question 11: What Are the Harmful Effects of Class III Orthopedic Appliances?

Evidence

Systematic Review
Watkinson/2013 [7]

This Cochrane systematic review has been discussed before. Only one included study [8] in this review reported on the adverse effects of FM on TMJ. According to this review, FM treatment was not associated with any signs or symptoms of TMJ as the prevalence of these effects was very low that preclude undertaking a statistical analysis.

Case Report
Parenti/2015 [29]

This case report highlighted periodontal side effects resulting from facemask treatment in Class III 7-year-old boy. The authors described gingival recession in the lower incisors that occurred during facemask treatment with a combination of plaque accumulation. They hypothesized that the chin pad applied pressure on the labiomental groove resulting in gingival recession. The researchers interpreted the gingival rescission by the traumatic pressure of the vertical chin pad extension along with bacterial factors and thin gingival biotype that evoked bone resorption and gingival retraction. The researchers reduced the vertical chin pad extension, which resulted in an improvement in gingival recession.

Evidence Summary

The available evidence suggests that TMJ signs and symptoms after FM thereby are trivial. Very low evidence in the form of the case report suggests lower incisor gingival recession while using FM, if the appliance design is not appropriate and other risk factors are present.

Evidence Interpretation

There is little or weak evidence for the harmful effects related to FM. Gingival recession on lower incisors can be avoided by modifying the chin pad. In most of the studies, the patients selected for Class III problems do not have pretreatment TMJ problems. Though the present evidence is low, the clinician should keep in mind that the absence of strong evidence does not mean the effect is absent.

Viewpoint

Watkinson review [7] has been discussed before.

Parenti et al. [29] case report provided important information regarding the adverse effects of FM. The current evidence is very low and long-term RCTs are needed to increase our confidence about the estimate of adverse effects.

Authors' Recommendations

- Facemask treatment is an effective method for correction of Class III malocclusion in children, and ideally should be initiated before 10 years of age. Successful treatment decreases the incidence of future orthognathic surgery.
- The success rate of the appliance is up to 70%, with an average treatment duration of 6–9 months. This information should be provided to the patients and their parents, and these information should also be included in the consent.
- Early treatment before 10 years is better than late treatment after 10 years due to the maturation of the maxillary sutures and cease in the growth of the cranial base. To overcome this biological limitation, late treatment after 10 years can be modified by FM-ALt-RAMEC or TSADs.
- In Class III malocclusion, traditionally patients with familial history are not treated with growth modification. However, none of the clinical trials to date have excluded such patients from the studies. As such, those patients should be treated with growth modification. Even if there is mandibular growth in them during the pubertal growth spurt, extent of future orthognathic surgery would be less in such patients.
- Functional appliances such as FR3, MJJ, or RTB are only effective in mild Class III cases. However, FM is superior to functional appliances in Class III treatment.
- With a facemask appliance usually, 300–500 gram/side protraction force is given with the help of extraoral elastics. A 15–30° downward directed force is usually given with daily wear of 12–16 hours.
- For appliance selection, a facemask or reverse pull headgear is the best choice. In young patients before 10 years of age, it can be given with or without rapid maxillary expansion depending upon maxillary constriction. While after 10 years of age, ALt-RAMEC protocol should be used with facemask, which may be combined with TSADs. If the patient has social issues with extraoral appliances, bone-anchored intermaxillary traction by Class III elastics can be used. BAIMT technique is usually used after 10 years of age as before this age the presence of permanent tooth buds hinders the insertion of bone-anchored appliances. Indications of other appliances such as chin cup are very limited and this appliance is usually not taken well by the patient.
- Greater overjet correction is achieved with tooth-supported extra oral appliances because both dental and skeletal changes will result. So ideal cases for these appliances should be low angle with retroclined upper incisors, proclined lower incisors, and with an increased overbite. But if the clinician wants to avoid dental effects, skeletal anchored appliances such as BAIMT should be used.
- There is little or weak evidence for the harmful effects of FM. The gingival recession of the lower incisor can be avoided by modifying the chin pad. In most of the studies, patients selected for Class III problems do not have pretreatment TMJ problems. However, the present evidence suggests no harmful effects on TMJ reported by FM.

References

1. Alhammadi MS, Halboub E, Fayed MS, Labib A, El-Saaidi C. Global distribution of malocclusion traits: a systematic review. Dental Press J Orthod. 2018;23(6):40.e1-e10. https://doi.org/10.1590/2177-6709.23.6.40.e1-10.onl.
2. Dehesa-Santos A, Iber-Diaz P, Iglesias-Linares A. Genetic factors contributing to skeletal class III malocclusion: a systematic review and meta-analysis. Clin Oral Investig. 2021;25(4):1587–612. https://doi.org/10.1007/s00784-020-03731-5.
3. Zere E, Chaudhari PK, Sharan J, Dhingra K, Tiwari N. Developing class III malocclusions: challenges and solutions. Clin Cosmet Investig Dent. 2018;10:99–116. https://doi.org/10.2147/ccide.S134303.
4. Kim JH, Viana MAG, Graber TM, Omerza FF, BeGole EA. The effectiveness of protraction face mask therapy: a meta-analysis. Am J Orthod Dentofac Orthop. 1999;115(6):675–85.
5. Woon SC, Thiruvenkatachari B. Early orthodontic treatment for class III malocclusion: a systematic review and meta-analysis. Am J Orthod Dentofacial Orthop: official publication of the American Association of Orthodontists, its constituent societies, and the American Board of Orthodontics. 2017;151(1):28–52. https://doi.org/10.1016/j.ajodo.2016.07.017.
6. Zhang W, Qu HC, Yu M, Zhang Y. The effects of maxillary protraction with or without rapid maxillary expansion and age factors in treating class III malocclusion: a meta-analysis. PLoS One. 2015;10(6):e0130096. https://doi.org/10.1371/journal.pone.0130096.
7. Watkinson S, Harrison JE, Furness S, Worthington HV. Orthodontic treatment for prominent lower front teeth (class III malocclusion) in children. Cochrane Database Syst Rev. 2013;(9):Cd003451. https://doi.org/10.1002/14651858.CD003451.pub2.
8. Mandall N, DiBiase A, Littlewood S, Nute S, Stivaros N, McDowall R, et al. Is early class III protraction facemask treatment effective? A multicentre, randomized, controlled trial: 15-month follow-up. J Orthod. 2010;37(3):149–61. https://doi.org/10.1179/14653121043056.
9. Mandall AN, Cousley R, DiBiase A, Dyer F, Littlewood S, Mattick R, et al. Is early class III protraction facemask treatment effective? A multicentre, randomized, controlled trial: 3-year follow-up. J Orthod. 2012;39(3):176–85. https://doi.org/10.1179/1465312512Z.00000000028.
10. Baccetti T, McGillis MG, Franchi L, McNamara JA Jr, Tollaro I. Skeletal effects of early treatment of class III malocclusion with maxillary expansion and face-mask therapy. Am J Orthod Dentofac Orthop. 1998;113(3):333–43.
11. Yavuz I, Halicioglu K, Ceylan I. Face mask therapy effects in two skeletal maturation groups of female subjects with skeletal class III malocclusions. Angle Orthod. 2009;79(5):842–8. https://doi.org/10.2319/090308-462.1.
12. Kim JH, Viana MAG, Graber TM, Omerza FF, BeGole EA. The effectiveness of protraction face mask therapy: a meta-analysis. Am J Orthod Dentofac Orthop. 1999;115(6):675–85. https://doi.org/10.1016/s0889-5406(99)70294-5.
13. Jäger A, Braumann B, Kim C, Wahner S. Skeletal and dental effects of maxillary protraction in patients with angle class III malocclusion a meta-analysis. J Orofac Orthop. 2001;62:275–84. https://doi.org/10.1007/s00056-001-0026-9.
14. Rongo R, D'Anto V, Bucci R, Polito I, Martina R, Michelotti A. Skeletal and dental effects of class III orthopaedic treatment: a systematic review and meta-analysis. J Oral Rehabil. 2017;44(7):545–62. https://doi.org/10.1111/joor.12495.
15. Abdelnaby YL, Nassar EA. Chin cup effects using two different force magnitudes in the management of class III malocclusions. Angle Orthod. 2010;80(5):957–62. https://doi.org/10.2319/022210-110.1.
16. Yang X, Li C, Bai D, Su N, Chen T, Xu Y, et al. Treatment effectiveness of Frankel function regulator on the class III malocclusion: a systematic review and meta-analysis. Am J Orthod Dentofacial Orthop. 2014;146(2):143–54. https://doi.org/10.1016/j.ajodo.2014.04.017.
17. Kilicoglu H, Ogutlu NY, Uludag CA. Evaluation of skeletal and dental effects of modified Jasper jumper appliance and Delaire face mask with Pancherz analysis. Turk J Orthod. 2017;30(1):6–14. https://doi.org/10.5152/TurkJOrthod.2017.016.

18. Seehra J, Fleming PS, Mandall N, Dibiase AT. A comparison of two different techniques for early correction of class III malocclusion. Angle Orthod. 2011;82(1):96–101. https://doi.org/10.2319/032011-197.1. Epub 2011 Aug 1

19. Fareen N, Alam MK, Khamis MF, Mokhtar N. Treatment effects of reverse twin-block and reverse pull face mask on craniofacial morphology in early and late mixed dentition children. Orthod Craniofac Res. 2017;20(3):134–9. https://doi.org/10.1111/ocr.12179.

20. Yepes E, Quintero P, Rueda ZV, Pedroza A. Optimal force for maxillary protraction facemask therapy in the early treatment of class III malocclusion. Eur J Orthod. 2014;36(5):586–94. https://doi.org/10.1093/ejo/cjt091.

21. Keles A, Tokmak EC, Erverdi N, Nanda R. Effect of varying the force direction on maxillary orthopedic protraction. Angle Orthod. 2002;72(5):387–96. https://doi.org/10.1043/0003-321 9(2002)072<0387:Eovtfd>2.0.Co;2.

22. Almuzian M, McConnell E, Darendeliler MA, Alharbi F, Mohammed H. The effectiveness of alternating rapid maxillary expansion and constriction combined with maxillary protraction in the treatment of patients with a class III malocclusion: a systematic review and meta-analysis. J Orthod. 2018;45(4):250–9. https://doi.org/10.1080/14653125.2018.1518187.

23. Liu W, Zhou Y, Wang X, Liu D, Zhou S. Effect of maxillary protraction with alternating rapid palatal expansion and constriction vs expansion alone in maxillary retrusive patients: a single-center, randomized controlled trial. Am J Orthod Dentofacial Orthop. 2015;148(4):641–51. https://doi.org/10.1016/j.ajodo.2015.04.038.

24. Vaughn GA, Mason B, Moon HB, Turley PK. The effects of maxillary protraction therapy with or without rapid palatal expansion: a prospective, randomized clinical trial. Am J Orthod Dentofac Orthop. 2005;128(3):299–309. https://doi.org/10.1016/j.ajodo.2005.04.030.

25. Rodriguez de Guzman-Barrera J, Saez Martinez C, Boronat-Catala M, Montiel-Company JM, Paredes-Gallardo V, Gandia-Franco JL, et al. Effectiveness of interceptive treatment of class III malocclusions with skeletal anchorage: a systematic review and meta-analysis. PLoS One. 2017;12(3):e0173875. https://doi.org/10.1371/journal.pone.0173875.

26. Aglarci C, Esenlik E, Findik Y. Comparison of short-term effects between face mask and skeletal anchorage therapy with intermaxillary elastics in patients with maxillary retrognathia. Eur J Orthod. 2016;38(3):313–23. https://doi.org/10.1093/ejo/cjv053.

27. Wu Z, Zhang X, Li Z, Liu Y, Jin H, Chen Q, et al. A Bayesian network meta-analysis of orthopaedic treatment in class III malocclusion: maxillary protraction with skeletal anchorage or a rapid maxillary expander. Orthod Craniofac Res. 2019;23(1):1–15. https://doi.org/10.1111/ocr.12339.

28. Mandall N, Cousley R, DiBiase A, Dyer F, Littlewood S, Mattick R, et al. Early class III protraction facemask treatment reduces the need for orthognathic surgery: a multi-Centre, two-arm parallel randomized, controlled trial. J Orthod. 2016;43(3):164–75. https://doi.org/10.108 0/14653125.2016.1201302.

29. Parenti SI, Checchi V, Molinari C, Bonetti GA. Periodontal side effect during orthopedic face mask therapy. IJO. 2015;26(4):49–51.

Maxillary Expansion 5

Contents

© The Author(s), under exclusive license to Springer Nature Switzerland AG 2023
S. Mheissen, H. Khan, *Orthodontic Evidence*,
https://doi.org/10.1007/978-3-031-24422-3_5

Abbreviations

BBE	Bone-borne expander/expansion
CS2	Cervical stage two
H	Holdaway angle
HARKing	Hypothesizing after the results are known
MARPE	Miniscrews-assisted rapid maxillary expansion
MPSM	Midpalatal suture maturation
PA	posteroanterior
QH	Quadhelix appliance
RA	Removable appliance
RME	Rapid maxillary expansion
RR	Root resorption
SARME	Surgical assisted maxillary expansion
TBE	Tooth-borne expander

Introduction

Maxillary constriction is a common orthodontic problem, with an 8–22% prevalence in early and mixed dentition [1]. It can clinically manifest as posterior crossbite, which can be unilateral or bilateral, with or without mandibular deviation.

The treatment of maxillary constriction depends on different factors; the severity and the extension of the crossbite, the structure involved, the buccal molar tipping, and the age of the patient. In young patients, the intermaxillary and circummaxillary sutures are easy to open. But, once the pubertal growth spurt ends, the suture becomes more interdigitated, and also resistance to expansion is provided by the lateral and medial pterygoid plates of the sphenoid bone, so some invasive interventions are needed to open the sutures.

Angell suggested maxillary expansion in 1860 [2]. In contemporary orthodontics, both removable and fixed expanders are used for maxillary expansion with the severity of the maxillary constriction and the case characteristics influencing the selection of appliance. Some of these appliances are activated by the clinician in the practice, while the vast majority are activated by the patient/parents according to the clinician's instructions. Three activation protocols can be used for maxillary expansion; the slow protocol with 1 mm/week of expansion, the semi-rapid protocol with 0.25 mm/day of expansion, and the rapid expansion with 0.5–1 mm/day of expansion (RME). Most of these expansion appliances are screw-based, with a one-quarter turn of the screw resulting in 0.20–0.25 mm of expansion. Clinicians prefer slow expansion in patients younger than 10 years because the anecdotal evidence is that doing rapid expansion in a young patient can distort the facial morphology [3]. While in patients older than 10 years of age, the rapid expansion protocol is favored, especially in late adolescents and adult patients.

In the last decade, miniscrews anchored rapid maxillary expansion appliances have been used with more effective results in late adolescent and adult patients compared to conventional RME. Moreover, surgical assisted maxillary expansion (SARME) is an alternative procedure in patients with transverse skeletal discrepancies where the maxillary sutures are fused and when the conventional expansion fails.

The most critical diagnosis in maxillary expansion is the patency of the maxillary suture. Conventional techniques are only successful if the sutures are open. Using conventional techniques in patients with fused midpalatal suture would lead to iatrogenic damages like root resorption, fenestration of alveolar bone, mobility of expander-supporting teeth, and pain. Five stages of midpalatal suture maturation have been identified by Angelieri [4]. In stage A, the suture line is straight with high density, with no or little interdigitation; in stage B, high-density sutural line with a scalloped appearance; in stage C, two parallel, scalloped, high-density lines are separated in some areas by small low-density spaces; stage D, two scalloped, high-density sutural lines with no evidence of a suture in the palatine bone; and stage E, sutural fusion has occurred in the maxilla. In late adolescents and adult patients where maturation of the suture is doubtful, radiographic diagnosis of suture maturation can be done before attempting maxillary expansion.

Effectiveness of Maxillary Expansion

Clinical Question 1: Is Maxillary Expansion Effective?

Evidence

Systematic Review and Meta-Analysis
Zhou/2014 [5]
This systematic review included 14 studies; 2 RCTs and 12 CCTs, to investigate the effects of rapid maxillary expansion (RME). The authors pooled six trials in the meta-analysis. There was a significant increase in the intermolar width in the RME group compared to non-treated controls (MD; 4.09 mm, 95%CI: 3.43–4.76, $I^2 = 78\%$, $P < 0.001$, six trials). Also, there was a significant increase in the maxillary intercanine width in the RME group when compared to non-treated controls (MD; 2.7 mm, 95%CI: 2.15–3.27, $I^2 = 77\%$, $P < 0.001$, six trials). The interpremolar width significantly increased in the RME group when compared to non-treated controls (MD; 3.86 mm, 95%CI: 3.10–4.62, $I^2 = 84\%$, $P < 0.001$).

Systematic Review
Lagravere/2005 [6]
This systematic review included three studies; one measured the transversal effects of rapid maxillary expansion, and two investigated the sagittal and vertical effects. The researchers found that there was a significant increase in the width of the maxilla

by 3 mm, in patients before the pubertal growth spurt, when compared to non-treated controls. For the sagittal changes, only A point retruded by 1.05° in the RME treatment group versus non-treated control without any statistically significant difference regarding the anterior and posterior position of the maxilla or mandible.

Evidence Summary

The best available evidence suggests that RME can expand the constricted maxilla by opening the sutures. There was a statistically significant increase of 4.09 mm in the intermolar width, 2.7 mm in the intercanine width, and 3.09 mm in the interpremolar width [5]. Furthermore, RME increased the maxillary width by 3 mm in pre-pubertal patients [6].

Evidence Interpretation

Maxillary expansion is an effective method for the correction of transverse maxillary deficiencies. The conventional method of rapid maxillary expansion can open the sutures and expand the maxilla with better results in pre-pubertal patients.

Viewpoint

Zhou review [5] was a well-conducted review. The reviewer authors performed a good sensitivity analysis and publication bias investigation. However, there are some issues with the methodology that should be kept in mind when interpreting the results. Firstly, the assessment of risk of bias was done using Cochrane risk of bias tool for randomized controlled trial for all included studies and it was better to use the appropriate tool for non-randomized controlled trials. Secondly, most of the included studies were assessed at low to moderate quality due to the lack of randomization, allocation concealment, and blinding. Nevertheless, there was a wide range of age between 7 and 17 years for the patients, which may indicate a clinical heterogeneity.

Lagravere review [6] provided good information with limited evidence. The included studies were of low to medium quality with methodological issues related to the sample size calculation and dropouts. Also, the authors reported that their quality score list was limited. Moreover, the measurements, such as the maxillary width were not clearly defined. These important issues may influence our confidence in the findings and the true effect of RME is likely to be substantially different from the estimate of this review.

Treatment Timing

Clinical Question 2: What Is the Best Time for Expanding the Maxilla?

Evidence

Systematic Review
Seif-Eldin/2019 [7]
This review included six studies in the qualitative analysis; five were prospective studies, and one was a retrospective study. The authors found that the short-term

skeletal effects of RME were statistically greater in the pre-pubertal group than in the post-pubertal group. There was a statistically significant increase in the latero-nasal width in the pre-pubertal group more than in the post-pubertal group by (MD; 1.1 mm) (3.3 and 2.2 mm, in the pre- and post-pubertal periods, respectively) [8]. The maxillary width increase was greater in the pre-pubertal group than in the post-pubertal group (3.4 mm vs. 2.8, in the pre- and post-pubertal period, respectively), but it was not statistically significant. The increase in the intermolar width was 9 mm in both groups [8].

Retrospective Study
Sayar/2019 [9]

This study comprised 32 patients (11 males and 21 females) with age 10–18 years. The authors devided the patients according to the skeletal maturation; 14 patients in the post-pubertal peak group and 18 patients in the pre-pubertal peak group. They used bonded hyrax for all patients with two turns daily for 3 weeks. After expansion, the hyrax appliance was used as a retainer for 6 months. Within groups, there was a statistically significant difference between pre and post-treatment. However, there was no statistically significant difference between the pre and post-pubertal groups regarding the maxillary expansion. The maxillary width increased by 2.91 ± 1.68 mm and 2.92 ± 2.12 mm in pre and post-growth peak, respectively. The nasal base width increased by 1.81 ± 1.56 mm and 1.83 ± 1.48 in pre- and post-growth peak, respectively. The palatal intermolar width increased 4.82 ± 1.29 and 4.82 ± 1.29, in pre and post-growth peak, respectively.

Jimenez-Valdivia/2019 [10]

This study comprised 200 CBCT scans of participants (95 males and 105 females); their ages ranged between 10 and 25 years. The researchers classified patients into three groups; 48 in the pre-adolescent group with an age range of 10–15 years, 52 in the post-adolescent group with an age range of 16–20 years, and 100 in the adults group with an age range of 21–25 years. They used the Angelieri [4] method to classify the midpalatal suture's maturation. They considered A, B, and C stages coincided with an open suture, while D and E have coincided with a fused suture. The authors found that the midpalatal suture was not fused in 63 subjects (31.5% of the sample). The prevalence of stage C in females was higher within the age of 10–15 years than at other ages. The prevalence of open sutures was 70.8% at age 10–15 years, 21.2% at age 16–20 years, and 17% at age 21–25 years. Males had more open sutures than females in the age range of 16–20 and 21–25 years.

Evidence Summary

The best available evidence suggests that the skeletal effects of the rapid maxillary expansion are greater in pre-pubertal patients than post-pubertal patients in the short term [7, 8]. Also, the open midpalatal suture prevalence was high (70.8%) in pre-pubertal patients (younger than 16 years). The open suture prevalence decreased after the age of 16 years to become 21.2 and 17%, at 16–20 and 21–25 years, respectively. There was no difference between groups after 6 months retention period.

Evidence Interpretation

In patients younger than 16 years of age, the likelihood of having an open midpalatal suture is high. Subsequently, the skeletal effects of expansion would also be higher in patients younger than 16 years, and all conventional expanders with any expansion protocol can work without any invasive intervention. However, in approximately 30% of the patients younger than 16 years, there is a possibility of fused midpalatal suture, which may lead to failure or only dental expansion by conventional expanders. Likewise, the suture's maturation occurs earlier in females than in males. The patient should be informed prior to treatment, during the planning process, as follows; if the suture does not respond, other methods of expansion would be used.

In patients older than 16 years of age, there is less probability of opening the midpalatal suture. Ideally, other diagnostic methods such as CBCT can help to predict the stage of suture maturation in such patients. But if there are legal limitations for using CBCTs in a specific country, mini-implant-supported expansion or surgical-assisted maxillary expansion is a viable option.

Viewpoint

Seif-Eldin review [7] included low-quality studies' due to the design and methodology, which is not enough to provide reliable evidence.

Sayar [9] study was a retrospective design with a small sample. It is more prone to selection bias as the patients who have a successful treatment will continue with their treatment, so the study may have full records only for the successfully treated patients. Moreover, with a lack of sample size calculation, it is unknown wether the study is powered or not.

Jimenez-Valdivia study [10] was a good retrospective study that used a valid assessment method. However, there are some points when we interpret the results. The cohort study design is considered weak in the hierarchy of evidence than the randomized controlled trials, and this design is more prone to selection bias. The study may not have enough power because the authors calculated the sample size according to the possibility of the open suture in adults older than 18 years, and that was 163 adults, while they only assessed 100 CBCT records for adults with no details for other groups. The groups' distribution was not equal, which could lead to a statistical issue with the prevalence of the maturation stages.

Expansion Pattern

Clinical Question 3: What Is the Pattern of Suture Opening During Maxillary Expansion?

Evidence

Systematic Review
Bazargani/2013 [11]
This systematic review included five trials investigating the pattern of the suture opening and concluded that there is no consistent evidence regarding the pattern of

the suture opening. Three included studies [12–14] revealed that the suture opened in a triangle pattern with a large opening in the anterior region. While one study [15]reported that the suture opening was parallel, and one study [16] found individual differences between patients in the suture opening pattern.

Randomized Controlled Trial
Weissheimer/2011 [13]
This trial was included in the aforementioned systematic review [11]. The authors randomly allocated 33 patients with transverse maxillary deficiency into two groups; 18 patients in the Haas expander group and 15 patients in a Hyrax expander group. The authors found that the expansion had taken a V shape in the horizontal plane, and the increase was greater in the anterior midpalatal suture region (MD ± SE; 4.00 ± 0.13 mm) than posterior midpalatal suture region (MD ± SE; 2.88 ± 0.09 mm). Also, the expansion had taken a V shape in the vertical plane, the increase was greater in the inferior apical base width (MD ± SE; 3.48 ± 0.23 mm) than in the superior apical base width (MD ± SE; 2.82 ± 0.23 mm) in the anterior region as well as the posterior region.

Evidence Summary
The best available evidence suggests that there is no uniform pattern of the suture opening. There were individual differences between patients in the pattern of the suture opening. In some trials, the suture opened in a V shape in the horizontal plane and in a V shape in the vertical plane. While other studies reported a parallel shape of the suture opening. The findings for the present evidence are low.

Evidence Interpretation
The vertical V-shaped pattern of expansion means there would be some hanging off the palatal cusp during expansion, resulting in an increase in the vertical dimension. Negative torque in posterior brackets can help to correct this problem later in the treatment. The horizontal V-shaped pattern of expansion means that less skeletal expansion would be achieved in the posterior region, so a greater amount of expansion would be required in that area. As such, the dental nature of expansion in the posterior maxillary arch increases the chances of relapse in this area.

Viewpoint
Bazargani review [11] is a well-conducted review that provides information about the skeletal and dental effects of rapid maxillary expansion. However, there were some shortcomings that should be kept in mind when interpreting the results of this study. Firstly, there was a restricted search to the English language, with a lack of gray literature search that may miss some relevant studies. The design of the included studies was mostly case series, with no blinding and lack of missing data reporting. So, the quality of the included studies was mostly low and moderate in a few studies.

Weissheimer trial [13] is a good trial that provides a lot of information about the effects of RME. However, there are some issues that may influence the interpretation of the findings. Firstly, there was a lack of sample size calculation, which may underpower the study. The authors did not report the randomization process in enough detail with a lack of allocation concealment. The females were more than males in this study, which may affect the suture's maturation as the suture's maturation occurs earlier in females than in males. The blinding was not possible for the operators or the patients in this study, but it was possible for the assessors to minimize the bias in measuring the data.

Dental Versus Skeletal Effects

Clinical Question 4: What Are the Skeletal and Dental Effects of Maxillary Expansion?

Evidence

Systematic Review and Meta-Analysis
Lagravère/2006 [17]

This systematic review and meta-analysis included 14 trials that measured the immediate effects of the rapid maxillary expansion. Of those, eight studies measured the dental and skeletal effects using the posterior-anterior cephalometric radiograph, three measured the skeletal and dental changes using the same radiographs and the dental casts, and three trials measured only the dental effects using the dental casts. The transverse changes were statistically significant; the intermolar width significantly increased by 6.74 mm (95%CI: 4.59–8.89 mm), and the intercanine width significantly increased by 5.35 mm (95%CI: 4.31–6.39). The skeletal transverse increase was statistically significant in the molar region (1.88 mm, 95%CI: 0.32–3.44), and in the nasal cavity region (2.14 mm, 95%CI: 1.56–2.72). Interestingly, rapid maxillary expansion led to a statistically significant vertical increase in the mandibular angle by 1.97° (95%CI: 1.75°–2.19°). Furthermore, there was a statistically significant maxillary protrusion by 0.87° (95%CI; 0.48°–1.25°) and significant retrusion of the mandible (−0.62, 95%C: −0.76 to −0.49).

Systematic Review
Bazargani/2013 [11]

This systematic review included 10 studies: two studies were randomized controlled trials and eight studies were case series studies. The age of the patients ranged between 6 and 14.5 years. The maxillary expansion was 7–8 mm screw opening. The researchers found that the midpalatal suture expansion was 1.6–4.33 mm in the posterior region, representing 22–53% of the total screw expansion.

Moreover, three studies reported that the nasal cavity expanded by 1.2 mm [16], 1.4 mm [14], and 2.73 mm [15] (17, 20, and 33% of the total screw opening).

The dental expansion was significantly larger than the skeletal expansion. The tipping of the first molar was 7° in three studies [13, 15, 18] and 1° in one study [16]. However, 30% of the total expansion was due to the bending of the alveolar bone.

Randomized Controlled Trial
Weissheimer/2011 [13]

In this trial, the investigators randomly allocated 33 patients with transverse maxillary deficiency into two groups: 18 patients in a Haas expander group and 15 patients in a Hyrax expander group. The age of patients ranged from 7.2 to 14.5 years, with a mean age of 10.7 years. The rapid expansion protocol was four initial quarter turns followed by two turns per day until achieving 8 mm of expansion. The authors used cone-beam computed tomography scans (CBCT) to assess the transversal changes.

There was a significant increase in the transverse dimension in the two groups with more dental changes (Intermolar width increased by 7.8 ± 0.15 mm) than skeletal changes (Posterior midpalatal suture width increased by 2.88 ± 0.09 mm). The posterior midpalatal suture width increased by 2.62 ± 0.31 mm in the Haas group and 3.14 ± 0.14 mm in the Hyrax group. The anterior midpalatal suture width increased by 3.63 ± 0.17 mm in Haas group and 4.37 ± 0.2 mm in Hyrax group. On the other hand, the molar tipping was lesser in Hyrax group but not statistically significant. The right first molar angulation was 6.80° ± 1.11 in Hyrax group vs. 8.25° ± 0.98 in Haas group ($P = 0.33$). The left first molar angulation was 6.19 ± 1.02 and 6.14 ± 0.9 in Hyrax and Haas groups, respectively ($P = 0.98$).

Evidence Summary

The best available evidence suggests that RME produces a significant increase in the width of the maxilla with dental and skeletal effects. The opening of the midpalatal suture in the posterior region is equal to 22–53% of the total expansion, while the bending of alveolar bone which was a part of the dental expansion, was 30% of the total expansion. The pure skeletal expansion is less than the dental expansion, with a total expansion of (6.74–7.8 mm in different SRs) in the occlusal plane between molars. There was an increase in nasal cavity width by 1.2–2.73 mm. Furthermore, RME has a statistically significant vertical effect, demonstrated by increase in ML-SN (MD; 1.97°, 95%CI: 1.75°–2.19°), and statistically significant sagittal effects which are demonstrated by increase in SNA angle (MD; 0.87°, 95%CI: 0.48°–1.25 °) and decrease in SNB (MD: −0.62, 95%CI: −0.76 to −0.49).

Evidence Interpretation

Maxillary expansion has both dental and skeletal effects. Skeletal effects involve opening of the midpalatal suture, while dental effects comprise the bending of alveolar bone, buccal teeth movement, and tipping of maxillary teeth, especially the molars. However, the skeletal changes are less than the dental changes. The dental tipping leads to an increase in the vertical dimension by downward and backward rotation of the mandible, and it may be the reason for the mandibular retrusion. Maxillary expansion also leads to some minor advancement of the maxilla.

Dental changes and bending of alveolar bone may increase the chances of post-expansion relapse. To prevent the relapse, palatal appliances are maintained for 6 months after expansion, and after treatment, long-term retention is required. Likewise, maxillary expansion results in minor improvement of Class III skeletal relationships by mild protraction of the maxilla and downward and backward rotation of the mandible. As the sagittal changes are not clinically significant, so these should not be considered during treatment planning. This increase in the vertical dimension usually results from the hanging of palatal cusps of posterior maxillary teeth. Negative posterior maxillary torque, which is present in almost all the bracket prescriptions, and some relapse, help to correct the increase in the vertical dimension.

Viewpoint

Although meta-analysis provides us with a useful quantitative synthesis of the results, there are some issues in Lagravère review [17]. First of all, the authors did not define the PICO question precisely. Secondly, the risk of bias assessment was not clear. The authors did not demonstrate the design of the included studies or the pooled studies in their meta-analysis, and hence there are some concerns in the pooled estimate from the cephalograms and the dental casts. Finally, the authors indicated that the included studies have flaws in the sampling and the statistical approaches, so the confidence is low in the skeletal/dental estimate of the expansion, and the real estimate may be different from the study's findings.

Rapid Versus Slow Expansion

Clinical Question 5: Which Is More Effective; Rapid or Slow Maxillary Expansion?

Evidence

Systematic Reviews
Algharbi/2018 [19]

In this review, two included studies investigated the skeletal and dental effects of rapid (RME) vs. slow maxillary expansion (SME). The results within groups were statistically significant, but the differences between groups' outcomes were not statistically significant [20, 21]. The sutural opening was statistically significant in the two groups (1.9 ± 1.0 and 2.4 ± 0.9, in SME and RME, respectively) [21]. The dental tipping was lesser in the SME than in the RME group (7.87° ± 6.80, and 12.88° ± 9.35 in SME and RME, respectively), but the differences between groups were not statistically significant thus, suggesting more bodily movement in the SME group.

Bastos/2019 [22]

This review included three trials that investigated the side effects of the SME and RME. The age of patients was between 6.3 and 13.2 years. The researchers found that two studies [23, 24] did not report any periodontal change between the two expansion groups. Only one included study [20] reported a bone loss involving the bone height and thickness in both SME and RME.

Agostino/2014 [25]

In this systematic review, one included study [21] compared SME versus RME and found that there is no statistically significant difference in the molar region expansion.

Randomized Controlled Trials
Martina/2012 [21]

In this trial, the authors recruited 41 patients with unilateral or bilateral posterior crossbites. They allocated 19 patients to the SME group and 22 patients to the RME group. The expansion screws were soldered only to the upper first molars bands. In the RME group, the activation was done eight times at the chair time and then three turns daily until overcorrection by 2 mm was achieved. However, in the SME group, the expansion was done two turns weekly until overcorrection by 2 mm also was achieved. The authors analyzed the results of 26 patients (14 in RME and 12 in SME). Expansion was noticed in both groups, with a statistically significant increase in the skeletal width of the maxilla in the anterior region (1.9 ± 1.3 mm in SME group vs. 2.5 ± 1.5 mm in RME group) and in the posterior region (1.9 ± 1 mm in SME group vs. 2.4 ± 0.9 mm in RME group). There was also a statistically significant difference in the expansion at the pterygoid processes level, which was greater in the RME group than in the SME group (1.2 ± 0.9 mm and 0.6 ± 0.6 mm in RME and SME, respectively, $P = 0.04$).

For the dental effects, there was a statistically significant molar tipping in the RME group (1.0 ± 1.2 mm), while the tipping in the SME group was not statistically significant (0.3 ± 0.9 mm). On the other hand, there was a more painful response in the RME group.

Baldini/2015 [26]

This randomized trial comprised 112 patients (54 males and 58 females) having a constricted maxillary arch with a mean age of 11 ± 1.8 years. The authors randomly assigned the patients for rapid maxillary expansion into two groups; one turn per day group (G1) and two turns per day group (G2). The researchers investigated the pain between groups after 15 min of activation using Numeric Rating and Faces Pain Scales. They found that the average pain in G1 ranged from 0.5 to 1, while it was 2.3 in G2, especially on the second day. There was a statistically significant difference in the pain between groups with a peak in the fifth to tenth activation, which means between third and fifth days in G2 and between the fifth and tenth days in G1. There were 10 patients who recorded pain scores of more than five in G2 and three patients in G1. There was no difference in the pain level between males and females in G1, but there was a difference in G2. Cervical vertebral maturation was correlated with the pain scores, where CS2 patients reported more pain scores than CS1 patients.

Evidence Summary

The best available evidence suggests that the rapid and the slow maxillary expansions have almost similar clinical skeletal effects in adolescents under 13 years of age; maxillary width increased by 1.9 mm in SME group and 2.4–2.5 mm in RME group, with the exception of the expansion at pterygoid processes level where more expansion was reported in RME group (1.2 ± 0.9 mm and 0.6 ± 0.6 mm in RME and SME, respectively, $P = 0.04$). Though RME is associated with slightly more expansion than SME, there was more tipping in the RME group (1.0 ± 1.2 mm, $P < 0.005$) than in the SME group (0.3 ± 0.9 mm), but this was not clinically significant. Pain during the expansion phase was statistically higher in the protocol of two turns daily (2.3) than the one turn daily (0.5–1), with a peak of pain in the fifth to tenth activation. Limited evidence suggests that both slow and rapid expansions were accompanied by bone loss.

Evidence Interpretation

Slow and rapid palatal expansion have similar results in patients under 13 years of age. RME has slightly greater dental and skeletal effects than SME but is also associated with more pain during treatment. So RME is a better choice if the crossbite has both dental and skeletal components, while SME is a better choice for patients with a low pain threshold.

In patients above 13 years of age, rapid expansion protocol is mostly used. Slow expansion, especially by wired appliances like quadhelix and W arch, is not used at this age as the anecdotal evidence is that more dental expansion is caused by these appliances at this age.

Viewpoint

Martina [21] trial has some shortcomings, and we should keep some points when we interpret the results of this study. There was an imbalance between the groups at the baseline, where the age of SME patients was 10.3 ± 2.5 years, and the age in the RME group was 9.7 ± 1.5 years, which means there are older patients in the SME group by 1 year. Even though the authors reported that they did block randomization with gender as a stratifying factor, they still have an imbalance regarding gender between groups. This may happen because of the high number of dropouts. Another point is the high number of missingness where the authors did not treat this issue, thus increasing the risk of attrition bias. However, it was a good trial with good potential applicability of slow expansion on patients with age younger than 13 years with a similar result to the rapid maxillary expansion at this age.

Baldini trial [26] was a good study that addressed an interesting question. There are some issues in this study that we should bear in mind when we interpret its results. The authors did not calculate the sample size to address the study's power, but they recruited a large number of patients. They did not clarify the randomization process, which resulted in imbalanced baseline groups, thus increasing the selection bias. Furthermore, the number of females was larger in group 1, and the higher maturation stage was more in group 2, which may increase the pain in group 2. Interestingly, the authors reported that the missingness happened more quickly in group 2, and they did not treat the missingness in their analysis. However, this study provides us with good information that the pain is correlated with activation protocol during rapid maxillary expansion. Algharbi [19] review has some issues that the clinician should keep in mind when she/he interprets the results: the search process was restricted by language filter and concise as only three search engines were used. The risk of bias tool was not a critical and not clear tool as they did not report the risk of bias arising from the randomization process, blinding, measures, and loss to follow-up patients in the included studies.

Bastos review [22] was a well-conducted review. Even though there were some shortcomings, the authors included studies that compared different expansion appliances (Hass versus quadhelix appliances). In one included RCT [20], there was a high number of patients who lost to follow-up; 39.9% and 48.4% in RME and SME groups, respectively, and this may increase the attrition bias and underpower the study. However, this missingness is not representative of the real-world settings, so what is the reason for the high missingness in this trial? The design of the appliance and the trial settings may play a vital role in this issue.

The included study in Agostino review [25] was a low-quality evidence with a high risk of bias and unclear missing data. Although this study was a randomized controlled trial, it analyzed only 10 patients, which means it was a very small study.

RME and TSADs

Clinical Question 6: Is Bone-Borne Rapid Maxillary Expansion More Effective Than Tooth-Borne Maxillary Expansion?

Evidence

Systematic Review and Meta-Analysis
Krüsi/2019 [27]
This review included 12 papers for 6 randomized controlled trials; 264 patients with an average age of 12.3 years. Two trials compared bone-borne expander (BBE) versus tooth-borne expander (TBE) and found that bone-borne expander had less dental expansion in the canine region (MD; −0.7 mm, 95% CI: −1.0 to −0.4, one trial), less buccal tipping of the first premolar (MD; −4.1°; 95% CI: −6.0 to −2.1°, two trials), and less buccal tipping in the first molar region (MD −5.4°; 95% CI: −8.0 to −2.7°) in comparison with conventional rapid expansion in the post-expansion phase.

After retention, the bone-borne expanders had more skeletal expansion effects at the incisal foramen level (MD; 1.8 mm, 95% CI: 1.3–2.3, one trial), more skeletal effects on the first premolar level (MD; 2.3 mm, 95% CI: 1.7–2.9), and more suture opening on the first molar level (MD; 2.0 mm, 95% CI: 1.4–2.6) than tooth-borne expanders.

Post retention, the authors found that Hybrid tooth-bone-borne RME showed a less intercanine width expansion (MD; −0.22 mm, 95% CI: −0.98 to 0.55, P=0.58, two trials) and more intermolar expansion (MD; 0.18, 95%CI: −0.40 to 0.76, P=0.55, two trials) than conventional rapid expansion, but not statistically significant. They found less expansion in the first premolars region (MD; −1.96 mm, 95% CI: −6.18 to 2.27, P=0.36, two trials), and in the second premolar region

(MD −3.3 mm, 95% CI: −6.2 to −0.5, one trial), with less buccal tipping of the first premolars (MD; −4.0°, 95% CI: −7.1 to −0.9, and MD; −0.79, 95% CI: −3.18 to 1.6, in the left and right sides, respectively, two trials) in hybrid expanders when compared to conventional rapid expansion, after retention.

Systematic Reviews
Algharbi/2018 [19]

Two included studies [28, 29], in this review, reported that the bone-borne expanders had more statistically significant skeletal expansion in the premolars' region with contradictory findings in regard to teeth tipping. However, one included study [28] found that the expansion was statistically greater in tooth-borne expanders without significant differences between the two appliances regarding dental tipping. Another study [29] found a statistically significant higher tipping in the tooth-borne expanders in the first premolars region.

Khosravi/2019 [30]

This systematic review included four RCTs that investigated the effects of bone- and tooth-borne expansion devices and found that the two expanders were effective in maxillary expansion. There was no statistically significant difference between the two devices regarding the dental and skeletal expansion in the molar region. There was no difference between devices regarding dental to skeletal changes ratio except for more dental tipping in tooth-borne devices that declined in the retention period. Also, no difference was reported between devices regarding pain except in the first activation, which was higher in the bone-borne devices. Furthermore, there were no differences between tooth- and bone-borne devices except for expansion in the pre-molar region, which was greater in the tooth-borne device, but this difference was not statistically significant.

Two included studies compared tooth- and bone-borne devices in combination with SARME. The researchers did not find differences between the two devices regarding intermolar and interpremolar expansion.

Evidence Summary

The best available evidence supports that there are contradictory findings regarding the difference between BBE and TBE. A systematic review [27] indicated that BBE has less dental expansion than TBE by (0.7 mm) from one included trial. While the other two reviews [19, 30] found no differences between tooth- and bone-borne devices except for expansion in the premolar region due to their inclusion criteria.

BBE has less tipping in the first premolars region by (4.1°) in comparison with conventional rapid maxillary expansion. Also, the buccal tipping of the first premolars was less in hybrid RME versus conventional RME by (0.8° to 4.0° one both sides).

Post retention, BBE can result in greater suture opening on incisal foramen level by 1.8 mm, first premolars level by 2.3 mm, and the first molars level by 2.0 mm in comparison with conventional rapid maxillary expansion. Furthermore, there was less expansion in hybrid tooth-borne RME after retention versus tooth-borne RME by 1.96 and 3.3 mm in first premolars and in second premolars regions, respectively.

Evidence Interpretation

Bone-borne rapid maxillary expansion is more effective than tooth-borne maxillary expansion in terms of skeletal effects. So if more skeletal effects are desired with less buccal tipping, bone-borne expanders are more favored than tooth-borne expanders. However, the cost-effectiveness and the extra exposure of invasive procedures to place the bone-borne expanders should be taken into account during the treatment planning as there is no major clinically significant difference between the two techniques.

Viewpoint

Krüsi review [27] is a well-conducted review. However, we should bear in mind during the results' interpretation that the included studies were of very low to moderate quality due to inadequate sample size calculation, lack of randomization, and lack of blinding. Interestingly, there was a difference between the table and the results section that may suggest selective reporting.

Algharbi [19] review has been discussed before.

In Khosravi [30] review, the risk of bias was high regarding the blinding and missing data. Also, the reporting was narrative without a cumulative effect measure values.

In conclusion, the evidence is based on a few trials with small sample sizes and inherent risk of bias, which may hamper the confidence in drawing clinical recommendations.

Success Rate of Suture Opening

Clinical Question 7: Does Miniscrews Assisted Rapid Maxillary Expansion (MARPE) Split the Suture in All Ages?

Evidence

A Retrospective Study
Shin/2019 [31]

This trial comprised records of 31 adult patients with an age range of (18–36) years. The protocol of expansion was one turn per day (0.2 mm/turn). The researchers found that the suture has been opened in 23 of 27 patients with age less than 30 years, while the suture has been opened in 2 of 4 patients with age more than 30 years. The rate of opening suture was 6/10 in males and 19/21 in females. The midpalatal suture opening ratio has a statistically significant negative correlation with age, palate length, and the midpalatal suture maturation (MPSM) stage ($r = -0.506$, -0.494, and -0.746, respectively). As such, the authors introduced this equation: Midpalatal suture opening ratio = $-0.346 \times$ age $- 0.325 \times$ palate length $- 0.4 \times$ dMPSM1 (dMPSM1 is a dummy variable equal to 1 in stages C and D, and equal to 0 in stage E).

Evidence Summary

The available evidence suggests that the efficacy of MARPE in opening the palatal suture is limited in adult patients. The suture did not open in 4/27 cases (14.8%) in adults with age under 30 years and in 2/4 cases (50%) in adults over 30 years. Also, this equation may be effective for adult patients' prediction: Midpalatal suture opening ratio = −0.346 × age − 0.325 × palate length− 0.4 × dMPSM1. There was a strong negative correlation between the MPSM stage and the suture opening ($r = -0.746$) and a moderate negative correlation with age ($r = -0.506$) and the palate length ($r = -0.494$).

Evidence Interpretation

The chance of suture opening decreases with age, especially after 30 years of age as the palatal suture becomes mature. In adult patients, the stage of suture maturation should be assessed before the intervention, and proper consent should be taken. There are fewer chances of suture opening in males if the midpalatal suture is fused and the palatal length is increased. Surgical assisted rapid palatal expansion (SARME) should be considered in patients older than 30 years of age due to less predictability of expansion by MARPE.

Viewpoint

Shin et al. trial [31] has some issues that should be borne in mind during the findings' interpretation. The design is retrospective, which is more prone to selection bias as we lose some data and exclude patients after the treatment. The sample was divided by an arbitrary cutoff point of age 30 years without a clear reason; thus, this led to an imbalance between the comparison group (27 patients in the group under 30 years and 4 patients in the group over 30 years). The non-opening suture rate was 0.17 in the age group under 30 and 0.50 in the age group over 30; hence, the risk ratio (RR) is 2.94, which means the patients older than 30 years are less likely to have suture opening with MARPE by three times than the patients younger than 30 years.

Expansion and Appliances

Clinical Question 8: Is There Any Difference in the Maxillary Expansion Outcome When Using Different Appliances?

Evidence

Systematic Review and Meta-Analysis
Agostino/2014 [25]

A Cochrane systematic review included 15 trials to compare the effectiveness of different types of appliances in correcting posterior crossbite. Two RCTs compared the efficacy of quadhelix (QH) appliance and removable appliance (RA) in correcting the crossbite. They found that the fixed QH is better than the RA (RR; 1.20, 95% CI: 1.04–1.37) in correcting the posterior crossbite. They also found that the molar expansion is statistically greater in the QH appliance (MD; 1.15 mm, 95% CI: 0.4–1.9) group than the RA group, but those studies were from low-quality evidence.

Two RCTs compared bonded versus banded Hyrax, and they found that there is no statistically significant difference in the molar expansion between the two groups. Two RCTs compared the tooth-tissue-borne Haas expander versus the tooth-borne Hyrax expander for 3 months after expansion and found that the molar expansion was greater in the Haas group (MD; 0.7 mm, 95%CI: −0.25 to 1.66), but this was not statistically significant. One RCT compared four-point banded Hyrax versus two-point banded Hyrax after 3 months of expansion and found no statistically significant difference between the two interventions. One RCT compared Hyrax tooth-borne expander versus bone-anchored expander after 6 and 12 months of expansion and found no statistically significant difference between the two groups.

Systematic Review
Algharbi/2018 [19]

This review included seven studies; only one of the included studies, Weissheimer trial [13], compared the Haas expander versus the Hyrax expander. They found that the skeletal effects are statistically higher in the Hyrax group when compared with the Hass group. The anterior midpalatal suture opening was 4.37 mm in the Hyrax group and 3.63 mm in the Haas group. The posterior midpalatal suture opening was 3.14 mm in the Hyrax group and 2.62 mm in the Haas group. There was no statistically significant difference between the two appliances regarding the intermolar width at the occlusal surface (7.7 ± 0.2 mm in Haas group versus 7.9 ± 0.23 mm in Hyrax group), but the intermolar width at palatal root apices was statically different between groups (2.15 ± 0.18 mm in Haas group versus 3.14 ± 0.21 mm in Hyrax group) that indicated more upper molar tipping in Haas appliance.

One included study [32] reported no difference between banded and bonded expanders in regard to the skeletal effects, and there was no statistically significant difference regarding the molar tipping.

Evidence Summary

Limited evidence suggests that the quadhelix appliance is 20% more likely to correct the posterior crossbite than a removable appliance. In regard to the choice of Hass versus Hyrax appliance, the evidence is controversial, but the latest available evidence suggests that a tooth-borne expander (Hyrax) has statistically higher skeletal effects than bone tissue expander (Haas). Also, limited evidence suggests no difference between banded and bonded appliances regarding skeletal changes with no significant difference in molar tipping.

Evidence Interpretation

In young patients, quadhelix is a better choice for slow expansion than removable expanders. Bonded, banded, tooth-borne, or tooth tissue-borne appliances are all effective in treating maxillary constriction with diverse outcomes. The clinician should make the decision for the selection of appliance according to his expertise and clinical indications as well as the cost, patients' characteristics and preferences. For example, in young patients aged 8–13 years where the chances of suture fusion are limited, any conventional expander can open the sutures. In such patients if the clinician wants to do slow expansion, quadhelix is the appliance of choice. In rapid or semi-rapid expansion, hyrax expander is mostly preferred. In patients between 13 and 15 hyrax expander is mostly given as suture starts to interdigitate and quadhelix like appliances mostly do dental expansion in this age group. The Hyrax expanders can be given in slow, semi-rapid, and rapid protocols in such patients. In patients above 15 years of age, a quadhelix appliance can only produce dental expansion, while bone-borne and hybrid expanders are more effective than conventional appliances.

Viewpoint

Agostino [25] review is a Cochrane systematic review with a rigorous methodology, but most included studies are from low-quality evidence due to unclear or high risk of bias, which may downgrade the evidence.

Algharbi [19] review has been discussed before.

Surgical Expansion

Clinical Question 9: What Are the Effects of Surgical Assisted Rapid Maxillary Expansion (SARME)?

Evidence

Systematic Reviews and Meta-Analyses
Bortolotti/2019 [33]

In this review, the authors included nine RCTs in the qualitative analysis and, finally, five RCTs in their meta-analysis. One RCT used both BBE and TBE alongside SARME, while the rest used TBE. Their main aim was to assess the dental and skeletal changes of SARME. The patients' age was 18 years or more. The review found that there was a statistically significant difference in both skeletal and dental effects after the SARME intervention. SARME, statistically and clinically, increased the skeletal width (MD; 3.3 mm, 95%CI: 2.8–3.9, $P < 0.001$, four trials) and dental intermolar width (MD; 7 mm, 95%CI: 6.1–7.8, $P < 0.001$, five trials) when compared to the initial measures.

Vilani/2012 [34]

This systematic review included five studies in a meta-analysis; those studies investigated the long-term effect of SARME. The increase in the posterior width of the molar alveolus was statistically significant (MD; 3.33 mm, 95%CI: 2–4.65, $P < 0.00001$, three trials) with no statistically significant relapse (MD; 0.01 mm, $P = 0.99$). The long-term alveolar width increase was statistically significant (MD;

3.3 mm, 95%CI: 1.96–4.64, $P < 0.00001$, three trials). The intermolar width increase was statistically significant (MD; 3.71 mm, 95%CI: 2.61–4.82, $P < 0.00001$, two trails). Also, there was a statistically significant increase in the intercanine width (MD; 5.62 mm, 95%CI: 4.17–7.08, $P < 0.00001$, three trials) with a statistically significant relapse (MD; -1.5 mm, 95%CI: -2.82 to -0.19, $P=0.02$, three trials). The long-term intercanine width increase was statistically significant (MD; 3.55 mm, 95%CI:2.76–4.33, $P < 0.00001$, four trials) after the relapse.

Evidence Summary

The best available evidence suggests that the SARME is an effective procedure in adult patients with maxillary transversal constriction. The post-treatment effects have both dental (intermolar width MD; 7 mm) and skeletal components (MD; 3.3 mm). Also, there was a significant skeletal effect of SARME on molars' alveolar width (MD; 3.3 mm), the intermolar width (MD; 3.71 mm), and the intercanine width (MD; 3.55 mm) in the long term with significant relapse in the intercanine region (-1.5 mm).

Evidence Interpretation

SARME is an effective treatment for constricted maxilla in adults. 53% of SARME effects are dental, while 47% are skeletal. In the long term, relapse occurs in the intercanine and intermolar regions. In this respect, the relapse should be taken into account at the treatment planning level, and the post-treatment retention should be maintained in the long term.

Viewpoint

Bortolotti [33] review has some issues that should be taken into account during the interpretation of findings. The studies were graded as low to moderate quality according to the GRADE approach. For the risk of bias, most of the included studies (seven studies) presented some concern, one at high risk and one at low risk of bias. The main issues were the lack of blinding, missingness, and inadequate randomization. However, SARME research always provides limited evidence as there are a few surgical cases, so this systematic review provides us with good information about SARME efficacy.

Vilani [34] review also has some issues that should be considered when the reader interprets the results. The included studies were low to moderate quality evidence. The included study design is either retrospective or prospective, and no RCTs were included in this review. Also, the authors pooled four studies, not five studies as they reported, in the meta-analysis. Interestingly, they pooled tooth- and bone-borne expanders in the same meta-analysis, and this may lead to clinical heterogeneity in the meta analysis. So, the result of this study should be interpreted carefully.

At last, further research with a golden standard design (RCT) is needed to bring confidence about the estimate of the SARME effect.

RME and Sagittal Changes

Clinical Question 10: What Is the Effect of Rapid Maxillary Expansion on the Sagittal Plane?

Evidence

Systematic Review
Feres/2015 [35]

This review included seven trials to investigate the effects of the maxillary expansion in Class II growing patients. Three included studies reported the molar relationship changes pre and post-RME; two trials [36, 37] showed a significant improvement in the Class II relationship, while one trial [38] revealed that there is no significant change in the Class II relationship. Interestingly, six studies investigated the mandibular changes after RME; one study [39] reported that there is no significant change in mandibular Class II parameters, while a trial [40] revealed that SNB angle statistically increased but this was not clinically relevant for all parameters. On the other hand, another trial [37] reported that there was a significant increase in mandibular length and advancement of the symphysis, while two studies [41, 42] revealed that there was a statistically significant anterior displacement of the mandible during the retention period.

Retrospective Study
Farronato/2011 [41]

This RCT was included in the aforementioned systematic review [35]. The authors included 183 patients with bilateral crossbite in this study with a mean age of 8.7 years. They divided the patients according to their skeletal classification into three groups; 65 patients with Class I, 55 patients with Class II, and 63 patients with Class III. After the expansion, there was insignificant advancement of both maxilla and mandible in Class I patients with a statistical decrease in ANB angle by 0.34°. In Class II patients, the mandible statistically advanced by 2.25° (SNB) with a decrease in ANB by 1.81°. However, patients with Class III malocclusion showed an advancement of the maxilla by 0.81° in SNA, and an increase in ANB by 2.16° with downward and backward rotation of the mandible by 0.84° (N-Me), leading to an increase in the anterior vertical dimension.

Evidence Summary

There is limited evidence to support the effects of the rapid maxillary expansion on the sagittal correction of Class II and Class III malocclusion. There are still contradictory findings in regard to this question. Limited evidence supports that there is a correction of the molar relationship, and there is a change in SNB and ANB angles after RME with suspected anterior mandibular displacement in Class II patients. In contrast, in Class III patients, advancement of the maxilla and backward rotation of the mandible may improve the Class III relationship.

Evidence Interpretation

According to low-level evidence, RME in Classes II and III patients may positively affect mandibular displacement, but this effect is still insignificant. As there is low and conflicting evidence, the clinician should not incorporate any provision in their treatment plan that, after RME, there would be an improvement in the sagittal skeletal and dental relationships.

Viewpoint

Feres [35] was a well-conducted review. However, there are some limitations; the included trials are of low to medium quality. There was a lack of sample size calculation in most of the included studies. The assessment or the measurements were biased with different measure points and a lack of blinding that may hamper the confidence in drawing clinical recommendations. As such, further well-conducted RCTs may substantially change the estimate of the RME effect on the sagittal plane. Farronato study [41] was a retrospective study. The design is more prone to selection bias as the cases with full records only might be included. The lack of sample size calculation may leave the study with not enough power for the significance of the findings. The authors included patients with only bilateral crossbites and excluded unilateral crossbite with midline deviation, which may restrict the generalizability of the findings and ignore a large category in the crossbite cases. The centric occlusion and the premature contacts may affect the sagittal changes during expansion and that should be borne in mind.

RME and Breathing

Clinical Question 11: What Is the Effect of Rapid Maxillary Expansion on Breathing?

Evidence

Systematic Review
Baratieri/2011 [43]

This systematic review included eight studies to investigate airway tract changes as a result of RME. The variation in the age range was from 7.8 to 16 years. The posteroanterior (PA) radiographic studies reported a significant increase of 2.2 mm in the nasal cavity width after palatal RME with long-term stability. One included study reported that this increase was greater in the pre-peak growth spurt (2.3 mm) than after the growth spurt (1.5 mm). A study also investigated the nasopharyngeal airway dimension and found that the increase was significant (5.3 mm) after 6 months of RME treatment versus (1.2 mm) in the control group. Included studies that evaluated airway tracts using acoustic rhinometry or rhinomanometry reported a significant effect of RME on the nasal cavity. However, cone-beam computed tomography did not show any significant increases in the nasal cavity volume.

Evidence Summary

The best available evidence suggests that the RME may affect the airway tracts, and may increase the width of the airway tracts on the nasal cavity level by 2.2 mm when measured on PA radiographs. These effects are observed more in pre-growth spurt patients. The nasopharyngeal airway dimensions increased by 5.3 mm in the RME group versus 1.2 in the control group.

Evidence Interpretation

RME may have an effect on the airway tracts but the evidence for this finding is very low. So RME should not solely be done for this purpose. In other words, increasing the airway tracts should not be a part of the orthodontic treatment plan. It would be considered as a positive effect of the RME that the breathing may improve, and this may lead the clinician to use RME instead of appliances with dental effects.

Viewpoint

Baratieri [43] is a well-conducted review; however, its findings should be interpreted with caution. Although the authors evaluated the included studies as moderate quality evidence, most of them have a high risk of bias due to a lack of blinding and inadequate randomization. The included study design was not the gold standard design as mostly it was non-randomized design. Some of the measurement's methods do not have validity in evaluating airway tracts. Hence, our certainty is low in this estimate and more valid RCTs are needed to be certain about the estimate of the RME effect on the airway tracts.

RME and Facial Profile

Clinical Question 12: What Are the Effects of the Rapid Maxillary Expansion on the Facial Profile?

Evidence

Retrospective Study
Aras/2017 [44]

In this trial, the researchers investigated the changes in soft tissue profile as a result of RME or SARME. They assessed the lateral cephalograms for 25 RME patients and 16 SARME patients before and after the expansion by 83.25 ± 3.51 days for SARME and 85.68 ± 4.37 for RME. The author found that the upper lip thickness decreased significantly in the SARME group by -0.61 ± 1.1 and decreased insignificantly by -0.33 ± 0.15 in the RME group. In contrast, there was a statistically significant increase in Holdaway (H) angle by $2.04° \pm 1.79$ and a decrease in soft tissue facial angle by -1.5 ± 1.49 leading to a more convex profile in the RME group. Nose prominence decreased in SARME and increased in RME by -0.24 ± 0.92 and 0.3 ± 1.49, respectively, but this was not statistically significant.

Evidence Summary

The available evidence suggests that there is no correlation between skeletal and soft tissue changes due to maxillary expansion. The effect of SARME on the soft tissue was limited, and only the thickness of the upper lip statistically decreased. While the RME statistically decreased the soft tissue profile and increased the H angle most of these changes were neither statistically nor clinically significant.

Evidence Interpretation

RME has some effects on the soft tissue profile while SARME has no such effects. The effects of RME on soft tissue are clinically insignificant.

Viewpoint

Aras [44] study provides us with good information about the effect of maxillary expansion on the soft tissue profile. However, this evidence is low-quality due to the study design, which is more prone to bias, especially selection bias. Also, the period of 85 days is not sufficient for soft tissue change investigation, particularly after a surgical procedure such as SARME. The mean age in the SARME group was 27.4 ± 4.6, while it was 13.7 ± 1.9 years in the RME group, and this may affect the results of this study. Interestingly, the authors analyzed 13 soft tissue variables which may increase the false results and Hypothesizing After the Results are Known (HARKing). So, further research is needed regarding this effect as we are concerned about the effect of the estimate.

Iatrogenic Effects

Clinical Question 13: What Are the Potential Side Effects of the Maxillary Expansion?

Evidence

Systematic Reviews
Forst/2014 [45]

This review included three studies that investigated root resorption (RR) after rapid maxillary expansion. Of those studies; two studies [46, 47] used 2D intraoral X-ray, and one study [48] used CBCT to assess the root resorption. The 2D studies reported that there are no radiographic signs of external root resorption, but the 3D study [48] revealed that there was a statistically significant volume loss of roots after expansion. The histological assessment of the root resorption in the 2D studies [46, 47] after premolar extraction found that anchored premolars exhibited RR, mostly on the buccal surface. Also, RR was noticed on the mesial, distal, and apical sides of the root. The difference between 2D radiographic and histological findings suggests that the 2D radiographs underestimate root resorption.

Khosravi/2019 [30]

One included study in this review investigated the effects of BBE and TBE in combination with SARME. The researcher reported that there was central incisor' discoloration after 3 weeks of surgery and two asymmetrical expansions in the bone-borne device group. However, one included trial [49], in this review, pointed out movement of the bone-borne device due to tongue pressure.

Randomized Controlled Trial
Baldini/2015 [26]

As mentioned before, this RCT comprised 112 patients with a constricted maxilla of mean age (11 ± 1.8) years. The patients were assigned into two groups; one turn per day group (G1) and two turns per day group (G2). After 15 min of activation, the average pain was 0.5–1 and 2.3 in G1 and G2, respectively. The pain peak was noticed in the fifth to tenth activation. Interestingly, 10 patients recorded pain scores of more than 5 in G2 and 3 patients in G1. Patients with cervical stage (CS2) reported more pain scores than CS1 patients, thus suggesting a correlation between pain and skeletal maturation of the patients.

Evidence Summary

The best available evidence suggests that there are iatrogenic effects (root resorption, pain, asymmetrical expansion) of rapid expansion in conventional, MARPE and SARPE techniques. In SARME, some studies reported asymmetrical expansion and tooth vitality-related side effects while in RME, some studies reported histological and volumetric root resorption. More pain is experienced as skeletal maturity increases.

Evidence Interpretation

RME may be associated with some iatrogenic effects such as root resorption, asymmetrical expansion, pain, bone loss, and loss of tooth vitality. Before the start of any expansion procedure, the patient should be informed of these iatrogenic damages, and written consent should be taken.

Viewpoint

Forst [45] review has a few limitations; this review included only two non-randomized trials and one retrospective study, which is a weaker design than randomized controlled trials. Interestingly, the authors used the ROB tool to assess the risk of bias, and this tool is used for RCTs, so it would be better to use ROBINS I or E for non-randomized and retrospective designs. External root resorption may interfere with the open apexes of roots that may be interrupted by expansion. As such, these issues may hamper the confidence in the available evidence and hinder drawing clinical recommendations.

Authors' Recommendations

- Rapid maxillary expansion is an effective method for correcting the maxillary transverse discrepancy by opening the midpalatal sutures.
- The conventional RME technique is effective in young patients under 16 years of age. In patients above 16 years of age, the midpalatal sutures maturation should be assessed and MARPE or SARME should be chosen depending upon the maturation of the sutures. In patients above 30 years of age, the chances of opening the suture decrease by 50%, so SARME is the only viable option for those patients. CBCT is a better choice in adult patients to assess the continuity of the suture.
- Both slow and rapid expansion protocols are effective, with quadhelix the appliance of choice for slow expansion in adolescents. In children above 13 years of age, RME is the treatment of choice. For cases requiring rapid expansion, the clinician should choose the appliance design according to case needs and clinical experience.
- Nearly half of the effects of expansion are dental, so long-term retention should be given. To increase skeletal effects, bone-borne expanders can be used.
- The midpalatal suture usually is opened in a triangular or V-shaped pattern in horizontal and vertical planes. This lead to more expansion in the anterior palate and hanging of palatal cusps of molars posteriorly. So there is more relief of crowding anteriorly than posteriorly. Also, the mandible backward rotation and bite opening occur due to the hanging of palatal cusps. Negative torque may be incorporated in the fixed appliances on maxillary molars to compensate this undesirable effect.
- Maxillary expansion should not be done for improvement of the airway space, correction of sagittal relations, or facial profile.
- Like every intervention procedure, expansion is also associated with side effects which should be considered in the treatment planning, and proper consent should be taken from the patients.

References

1. Andrade Ada S, Gameiro GH, Derossi M, Gavião MB. Posterior crossbite and functional changes. A systematic review. Angle Orthod. 2009;79(2):380–6. https://doi.org/10.231 9/030708-137.1.
2. Timms DJ. The dawn of rapid maxillary expansion. Angle Orthod. 1999;69(3):247–50.
3. Proffit WR, Fields HW, Larson B, Sarver DM. Contemporary orthodontics-e-book. Elsevier Health Sciences; 2018.
4. Angelieri F, Cevidanes LH, Franchi L, Gonçalves JR, Benavides E, McNamara JA Jr. Midpalatal suture maturation: classification method for individual assessment before rapid maxillary expansion. Am J Orthod Dentofac Orthop. 2013;144(5):759–69. https://doi. org/10.1016/j.ajodo.2013.04.022.

 5. Zhou Y, Long H, Ye N, Xue J, Yang X, Liao L, et al. The effectiveness of non-surgical maxillary expansion: a meta-analysis. Eur J Orthod. 2014;36(2):233–42. https://doi.org/10.1093/ejo/cjt044.
 6. Lagravere MO, Majorb PW, Flores-Mirc C. Long-term skeletal changes with rapid maxillary expansion: a systematic review. Angle Orthod. 2005;75(6):1046–52.
 7. Seif-Eldin NF, Elkordy SA, Fayed MS, Elbeialy AR, Eid FH. Transverse skeletal effects of rapid maxillary expansion in pre and post pubertal subjects: a systematic review. Open Access Maced J Med Sci. 2019;7(3):467–77. https://doi.org/10.3889/oamjms.2019.080.
 8. Baccetti T, Franchi L, Cameron CG, McNamara JA Jr. Treatment timing for rapid maxillary expansion. Angle Orthod. 2001;71(5):343–50. https://doi.org/10.1043/0003-3219(2001)071<0343:Ttfrme>2.0.Co;2.
 9. Sayar G, Kilinc DD. Rapid maxillary expansion outcomes according to midpalatal suture maturation levels. Prog Orthod. 2019;20(1):27. https://doi.org/10.1186/s40510-019-0278-9.
10. Jimenez-Valdivia LM, Malpartida-Carrillo V, Rodriguez-Cardenas YA, Dias-Da Silveira HL, Arriola-Guillen LE. Midpalatal suture maturation stage assessment in adolescents and young adults using cone-beam computed tomography. Prog Orthod. 2019;20(1):38. https://doi.org/10.1186/s40510-019-0291-z.
11. Bazargani F, Feldmann I, Bondemark L. Three-dimensional analysis of effects of rapid maxillary expansion on facial sutures and bones. Angle Orthod. 2013;83(6):1074–82. https://doi.org/10.2319/020413-103.1.
12. Lione R, Ballanti F, Franchi L, Baccetti T, Cozza P. Treatment and posttreatment skeletal effects of rapid maxillary expansion studied with low-dose computed tomography in growing subjects. Am J Orthod Dentofac Orthop. 2008;134(3):389–92. https://doi.org/10.1016/j.ajodo.2008.05.011.
13. Weissheimer A, de Menezes LM, Mezomo M, Dias DM, de Lima EM, Rizzatto SM. Immediate effects of rapid maxillary expansion with Haas-type and hyrax-type expanders: a randomized clinical trial. Am J Orthod Dentofac Orthop. 2011;140(3):366–76. https://doi.org/10.1016/j.ajodo.2010.07.025.
14. Ballanti F, Lione R, Baccetti T, Franchi L, Cozza P. Treatment and posttreatment skeletal effects of rapid maxillary expansion investigated with low-dose computed tomography in growing subjects. Am J Orthod Dentofac Orthop. 2010;138(3):311–7. https://doi.org/10.1016/j.ajodo.2008.10.022.
15. Christie KF, Boucher N, Chung CH. Effects of bonded rapid palatal expansion on the transverse dimensions of the maxilla: a cone-beam computed tomography study. Am J Orthod Dentofac Orthop. 2010;137(4 Suppl):S79–85. https://doi.org/10.1016/j.ajodo.2008.11.024.
16. Podesser B, Williams S, Crismani AG, Bantleon HP. Evaluation of the effects of rapid maxillary expansion in growing children using computer tomography scanning: a pilot study. Eur J Orthod. 2007;29(1):37–44. https://doi.org/10.1093/ejo/cjl068.
17. Lagravere MO, Gamble J, Major PW, Heo G. Transverse dental changes after tooth-borne and bone-borne maxillary expansion. Int Orthod. 2013;11(1):21–34. https://doi.org/10.1016/j.ortho.2012.12.003.
18. Lagravère MO, Heo G, Major PW, Flores-Mir C. Meta-analysis of immediate changes with rapid maxillary expansion treatment. JADA. 2006;137:44–53.
19. Algharbi M, Bazargani F, Dimberg L. Do different maxillary expansion appliances influence the outcomes of the treatment? Eur J Orthod. 2018;40(1):97–106. https://doi.org/10.1093/ejo/cjx035.
20. Brunetto M, Andriani Jda S, Ribeiro GL, Locks A, Correa M, Correa LR. Three-dimensional assessment of buccal alveolar bone after rapid and slow maxillary expansion: a clinical trial study. Am J Orthod Dentofac Orthop. 2013;143(5):633–44. https://doi.org/10.1016/j.ajodo.2012.12.008.
21. Martina R, Cioffi I, Farella M, Leone P, Manzo P, Matarese G, et al. Transverse changes determined by rapid and slow maxillary expansion – a low-dose CT-based randomized controlled trial. Orthod Craniofac Res. 2012;15(3):159–68. https://doi.org/10.1111/j.1601-6343.2012.01543.x.

22. Bastos R, Blagitz MN, Aragon M, Maia LC, Normando D. Periodontal side effects of rapid and slow maxillary expansion: a systematic review. Angle Orthod. 2019;89(4):651–60. https://doi.org/10.2319/060218-419.1.

23. Greenbaum KR, Zachrisson BU. The effect of palatal expansion therapy on the periodontal supporting tissues. Am J Orthod. 1982;81(1):12–21. https://doi.org/10.1016/0002-9416(82)90283-4.

24. Mummolo S, Marchetti E, Albani F, Campanella V, Pugliese F, Di Martino S, et al. Comparison between rapid and slow palatal expansion: evaluation of selected periodontal indices. Head Face Med. 2014;10:30. https://doi.org/10.1186/1746-160x-10-30.

25. Agostino P, Ugolini A, Signori A, Silvestrini-Biavati A, Harrison JE, Riley P. Orthodontic treatment for posterior crossbites. Cochrane Database Syst Rev. 2014;(8):CD000979. https://doi.org/10.1002/14651858.CD000979.pub2.

26. Baldini A, Nota A, Santariello C, Assi V, Ballanti F, Cozza P. Influence of activation protocol on perceived pain during rapid maxillary expansion. Angle Orthod. 2015;85(6):1015–20. https://doi.org/10.2319/112114-833.1.

27. Krusi M, Eliades T, Papageorgiou SN. Are there benefits from using bone-borne maxillary expansion instead of tooth-borne maxillary expansion? A systematic review with meta-analysis. Prog Orthod. 2019;20(1):9. https://doi.org/10.1186/s40510-019-0261-5.

28. Lagravere MO, Carey J, Heo G, Toogood RW, Major PW. Transverse, vertical, and anteroposterior changes from bone-anchored maxillary expansion vs traditional rapid maxillary expansion: a randomized clinical trial. Am J Orthod Dentofac Orthop. 2010;137(3):304 e1–304 e12; discussion 5. https://doi.org/10.1016/j.ajodo.2009.09.016.

29. Mosleh MI, Kaddah MA, Abd ElSayed FA, ElSayed HS. Comparison of transverse changes during maxillary expansion with 4-point bone-borne and tooth-borne maxillary expanders. Am J Orthod Dentofac Orthop. 2015;148(4):599–607. https://doi.org/10.1016/j.ajodo.2015.04.040.

30. Khosravi M, Ugolini A, Miresmaeili A, Mirzaei H, Shahidi-Zandi V, Soheilifar S, et al. Tooth-borne versus bone-borne rapid maxillary expansion for transverse maxillary deficiency: a systematic review. Int Orthod. 2019;17(3):425–36. https://doi.org/10.1016/j.ortho.2019.06.003.

31. Shin H, Hwang CJ, Lee KJ, Choi YJ, Han SS, Yu HS. Predictors of midpalatal suture expansion by miniscrew-assisted rapid palatal expansion in young adults: a preliminary study. Korean J Orthod. 2019;49(6):360–71. https://doi.org/10.4041/kjod.2019.49.6.360.

32. Pangrazio-Kulbersh V, Wine P, Haughey M, Pajtas B, Kaczynski R. Cone beam computed tomography evaluation of changes in the naso-maxillary complex associated with two types of maxillary expanders. Angle Orthod. 2012;82(3):448–57. https://doi.org/10.2319/072211-464.1.

33. Bortolotti F, Solidoro L, Bartolucci ML, Incerti Parenti S, Paganelli C, Alessandri-Bonetti G. Skeletal and dental effects of surgically assisted rapid palatal expansion: a systematic review of randomized controlled trials. Eur J Orthod. 2019;42(4):434–40. https://doi.org/10.1093/ejo/cjz057.

34. Vilani GN, Mattos CT, de Oliveira Ruellas AC, Maia LC. Long-term dental and skeletal changes in patients submitted to surgically assisted rapid maxillary expansion: a meta-analysis. Oral Surg Oral Med Oral Pathol Oral Radiol. 2012;114(6):689–97. https://doi.org/10.1016/j.oooo.2012.01.040.

35. Feres MF, Raza H, Alhadlaq A, El-Bialy T. Rapid maxillary expansion effects in Class II malocclusion: a systematic review. Angle Orthod. 2015;85(6):1070–9. https://doi.org/10.2319/102514-768.1.

36. McNamara JA Jr, Sigler LM, Franchi L, Guest SS, Baccetti T. Changes in occlusal relationships in mixed dentition patients treated with rapid maxillary expansion. A prospective clinical study. Angle Orthod. 2010;80(2):230–8. https://doi.org/10.2319/040309-192.1.

37. Guest SS, McNamara JA Jr, Baccetti T, Franchi L. Improving Class II malocclusion as a side-effect of rapid maxillary expansion: a prospective clinical study. Am J Orthod Dentofac Orthop. 2010;138(5):582–91. https://doi.org/10.1016/j.ajodo.2008.12.026.

38. Volk T, Sadowsky C, Begole EA, Boice P. Rapid palatal expansion for spontaneous Class II correction. Am J Orthod Dentofac Orthop. 2010;137(3):310–5. https://doi.org/10.1016/j.ajodo.2008.05.017.

39. Cozza P, Giancotti A, Petrosino A. Rapid palatal expansion in mixed dentition using a modified expander: a cephalometric investigation. J Orthod. 2001;28(2):129–34. https://doi.org/10.1093/ortho/28.2.129.
40. Lambot T, Van Steenberghe PR, Vanmuylder N, De Maertelaer V, Glineur R. Early treatment with rapid palatal expander and 3D Quad Action mandibular appliance: evaluation of a comprehensive approach in 22 patients. Orthod Fr. 2008;79(2):107–14. https://doi.org/10.1051/orthodfr:2008005.
41. Farronato G, Giannini L, Galbiati G, Maspero C. Sagittal and vertical effects of rapid maxillary expansion in Class I, II, and III occlusions. Angle Orthod. 2011;81(2):298–303. https://doi.org/10.2319/050410-241.1.
42. Baratieri C, Alves M Jr, Sant'anna EF, Nojima Mda C, Nojima LI. 3D mandibular positioning after rapid maxillary expansion in Class II malocclusion. Braz Dent J. 2011;22(5):428–34. https://doi.org/10.1590/s0103-64402011000500014.
43. Baratieri C, Alves M Jr, de Souza MM, de Souza Araujo MT, Maia LC. Does rapid maxillary expansion have long-term effects on airway dimensions and breathing? Am J Orthod Dentofac Orthop. 2011;140(2):146–56. https://doi.org/10.1016/j.ajodo.2011.02.019.
44. Aras I, Olmez S, Akay MC, Gunbay T, Aras A. The effects of maxillary expansion on the soft tissue facial profile. J Istanb Univ Fac Dent. 2017;51(3):1–10. https://doi.org/10.17096/jiufd.85884.
45. Forst D, Nijjar S, Khaled Y, Lagravere M, Flores-Mir C. Radiographic assessment of external root resorption associated with jackscrew-based maxillary expansion therapies: a systematic review. Eur J Orthod. 2014;36(5):576–85. https://doi.org/10.1093/ejo/cjt090.
46. Barber AF, Sims MR. Rapid maxillary expansion and external root resorption in man: a scanning electron microscope study. Am J Orthod. 1981;79(6):630–52. https://doi.org/10.1016/0002-9416(81)90356-0.
47. Odenrick L, Karlander EL, Pierce A, Kretschmar U. Surface resorption following two forms of rapid maxillary expansion. Eur J Orthod. 1991;13(4):264–70. https://doi.org/10.1093/ejo/13.4.264.
48. Baysal A, Karadede I, Hekimoglu S, Ucar F, Ozer T, Veli I, et al. Evaluation of root resorption following rapid maxillary expansion using cone-beam computed tomography. Angle Orthod. 2012;82(3):488–94. https://doi.org/10.2319/060411-367.1.
49. Koudstaal MJ, Smeets JB, Kleinrensink GJ, Schulten AJ, van der Wal KG. Relapse and stability of surgically assisted rapid maxillary expansion: an anatomic biomechanical study. J Oral Maxillofac Surg. 2009;67(1):10–4. https://doi.org/10.1016/j.joms.2007.11.026.

6

Temporary Skeletal Anchorage Devices in Orthodontics

Contents

© The Author(s), under exclusive license to Springer Nature Switzerland AG 2023
S. Mheissen, H. Khan, *Orthodontic Evidence*,
https://doi.org/10.1007/978-3-031-24422-3_6

Abbreviations

CADs	Conventional anchorage devices
MIs	Miniscrews, mini or micro implants
MIT	Maximum insertion torque
PCS	Prospective cohort studies
PS	Pull-out strength
PTV	Periotest value
TSADs	Temporary skeletal anchorage devices
VBH	Vertical palatal bone height

Introduction

Orthodontic anchorage, which is the prevention of unwanted tooth movement, is one of the core components of orthodontic treatment mechanics. It is conventionally provided by various intra and extraoral appliances. These appliances include extraoral appliances such as headgears and intraoral appliances such as Nance, transpalatal or lingual arches, tip back bends, and differential tooth movement. All these appliances have limitations and are always related to unwanted tooth movement. To search for a better alternative method, mini-implants/screws were first proposed for orthodontic anchorage by Kanomi [1]. Hence, temporary skeletal anchorage devices (TSADs) have gained enormous popularity in the last decade and become a fundamental part of the daily orthodontic practice to provide orthodontic anchorage and enable simple biomechanics for orthodontic tooth movement. TSADs can be used to enhance anchorage, which may decrease the side effects on the anchoring teeth [2]. Also, it can be used for establishing more control over the teeth by delivering force/moments to specific teeth that yield effective biomechancis during different orthodontic tooth movements; such as intrusion, expansion, and extrusion. Additionally, TSADs can be used to increase skeletal effects in some treatment modalities [3, 4].

TSADs are intraoral anchorage devices, fixed to bone either biochemically (osseointegrated; dental implants) or mechanically (cortically stabilized; miniscrews). The term TSADs comprises of multiple designs of screws, which are used for different purposes in clinical practice. The first group comprises of *miniscrews, mini or micro implants (MIs)* which are the simple design of TSADs and consist of a small screw with different dimensions (length 5–16 mm, diameter 1–2 mm). These small MIs provide the clinician the leverage to place them at various locations as dictated by the biomechanics. These anatomical locations include inter radicular areas both buccally and palatally, hard palate, maxillary tuberosity, infra zygomatic crest, buccal shelves, and retromolar pads. The miniscrews can be self-drilling or self-taping. The self-taping miniscrews need a predrilling for their insertion. The majority of these MIs used in contemporary orthodontics are non-osseointegrated and are mostly of self-drilling type. So, they give the ease of simple insertion, immediate loading, and removal without any complex armamentarium. Some important characteristics of MIs are threads, flutes, pitch, taper, and the head design. The threads are cutting parts of the screws and the pitch is the distance between two threads. The flutes are recessed areas in the cross-sectional threads that help to carry bone chips away from the cutting edge of the screws. The head design which can be shaped like a mushroom, hook, or a bracket slot (Fig. 6.1).

The second group of TSADs consists of *miniplates* which are a type of surgical plates available in different designs for orthodontic purposes. These miniplates are mostly placed intraorally with the help of an oral surgeon after a flap surgery procedure. Also, their removal needs a surgeon's help. Various orthodontic force systems are attached to one end of these miniplates which is exposed from the gingiva, especially the attached gingiva. Miniplates are mostly used when heavy forces are required, such as orthopedic forces for growth modification in both skeletal Class II and Class III cases.

The third group of TSADs is osseointegrated *palatal implants, dental implants, and onplants*. Osteointegrated palatal implants are self-taping implants and are mostly used for maxillary distalization. Their use has declined over the years due to difficulty placing and especially removing them. Onplants are disks that are placed subperiosteal in the palate after a minor surgical procedure. Like palatal osseointegrated implants, onplants are also not popular these days due to the surgical procedure involved. Dental implants can be used for orthodontic anchorage but are not

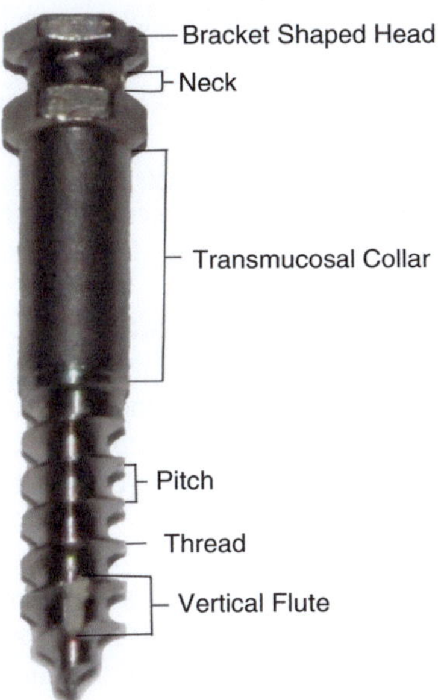

Fig. 6.1 A photo of miniscrew showing the different parts of the miniscrews

solely placed for this purpose. Anchorage can be utilized by them whenever they are present or justified in a case.

Anchorage and Miniscrews

Clinical Question 1: Do Miniscrews or Miniplates Provide Absolute Anchorage?

Evidence

Systematic Review and Meta-Analysis
Alharbi/2018 [2]

In this systematic review, the authors included seven RCTs to compare the effectiveness of mini-implants/screws (MIs) versus the conventional anchorage devices (CADs; headgear and transpalatal arch) in reinforcing the anchorage during enmasse retraction. Those studies included 271 orthodontic patients with 310 MIs and 149 CADs. Two included RCTs reported a small amount of anchorage loss by 0.89 mm [5] and 0.78 mm [6] using MIs for enhancing anchorage, two studies [7, 8] found no anchorage loss in the MIs group, while two trials found a minor gain of space by −0.89 [9] and −0.06 [10].

Randomized Clinical Trials
Genzer/2018 [11]

This RCT randomly assigned 80 adolescent patients into two groups; one group used MIs for anchorage, while another group used molar blocks after the first premolar extraction for anchorage reinforcement. The anchorage loss was 0.2 ± 0.2 mm in MIs group, and 2.4 ± 0.2 mm in the molar blocks group, and the difference between the two groups was clinically significant.

Evidence Summary

Looking at the evidence collectively, the best available evidence indicates that the anchorage loss ranged from −0.89 to 0.89 mm using MIs.

Evidence Interpretation

The evidence about absolute anchorage is controversial. Studies have reported space gain, absolute anchorage, or minimal anchorage loss using TSADs mainly MIs. This may be related to the type of anchorage that is direct versus indirect anchorage or the nature of biomechanics and the amount of force.

Viewpoint

Alharbi review [2] was a well-conducted review with some limitations. There was a high risk of bias in four of the seven studies. The statistical heterogeneity was very high, which may mislead the interpretation of the results. The differences in conventional methods in the primary studies may be considered as a clinical heterogeneity.

Genzer et al. [11] trial was a well-conducted trial. There were seven dropouts in the MIs group, and two dropouts in the molar block group, and the authors used intention to treat analysis to overcome this problem. However, the difference in missing data between the two groups may suggest a problem related to one group more than the other and subsequently suggest a bias due to deviations from the intended interventions. The random generation was not reported in detail. Furthermore, the authors acknowledged that there was uneven sex distribution in the total sample, which may limit the generalizability of the results. The blinding of the patients and clinicians was not possible in this study, but the assessor was blinded to reduce the bias.

Clinical Question 2: Are TSADs More Effective in Providing Anchorage Than Conventional Appliances?

Evidence

Systematic Reviews and Meta-Analyses
Papadopoulos/2011 [12]
This review included eight studies; three RCTs and five CCTs. The researchers assessed one study as high quality, four as medium quality, and three as low quality. The included studies compared the conventional anchorage devices (CADs) with the MIs enhanced anchorage. The researchers found that the MIs were significantly better than CADs in enhancing the anchorage (MD; 2.39 mm, 95%CI: 1.84–2.94, $P < 0.001$, $I^2 = 80\%$, eight trials). The MIs anchorage loss was statistically lesser in the mandible than in the maxilla (−0.6 vs. 0.2 mm). In the maxilla, the MIs anchorage loss was lesser when MIs when inserted on the buccal side between the second premolar and first molar rather than when inserted on the palatal side (−0.2 vs. 1.3 mm). Direct anchorage to MIs showed a statistically less anchorage loss than indirect anchorage (−0.2 vs. 0.8 mm). Two MIs per patient were more effective than one in enhancing anchorage (−0.2 vs. 1.3 mm).

Alharbi/2018 [2]
In this systematic review, the authors included seven RCTs to compare the effectiveness of mini-implants/screws (MIs) versus the CADs (headgear and transpalatal arch) in reinforcing the anchorage during enmasse retraction. Those studies included 271 orthodontic patients with 310 MIs and 149 CADs. The authors pooled six studies in the meta-analysis and found that the MIs provided more anchorage than CADs (SMD: −2.07 mm, 95% CI: −3.05 to −1.08, $P < 0.001$, $I^2 = 88\%$). The comparison between TPA and MIs, depicted that the anchorage loss was higher in the TPA group than in the MIs group (SMD; −3.13 mm, 95% CI: −4.72 to −1.55, $P < 0.001$, $I^2 = 88\%$, four trials). There was no statistically significant difference between MIs and TPA in regard to the total treatment duration (25.65 ± 5.06 months and 26.88 ± 6.54 months in MIs and TPA groups, respectively). Regarding the time needed for space closure, there was no statistically significant difference between TPA and MIs. However, the

number of visits to complete the treatment was statistically lesser in MIs group (18.38) than the headgear (19.24) or the Nance appliance group (21.77). The authors reported that this evidence was of low to moderate quality.

Antoszewska-Smith/2017 [13]

This review included 14 studies; 7 CCTs and 7 RCTs, to compare the effectiveness of TSADs versus CADs. Only one included trial compared miniplates with conventional appliances, while the rest compared MIs with CAD. The authors found that TSADs had significantly less anchorage loss than CADs (MD; 1.86 mm, 95%CI: 1.5–2.22, $P < 0.001$, $I^2 = 65\%$, 13 trials). The molar tipping was less in TSADs than CADs (MD; $-1.69°$, 95%CI: -3.69 to 0.31, $P = 0.1$, $I^2 = 89.8\%$, 5 trials), but not statistically significant. The incisors' retraction was statistically higher in TSADs than in conventional devices (MD; -1.37, 95%CI: -1.91 to -0.83, $P < 0.001$, 12 trials). The treatment duration was statistically shorter in TSADs group when compared with the CADs group (MD;-4 months, 95%CI: -5.79 to -2.21, $P < 0.001$, five trials).

Evidence Summary

Looking at the evidence collectively, the best available evidence suggests that TSADs provide more anchorage enhancement than CADs by 1.86–2.4 mm. There was better control on molar tipping (1.69°) and more incisors' retraction (1.37 mm) by TSADs than CADs. There was no consensus on the time duration of treatment, with more robust evidence supporting that anchorage provided by TSADs decreased treatment time by 4 months from a pooled effect of five trials [13]. Notwithstanding that there was no statistically significant difference in acquired time for space closure, the number of visits were statistically lesser in TSADs than in CADs, but this was a small difference. Interestingly, one study [12] reported that enhancing the anchorage is better when MIs placed in the mandible (space gain of 0.6 mm) rather than the maxilla and on the buccal side between the second premolar and first molar using direct anchorage. Also, two MIs per patient is more effective in providing anchorage.

Evidence Interpretation

Miniscrews and miniplates provide better anchorage than conventional anchorage appliance. TSADs may provide absolute anchorage with some distal molar movement, especially in the case of direct anchorage, buccal placement, and lower arch or when two MIs are used to provide traction force. Some anchorage loss should be anticipated when placing TSADs in the palate or in the maxilla in general. Indirect anchorage by TSADs and single MI per patient may be associated with a minor anchorage loss. Furthermore, TSADs enable more retraction of maxillary incisors, decrease the treatment time, and provide better control of molar tipping.

Viewpoint

Although Papadopoulos [12] review was a well-conducted review, its findings should be interpreted with caution because of the high statistical heterogeneity and the quality of the included studies.

In Antoszewska-Smith review [13], the authors included a rather high number of studies in the meta-analysis, and they mentioned that the risk of bias was high in the included studies due to the lack of blinding. However, including non-randomized trials may reduce the quality of the evidence. Two reviews [2, 13] reported contradictory findings regarding the treatment duration, due to inclusion of five studies in Antoszewska-Smith review [13] versus one study in the Alharbi review [2] of different designs.

Failure Rate

Clinical Question 2: What Is the Failure/Success Rate of Miniscrews?

Evidence

Systematic Reviews and Meta-Analyses
Papageorgiou/2012 [14]
The authors included 52 studies in the meta-analysis. 4987 MIs were placed in 2281 orthodontic patients for anchorage reinforcement. The researchers found that the overall failure rate was 13.5% (95% CI: 11.5–15.8). Subgroup analysis for trials with more than 100 MIs, showed that the overall failure rate was 14%. The authors found that there is no association between failure rate and gender or age. However, the authors found that the jaw of insertion has a statistically significant impact on the success rate of MIs. The failure rate in the maxilla was 12%, while it was 19.3% in mandible (RR: 1.56; 95% CI: 1.13–2.15; $P = 0.007$, 17 trials). There was no difference between self-drilling and non-self-drilling MIs in the failure rate.

Alharbi/2018 [15]
This review included 46 studies; 16 RCTs, and 30 prospective cohort studies (PCS). The authors pooled 41 studies with 3250 MIs in meta-analysis. They found that the failure rate was 13.5% (95% CI: 11.5–15.9, $P = 0.001$, $I^2 = 57.1\%$). For the effect of the length of MIs on the failure rate, they found that the failure rate in MIs longer than 8 mm was 12.2% (95% CI: 6.7–21.4, $P < 0.001$, $I^2 = 67.2\%$) and this was slightly less than the failure rate in MIs shorter than 8 mm (12.7%, 95% CI: 10.5–15.4, $P < 0.001$, $I^2 = 44.9\%$). Also, in 11 included studies, they found that the failure rate was slightly higher in non-self-drilling MIs (14.9%, 95% CI: 10.4–20.8, $P < 0.001$, $I^2 = 88.9\%$) than the self-drilling MIs (14.2%, 95% CI: 5.6–31.8, $P < 0.001$, $I^2 = 71.41\%$). The authors assessed that most RCTs were having a high risk of bias, and most of PCS were having a moderate risk of bias.

Cunha/2017 [16]
This review included 27 studies; 5 RCTs, 8 prospective clinical studies, and 14 retrospective studies. The five RCTs were assessed as having an unclear risk of bias, 21 trials were having a moderate risk of bias, and one study was having a serious

risk of bias. The authors reported that the success rate of MIs was 85% (95% CI: 82–88) for 6–12 months of follow up and 88% (95% CI: 81–92) for more than 12 months. The success rate was 89% (95% CI: 86–92) for the maxilla and 82% (95% CI: 77–86) for the mandible. For the small and short MIs, the success rate was 71%, while it was 87.9% for the medium and small MIs. Also, the success rate was 81% and 88% for the cylindrical MIs in the mandible and maxilla, respectively. For the thread design, the success rate was 87% and 90% for the self-drilling and pre-drilling designs, respectively.

Systematic Reviews
Tsui/2012 [17]
This review included 54 studies investigating TSADs failure rate; 10 miniplates studies, 12 palatal implants (Orthosystem, Straumann), and onplants (Nobel Biocare) studies, 32 MIs studies, and 2 dental implants studies. The authors found that the success rate ranged from 91.4 to 100% for miniplates, 74–93.3% for palatal implants and 82.8% for onplants, 61–100% for miniscrews, and 100% for dental implants.

Kakali/2019 [18]
This review included 27 studies from different designs; 4 RCTs, 12 prospective studies, and 11 retrospective studies. The methodological qualities of the included studies were diverse as 13 studies had unclear risk of bias, 8 were at high risk of bias, and the rest of them were at low risk of bias. Seventeen studies assessed the failure rate using palatal implants (such as Orthosystem, Straumann), and nine studies assessed the palatal MIs failure rate. The failure rate in palatal implants ranged from 0 to 26%, with a median of 6% in a median follow-up period of 17.9 (2.0–35.6) months. However, the failure rate of palatal MIs ranged from 0 to 33%, with a median value of 6.1%, in a median of 6 months follow up (4–26 months). The success rate of MIs ranged from 61 to 100%. For dental implants, the number of cases was limited, with a success rate of 100%.

Mecenas/2020 [19]
This systematic review included six studies; one RCT and five non-randomized trials to investigate the differences between stainless steel and titanium miniscrews. The authors found that the evidence is high for the RCT and medium for the non-randomized trials, with a range of low risk of bias in the RCT to medium or high risk of bias in the non-RCT. The success rate ranged between 74.6 and 100% for stainless steel MIs and 80.9–100% for titanium MIs. Only one low-quality non-RCT reported that the success rate was significantly higher in titanium MIs than stainless steel MIs; 90% Vs. 50% for titanium and stainless steel MIs, respectively.

Evidence Summary
The best available evidence suggests that the overall failure rate of miniscrews was 13.5%, with a range of 0–40% in the included studies. The median failure rate for

palatal miniscrews was about 6.1% with a range of 0–33%. The failure rate of miniscrews was slightly higher in non-self-drilling MIs in one review [15] and without clear differences in another review [14], while it was higher in self-drilling in another review [16]. We may interpret that by different inclusion criteria and different included studies in design and methodology. The failure rate was slightly higher in short miniscrews and it can be influenced by the jaw of insertion. There was no association between the failure rate of MIs and gender or age. One review [19] reported that there is no significant difference between SS and titanium MIs regarding success rate. The failure rate of miniplates was less than 9%, and the failure rate of palatal implants was 6% [17].

Evidence Interpretation

In general, the success of miniscrews and miniplates is very good. The success of miniscrews is multifactorial. Higher success is reported for long MIs and lower jaw without any gender predisposition. There is controversy about superior success rate between self-drilling and non-self-drilling MIs.

Factors like cortical bone thickness, bone density, adjacent roots proximity, sinuses, amount of attached gingiva, oral hygiene, and amount of force applied may place a role in the success of MIs.

Viewpoint

Papageorgiou review [14] was a well-conducted review. The quality of the included studies should be considered during the interpretation of the findings. The authors included non-randomized studies in a meta-analysis which may reduce the quality of the evidence.

Alharbi review [15] was a well-conducted review, but including non-randomized trials may reduce the quality of the evidence. The high risk of bias was an issue in the primary studies. The authors reported that there was a publication bias in the included studies, and there was significant methodological and statistical heterogeneity between them.

Tsui review [17] has no information about the quality assessment of the primary studies. Also, there was no adherence to rigorous guidelines in conducting and reporting. In Kakali review [18] the authors reported that the risk of bias was unclear to high, in most of the included studies. Also, methodological heterogeneity may reduce the quality of the evidence. Another limitation of this review was the assessment of failure rate of MIs only for 6 months and not for the total orthodontic treatment duration.

In Mecenas review [19], the authors assessed the quality of the evidence based on the design of the included studies, while it should be based on the outcomes.

The differences between the aforementioned studies' findings may be due to many variables as follows; the number and the design of included studies, and the inclusion criteria. There were many uncontrolled factors like the operator's experience and patients' oral hygiene. Interestingly, two reviews [14, 15] reported a publication bias, meaning that unpublished studies may change the estimate of the effect, which may increase the failure rate of MIs.

Clinical Question 3: What Is the Success Rate of the Reinserted Miniscrews/Secondary Insertion?

Evidence

Cohort Study
Uesugi/2017 [20]

In this study, the researchers inserted 500 MIs in 240 orthodontic adults patients (61 males; 179 females, age; 28.1 ± 9.8 years). The diameters of these MIs were either 1.4 or 1.6 mm and lengths were 6.0 or 8.0 mm. If a miniscrew failed, the authors reinserted a new MI with the same or different size in the same location with a slight change (in the mesiodistal position, height, and insertion angle) or in another location. All miniscrews were inserted by flapless surgery with the self-drilling procedure. The researchers found that the success rate was 80.4% for the first inserted MIs (402 of 500 screws) and 44.2% for the reinserted 77 MIs.

Uesugi/2018 [21]

The authors recruited 238 patients with an age of 27.9 ± 8.4 years. They inserted 387 MIs in the maxillary buccal area between the second premolar and first molar and 84 MIs in the palatal area. Eighty-one buccal MIs failed, as they lacked stability, and the researchers reinserted new MIs from the same or different sizes in the same location or more distally after the failure by 1–2 months. Thirteen out of 84 MIs in the midpalatal suture failed, and they reinserted them in the midpalatal suture area again with a change in mesiodistal position. The primary insertion success rate was 79.1 and 84.5% for the buccal and palatal side, respectively. For the reinserted MIs, the success rate was 58.1% for the buccal MIs placed between the second premolar and first molar, 60.0% for the buccal MIs placed between the first and second molars, and 88.9% for the midpalatal MIs.

Evidence Summary

The best available evidence suggests that the reinsertion (secondary insertion) success rate was significantly lower than the primary insertion success rate. The overall secondary success rate was 44.2% [20]. The secondary success rate on the buccal side ranged from 58.1 to 60%, and the secondary insertion success rate in the midpalatal area was 88.9% [21].

Evidence Interpretation

There is a lack of high-quality evidence regarding the secondary success rate of MIs. However, the available evidence indicates a low success rate for the reinserted MIs. In other words, the reinsertion of new MIs in the same location or different location after a rest period of 1–2 months can be done but with a low success rate. Palatally reinserted MIs have more success than buccally reinserted MIs. This can be explained by the fact that repositioning in palatal area provides greater leeway to the orthodontist than between two roots on the buccal side.

The primary MIs failure should be considered a risk factor for MIs reinsertion, as it may be related to factors such as the cortical bone thickness, bone density, oral hygiene, tooth proximity, sinus, and attached gingiva.

Viewpoint

The two studies [20, 21] are of cohort study design which is more prone to selection bias and confounding factors. Though this is not high-quality evidence, those studies provide the clinician with good information. Further research from RCT design with a large sample size is needed to be more confident about the estimate.

Anatomical Sites for MIs

Clinical Question 4: What Is the Role of the Anatomical Sites in MIs Success Rate?

Evidence

Systematic Review and Meta-Analysis
Mohammed/2018 [22]

This systematic review included 63 studies; 28 studies were RCTs, 9 were prospective controlled clinical trials (CCT), and 26 were prospective cohort studies (PCS). Eight RCTs were at low risk of bias, 45 studies were at unclear risk of bias, and 10 were at high risk of bias. The overall failure rate of the palatal MIs was 4.7% (95% CI: 2.7–8.1). Three studies evaluated the failure rate of the midpalatal suture MIs and found that the failure rate was 1.3% (95% CI: 0.3–6). In the paramedian region, the failure rate was 4.8% (95% CI: 1.6–13.4, six trials), while the parapalatal MIs failure rate was 5.5% (95%CI: 2.8–10.7, 5 trials).

The overall failure rate of the buccal aspect for maxillary MIs was 9.6% (95% CI: 7.6–12.1). Thirty-seven studies investigated the failure rate of the interradicular MIs and reported that the failure rate was 9.2% (95% CI: 7.4–11.4) in the region between the first molar and the second premolar, 9.7% (95% CI: 5.1–17.6) in the region between lateral and canine, and 16.4% (95% CI: 4.9–42.5) in the zygomatic buttress area.

The overall failure rate in the mandible was 12.3% (95% CI: 7.3–20.1). Eight studies reported that the failure rate in the region between first molar and second premolar was 13.5% (95% CI: 7.3–23.6). The failure rate was 9.9% (95% CI: 4.9–19.1, three trials) in the region between first premolar and canine. Only one study reported the failure rate of the area between first and second molars by 25.9%.

In this systematic review, the authors also investigated the effect of different factors on the success rate of MIs. The risk ratio (RR) of MIs failure rate was higher on the right buccal side by 1.57(95%CI: 1.05–2.35, $P < 0.05$, 15 trials) than on the left side. The risk ratio of failure was higher in MIs perforating the sinus by 5.26 (95%CI: 1.48–18.75, $P < 0.05$, three trials) than in non-perforating MIs. The root contact increased the RR of failure by 8.71(95%CI:5.13–14.77, $P < 0.05$, eight trials).

Systematic Review
Winsauer/2014 [23]
In this review, the authors included 16 studies investigating the vertical palatal bone height (VBH) by using CBCT or CT scans. The VBH in the paramedian region varied between studies. Male patients showed higher values of VBH than females. The authors found that the region 3–4 mm behind the incisive foramen and 3–9 mm lateral to the midpalatal suture normally provides sufficient VBH to anchor molar distalizers. This area is located between the mesial of the first premolar to the distal of the second premolar which may provide a VBH of 5 mm or more.

Evidence Summary

The best available evidence suggests that the failure rate is lesser in the palatal region (4.7%) than the buccal region (9.6%) as the MIs in the buccal region are interradicular MIs and there is a difference in the bone density between the two regions. The higher success rate was reported in midpalatal region (98.7%) followed by the paramedian region (95.2%). As such, the best region in the palate is the area 3–4 mm behind the incisive foramen and 3–9 mm lateral to the midpalatal suture. In maxilla, the best buccal insertion site is between first molar and second premolar, then between lateral and canine, and the lowest success rate is in the zygomatic buttress area. In the mandible, the best insertion site was in the region between first premolar and canine then the region between first molar and second premolar. The highest failure rate was reported in one individual study between first and second molars by 25.9% [24].

There was a higher risk of failure in the maxillary right buccal side than the left side by 1.57 times, when the MIs perforate the sinus than non-perforating MIs by 5.26 times, and when the MIs contact the root by 8.71 times than non-contact MIs.

Evidence Interpretation

In the maxilla, the palatal side is a better insertion area than the buccal side, the closer to the midpalatal suture, the higher the success rate of MIs. From the buccal aspect, the first choice for MIs insertion is between the first molar and the second premolar, then between lateral and canine. Zygomatic buttress area has the least success rate. Perforating the maxillary sinus and the root proximity are risk factors for MIs failure.

In the mandible, the first choice for MIs insertion is between first premolar and canine, then between first molar and second premolar.

In general, the clinician should use the available tools to assess the interradicular space and its appropriateness for the MIs insertion, which may help in choosing the best place for MIs.

Viewpoint

Mohammed review [22] was a well-conducted review. However, most of the included studies were non-randomized studies which may suffer from an inherent risk of bias. Moreover, the inconsistency and the indirectness between studies may reduce the level of evidence.

In Winsauer's review [23], there was a lack of quality assessment of the included studies, which definitely reduces the quality of the evidence. The different radiographical methods may increase the clinical heterogeneity as well as it may limit the generalizability of the findings of this study.

Primary Stability of MIs

Clinical Question 5: What Are the Factors That Affect the Primary Stability of MIs?

Evidence

Systematic Review and Meta-Analysis
Marquezan/2014 [25]

This review included 12 studies of different designs; observational, ex vivo, and in vivo. Most of the included studies found a positive correlation between cortical thickness and primary stability. This correlation coefficient ranged from moderate to high (0.32–0.91). Three included studies used pull-out strength (PS) and found a significant moderate correlation between MIs primary stability and cortical thickness ($r = 0.409$, 95%CI: 0.25–0.54, $P < 0.001$, MIs: 134, 3 trials), while a weaker correlation was found in three human studies ($r = 0.338$, 95%CI: 0.08–0.56, $P = 0.01$, MIs: 269, 3 trials). The evidence was weak.

Systematic Review
Meursinge Reynders/2012 [26]

This systematic review included seven non-randomized cohort studies. One included study reported that a higher success rate was associated with torque values above 15 Ncm. In contrast, three included studies recommended torque values between 5 and 10 Ncm. However, the remaining three studies did not correlate the insertion torque with the stability of MIs. The evidence was low.

Meursinge Reynders/2013 [27]

This systematic review included 23 studies that investigated the insertion torque of MIs in the artificial bone. The range of the maximum insertion torque (MIT) was different between studies, from 3 to 81 Ncm. The correlation between MIT and MIs dimensions was positive, in other words, MIT increased when the length or the diameter of MIs increased. The MIT was higher in bone with a cortical thickness of 1 mm when compared with bone without cortex. The MIT decreased in the case of predrilled holes.

Cunha/2017 [16]

This review included 27 studies; 5 RCTs, 8 prospective clinical studies, and 14 retrospective studies. The MIT ranged from 7.05 Ncm in the maxilla for the cylindrical shape MIs to 13.28 Ncm in the mandible for tapered shape MIs. The MIT was 7.14

and 10.08 Ncm for the predrilling and self-drilling MIs in the maxilla, respectively. The removal torque was similar between tapered and cylindrical MIs in the mandible, while the cylindrical MIs showed a higher removal torque (10.01 Ncm) than tapered ones (7.35 Ncm) in the maxilla.

Evidence Summary

The best available evidence suggests that the primary stability of the MIs and the success rate are multifactorial. The most advocated value of insertion torque MIT ranged between 5 and 15 N cm. There were conflicting data in the literature regarding the correlation between the success rate and the insertion torque values. One review [26] recommended that the best MIT range is between 5 and 10 Ncm. In contrast, Cunha et al. [16] reported that the MIT ranged between 7 and 13.28 Ncm with differences related to the shape, the thread, and the jaw of insertion. Also, low-level evidence revealed that the correlation between cortical thickness and primary stability was positive but not crucial for making a definite conclusion on the pure correlation between primary stability and cortical thickness.

Evidence Interpretation

The bone density, the cortical bone thickness, as well as the insertion torque can play a role in the primary stability and the success rate of MIs. At present, there is a lack of conclusive evidence on this aspect of MIs.

Viewpoint

The evidence in Marquezan review [25], Reynders review [26], and Cunha review [16] was low due to the design limitation and the low quality of the included studies, as well as, the substantial heterogeneity between them. Reynders review [27] does not have applicability as they investigated the insertion torque in vitro and not clinically. Furthermore, the high risk of bias, the high heterogeneity between studies, and the methodological differences across studies led to a vague clinical answer.

Loading Protocols

Clinical Question 6: What Is the Best Loading Protocol for MIs?

Evidence

Systematic Review
Ohashi/2006 [28]

This systematic review investigated the loading time of MIs. Six included studies with a poor methodology evaluated the time of loading. Four studies applied a force range between 150 and 500 g immediately after MIs insertion, while two studies applied 100–400 g of force after 2 weeks of waiting period. The loading time either immediately or after 2 weeks of MIs insertion has no significant effect on the MIs success rate.

Clinical Trial
Motoyoshi/2007 [29]

This study aimed to determine the effect of the latent period on the success rate of MIs. The authors recruited 57 patients (30 adolescents and 27 adults) for the insertion of 169 MIs. The average latent period was 2.6 weeks in the early-load group of adolescents, 13.2 weeks in the late-load group of adolescents, and 2.2 weeks in the adult group. The authors found that the success rate was 63.8% in the early-load group (less than 1-month latent period) of adolescents, 97.2% in the late-load group (3-month latent period) of adolescents, and 91.9% in the adult group. The placement torque ranged from 7.6 to 9.2 Ncm, with the best success rate for placement torque of 5–10 Ncm in early-load group of adolescents and adults.

Evidence Summary

Low-level evidence suggests that there is no significant difference between immediate or delayed loading of MIs in adults, but delayed loading for approximately 3 months was significantly better in adolescents. The applied force ranged between 150 and 500 g without significant reported differences.

Evidence Interpretation

There is a lack of evidence regarding the best loading protocol or the ideal applied force. The acceptable force ranges between 150 and 500 g with immediate or delayed loading in adults. Also delayed loading >3 months is prefered in adolescents.

With the lack of conclusive evidence, the clinician's experience may play a role for deciding the latent period and the applied force.

Viewpoint

The included studies in Ohashi review [28] were low-quality studies with a high risk of bias. So, there is high uncertainty in this evidence. However, the lack of blinding and randomization may increase the selection bias and other biases in the outcomes of Motoyoshi study [29].

Miniscrews Design

Clinical Question 7: What Should Be the Ideal Design Features of Miniscrews?

Evidence

In Vitro Study
Brinley/2009 [30]

In this experimental study, the authors investigated the maximum placement torque and pull-out strength in different designs of 60 MIs using synthetic and cadaver bone. They compared 1 mm pitch with 0.75 and 1.25 mm pitch, and three longitudinal flutes with the same MIs without flutes. In synthetic bone, the placement torque was higher in 0.75 mm pitch than in others but not statistically significant, and the maximum pull-out force at failure was significantly higher in 0.75 mm pitch MIs than in others, with no significant difference between 1 and 1.25 mm pitch. In cadaver bone, there was no significant difference between the three pitch MIs regarding the placement torque or pull-out strength. However, the placement torque and pull-out strength were significantly greater ($P < 0.001$) for MIs with flutes than MIs without flutes.

Chang/2012 [31]

The study mechanically tested the effect of four types of MIs with different designs (the thread depth, degree of taper, and taper length) of MIs on the insertion torque, the pull-out strength, and stiffness. Finite element analysis showed that MIs with greater thread depths, smaller tapers, and shorter taper lengths generated higher maximum stresses on the bone with larger relative displacements. Pull-out resistance increased as the thread depth increased from 0.16 to 0.32 mm, but decreased when the thread depth exceeded 0.32 mm. Also, higher maximum bone stress is generated by the smaller taper degrees and shorter taper lengths.

Gracco/2012 [32]

This in vitro study investigated the effect of the variation in the thread design on the pull-out strength of MIs. The author tested 35 MIs in five groups; Buttress reverse (control), Buttress, 75° joint profile, Rounded, and Trapezoidal thread by using synthetic bone. The findings of this study reported that there was a statistically significant difference between the groups. The average pull-out tests ranged from 170.0 ± 10.3 N (buttress thread) to 192.8 ± 13.3 N (buttress reverse thread) and this was statistically significant. The mean difference was 22.8, 11.6, 4.4, and 8.1 N between the control thread and each one of buttress, 75° joint profile, rounded, and trapezoidal groups, respectively.

Evidence Summary

The best available evidence from in vitro studies suggests that the design of MIs plays a critical role in the mechanical characteristics of the MIs. The smaller pitch MIs (0.75 mm) has a higher pull-out force and a higher insertion torque than MIs with 1 and 1.25 mm pitch in the synthetic bone. MIs with flutes have higher placement torque and pull-out strength than MIs without flutes [30]. The greater the thread depth, the higher the pull-out resistance, and the less the taper degrees or length, the less the pull-out resistance [31]. The buttress reverse thread has a higher pull-out strength than other thread designs.

Evidence Interpretation

For the best mechanical characteristics, the best design should have 0.75 mm pitch with flutes, thread depth between 0.16 and 0.32 mm, smaller taper degrees and shorter taper lengths, and buttress reverse thread.

Viewpoint

These in vitro studies [30–32] do not fully represent the oral environment and the living bone, as well as the bone response to the MIs. Apart from the methodological issues, the differences in material properties, interface conditions, boundary conditions, and loading conditions lead to major differences between in vitro studies and living body studies. So, the available evidence answers only the mechanical characteristics of MIs without their biological interaction with living bone.

Miniscrews Versus Headgear

Clinical Question 8: Which Is Better for Anchorage Purposes, Headgear or Miniscrews?

Evidence

Systematic Review
Li/2011 [33]

This review included eight studies investigating the anchorage loss during anterior segment retraction; two trials with a low risk of bias, two trials with a medium risk of bias, and four trials with a high risk of bias. Three studies assessed miniscrews versus headgear and reported significantly greater retraction with miniscrews than with HG. Two studies revealed a less mesial molar movement in MIs group. There was contradictory data between studies regarding the incisors' inclination in MIs and HG. The treatment duration was significantly shorter in MIs groups.

Randomized Controlled Trial
Sandler/2014 [5]

The authors randomly assigned adolescents with a need for maximum anchorage into three groups; 25 patients in HG group, 26 patients in Nance group, and 27 patients in MIs group. The mean age of the patients was 14.22 years, with no significant difference between groups. The maxillary right molar anchorage loss was 1.36 ± 1.83 mm in HG group, 1.84 ± 1.32 mm in Nance group, and 0.80 ± 1.60 mm in MIs group. While, the maxillary left molar anchorage loss was 1.99 ± 2.09 in HG group, 2.09 ± 1.32 mm in Nance group, and 0.99 ± 1.15 mm in MIS group.

After adjusting the results for the sex and the comparator groups in HG, the anchorage loss was 0.62 mm (−4.68 to 3.52) and −0.58 (−1.53 to 0.36 mm) in Nance and MIs, respectively, for the maxillary right molar, while it was −0.09 (−1.00 to 0.83 mm) and −0.96 (−1.89 to −0.04 mm) in Nance and MIs, respectively, for the maxillary left molar.

Evidence Summary

The best available evidence suggests that miniscrews provide more retraction of incisors with less anchorage loss than HG and within shorter treatment duration. There was no crucial evidence about the favorable method regarding incisors' inclination during retraction. The molar anchorage loss was lesser in MIs group when compared with HG by 0.58 mm and 0.96 mm in the right and left molars. But this difference was minimal; and statistically insignificant on the right side.

Evidence Interpretation

Miniscrews are better than headgears in providing anchorage. MIs can be a choice if absolute or critical anchorage is required and there is a need for more incisor retraction. Headgears can be given if patient compliance is good and maximum anchorage is required.

Viewpoint

Li review [33] has some limitations which may reduce the quality of this evidence. The search was limited by terms without using Medical Subject Headings (MeSH) terms that may miss some search results. The clinical and statistical heterogeneity are important points in this review. The included studies were having a high risk of bias. Finally, the authors reported a limitation related to measurement differences between studies that may increase the bias across studies.

Sandler et al. RCT [5] was a well-conducted study that provides us with useful information. The results should be interpreted with caution as five patients were lost to follow up in MIs group and two patients in HG group, while the authors used per protocol analysis which is less optimal than the intention to treat analysis. The females were more than males in this trial but the authors adjusted the results according to the sex.

Intrusion and TSADs

Clinical Question 9: How Much Maxillary Incisors' Intrusion Can Be Done? Which Is a Better Modality- Conventional or MIs?

Evidence

Systematic Reviews and Meta-Analyses
Sosly/2020 [3]

This systematic review included seven RCTs in the qualitative analysis and the meta-analysis. They compared the effectiveness of MIs and intrusion archwires in the intrusion of the upper incisors. The intrusion using MIs has a statistically significant higher reduction of the deep bite when compared with the intrusion archwires (MD; -1.5, $P = 0.025$, 5 trials). There was a statistically significant difference between MIs group and the intrusion arch group regarding the true incisor intrusion (SMD; -0.95, 95%CI: -1.41 to -0.49, $P<0.001$, five trials) favoring the MIs group. There was no statistically significant difference in root resorption between the MIs group and the intrusion arch group by using the two-dimensional radiographs. Six studies concluded that the molar extrusion was statistically higher in the intrusion arch group than in the MIs group (SMD; -0.86, 95% CI: -1.46 to -0.27, $P < 0.001$). In this respect, one RCT [34] used J-hook headgear (J-HG) in one group and reported that there was no statistically significant difference between J-HG group and MIs group regarding molar extrusion during incisors intrusion. However, the quality of the evidence was very low to low.

Atalla/2020 [35]

This review compared the effectiveness of upper incisors' intrusion using TSADs versus using conventional segmented arch (CSA). The authors included six studies; two were RCTs, and four were CCTs. Three pooled studies in a meta-analysis found that the mean difference between TSADs and CSA in the incisors' intrusion amount was statistically significant (MD; 0.78 mm, 95% CI: 0.28–1.29, $P = 0.002$, 3 trials), favoring the TSADs group. In regards to the inclination of the incisors, there was no statistically significant difference between the two groups (MD; $4.72°$, 95% CI: -1.09 to 10.53, $P = 0.11$, 4 studies). There was no statistically significant difference between the two groups in terms of the treatment duration (MD; -0.27; 95% CI: -0.78 to 0.23, $P = 0.29$, 3 trials). The molar tipping was statistically higher in the CSA group (MD; $-1.03°$; 95% CI: -1.79 to -0.27, $P = 0.008$).

Evidence Summary

Looking into the evidence collectively, the available evidence suggests that the MIs are more effective than intrusion archwires in intruding the upper incisors; the mean difference ranged between 0.78 and 1.5 mm in two reviews due to the differences in the inclusion criteria and the search strategy [3, 35]. There was no statistically significant difference between the two groups in regard to root resorption, the inclination of the incisors, and the treatment duration. The reactionary molar extrusion was statistically higher in the archwire group, as well as, the molar tipping by $1.03°$.

Evidence Interpretation

Miniscrews are more effective than conventional techniques for incisors' intrusion. Greater amount of incisors' intrusion by 0.78–1.5 mm can be achieved using MIs, with no reactionary effects on the molars as the MIs are the anchorage units. Root resorption usually occurs in both MIs and archwire techniques, with a trivial difference between the two treatment modalities in terms of treatment duration and inclination of the incisors.

Viewpoint

Sosly review [3] was a well-conducted review that included only RCTs, but all of the included RCTs were at high risk of bias; there was a lack of randomization with a bias in the reported results. The aforementioned limitations may reduce the level of confidence in the evidence.

In Atalla review [35], the reader should bear in mind the limitations of this study; the risk of bias in the included studies ranged from serious to moderate in CCTs and was high in RCTs. The clinical and methodological heterogeneity represents the dissimilarity between included studies regarding the clinical procedures and the treatment modality as well as the methodology of the studies. There was high heterogeneity in some forest plots, so the interpretation of the results should be taken with caution.

Clinical Question 10: How Much Molars Intrusion Can Be Done Using TSADs?

Evidence

Systematic Review
Alsafadi/2016 [36]
In this review, the researchers included 12 studies to investigate the effectiveness of TSADs in the upper molars' intrusion in patients with an anterior open bite. Five included studies used miniplates, and seven studies used miniscrews. The authors found that the mean amount of the mandible autorotation was 2° in six studies, with a range of 1.1° to 3.9° in the included studies. Most included studies reported molar intrusion by 1.6–3.6 mm, but only one included study [37] reported upper molar extrusion by 1 mm where the TSADs were placed in the lower jaw with lower molar intrusion by 1.8 mm. The authors considered the evidence as low due to the inherent risk of bias in the included studies. One study [37] reported a relapse of 27% of the intruded first molar, while another study [38] reported a relapse of 10.36%.

Prospective Clinical Study
Marzouk/2016 [39]
The authors recruited 28 patients with an anterior open bite in this study. The mean age of patients was 22 years 5 months, and the mean open bite was −4.75 ± 2.27 mm. The researchers used miniplates to intrude the upper two molars and premolars by force of 450 g per side. The duration of intrusion was 7.5 ± 2.3 months. They found that there was a mobility of miniplates in three patients. The magnitude of molar intrusion was 3.04 ± 0.79 mm, and the increase in the overbite was 6.93 ± 1.99 mm, with long-term stability for 4 years without statistically significant relapse (13.37% of the intrusion).

Evidence Summary
The best available evidence suggests that TSADs are effective in molars' intrusion with a mean of 3 mm, which closes the anterior bite by 7 mm. The average duration for intrusion was 7.5 ± 2.3 months. The mean amount of mandibular autorotation was 2° which contributed to closing the bite and reducing the overjet. One trial [39] followed the treated patients for 4 years and reported that the relapse was not significant and was 13.37% of the intrusion magnitude.

Evidence Interpretation

Miniscrews and miniplates can intrude the posterior teeth by 3 mm, with treatment duration ranging from 5 to 10 months. Intrusion of molars, especially the maxillary molars can lead to autorotation of the mandible and subsequently increase the overbite. This treatment is beneficial in openbite Class II cases as both the bite and skeletal relationship are corrected at the same time. So, these mechanics should be avoided in Class III or some Class I malocclusions where the sagittal skeletal relationship change might not be favorable and may increase the need for further mechanotherapy. There is some relapse after the molar intrusion, so overcorrection should be implemented whenever possible.

Viewpoint

Alsafadi review [36] reported that the design and the methodology of the included trials had drawbacks. Also, the heterogeneity in the included studies and the different types of TSADs represent clinical heterogeneity. As such, meta-analysis was not possible.

Marzouk study [39] was an ambitious study. The design was a cohort study, so the lack of blinding was a limitation in this design. Two patients (2/28) were lost to follow up and this represents 7% of the recruited patients. Although the study still has enough power by 80%, it would be better to analyze all the data, as the missing data are part of the results. The mobility of miniplates in three patients represents the failure rate and should be taken into account during the interpretation of the study.

Soft Tissue and MIs

Clinical Question 11: What Is the Effect of MIs on the Facial Soft Tissues in Premolars Extraction Cases?

Evidence

Systematic Review
Liu/2019 [40]

This review included five studies; two RCTs, and three CCTs, comparing the soft tissue changes after four premolars extraction and anterior retraction, between MIs and conventional anchorage devices (CADs). The change in the nasolabial angle was statistically greater in the MIs group than in the conventional group (SMD; 0.68, 95% CI: 0.39–0.97, $P < 0.0001$, five trials). The facial convexity angle decreased more in MIs when compared with the conventional group (SMD; 0.34, 95% CI: −0.07 to 0.76, $P = 0.1$, 3 trials) without a statistically significant difference. In four included studies, the change in labial superioris (Ls) to E line was significantly higher in MIs group (SMD; 0.51, 95% CI: 0.18–0.84, $P = 0.0025$). The differences between groups were not statistically significant regarding labial inferior is (Li) to E line (SMD; −0.28, 95% CI: 1.72 to −2.28, $P = 0.78$).

Evidence Summary

The best available evidence suggests that MIs have a statistically greater changes than conventional anchorage in nasolabial angle, and in the upper lip expressed by linear measures from Ls to E line. The difference between MIs and CADs was insignificant in terms of the facial convexity angle and Li to E line.

Evidence Interpretation

Greater soft tissue changes are produced when MIs are used for anchorage purpose compared to conventional anchorage. Most of these differences were apparent in the greater divergence of the nasolabial angle and more upper lip retraction.

Viewpoint

In Liu review [40], the RCTs were at moderate risk of bias, and the non-RCTs were at low risk of bias. As such, the methodological heterogeneity and the inherent risk of bias in the included studies may reduce the quality of the evidence.

Iatrogenic Effects and TSADs

Root Proximity and MIs

Clinical Question 12: What Is the Rate of MIs Contact With Roots, and Does This Affect the Success Rate?

Evidence

Clinical Trial
Motoyoshi/2016 [41]

In this trial, the authors recruited 110 patients; 31 males and 79 females with an average age of 21.3 ± 6.9 years. They inserted 202 miniscrews in the buccal alveolar bone of the maxilla. The MIs were self-drilling with a length of 8 mm and a diameter of 1.6 mm. The researchers tested the placement torque using a digital torque tester. The damping capacity was measured by Periotest device, and the root proximity was judged from CBCT images. The authors found that the rate of root contact with MIs was 18.3%, without significant differences between right and left sides or between males and females. The success rate was significantly higher in the non-contact group (98.9%) when compared with the contact group (81.1%). There was a statistically significant difference ($P < 0.05$) in the placement torque between contact and non-contact groups, with a higher value for the contact group (8.9 ± 3.3) than the non-contact group (7.5 ± 3.3). Also, the Periotest value (PTV)was statistically higher in the contact group (6.0 ± 4.3) than in the non-contact group (3.3 ± 3.5) ($P < 0.01$).

Evidence Summary

The best available evidence suggests that the root contact rate is 18.3%, with less success rate when MIs contact the root. The placement torque and the damping capacity can indicate the MIs root contact. The placement torque was statistically higher in the contact group (8.9 ± 3.3 and 7.5 ± 3.3 for the contact group and non-contact MIs group, respectively). Also, PTV was statistically higher in the contact group (6.0 ± 4.3 and 3.3 ± 3.5 for the contact and non-contact MIs group, respectively).

Evidence Interpretation

Root contact is a risk factor for MIs success. If there is root contact during the insertion of miniscrew the clinician would feel an increase in the insertion torque and in the damping capacity of MIs. Both two- and three-dimensional radiographs may be considered if the clinician suspects root contact after the insertion of MIs. The clinical experience and the use of intraoral radiographs can play a critical role in avoiding root contacts during MIs placement.

Viewpoint

In this clinical study [41] the external validity of the findings is poor because of many points; this study was done in a university hospital setting, the placement of MIs was between the second premolar and the first molar, the expertise of the clinician who inserted the MIs, and the characteristics of the ethnic group. Likewise, the lack of randomization, blinding, and sample size calculation may increase the risk of bias, and the findings of this study should be interpreted with caution.

Clinical Question 13: Is There Any Root Repair After MIs Contact?

Evidence

Prospective Clinical Trial
Ahmed/2012 [42]

In this study, the researchers recruited 17 patients (8 male, 9 females; mean age, 16.2 years; range, 13.5–21.6 years) undergoing orthodontic treatment and requiring a premolars extraction. They intentionally inserted a miniscrew in the root of 68 premolars under X-ray vision, and removed the MIs after establishing contact with the root. The authors extracted the premolars after three different observation periods; 17 teeth after 4 weeks, 17 teeth after 8 weeks, and 14 teeth 12 weeks. The damaged surfaces were then scrutinized under a stereomicroscope. The stereomicroscopic examinations confirmed root injuries and healing in all the groups. 50% of the patients showed repair greater than 50% by weeks 4 and 8. In 48 teeth examined histologically, the dentine in all specimens was damaged without root resorption or pulp damage. The periodontal ligament thickness increased in week 8 compared with week 4 and decreased by week 12. The repair of cementum was 59.6% and

73.1% by the end of week 4 and the end of week 12, respectively. The histological repair was 57.31% ± 20.22, 71.15% ± 14.09, and 73.12% ± 11.71 in weeks 4, 8, and 12, respectively. Furthermore, the histological repair between weeks 4 and 8 has a statistically significant difference (MD; 13.85, 95%CI: 0.21–27.48, P = 0.046). In contrast, there was no statistically significant difference between week 8 and week 12 (MD; 1.97, 95%CI: 12.38–16.31, P = 1).

Evidence Summary

The best available evidence suggests that more than 50% of root injuries after MIs contact may heal by weeks 4 and 8, with more healing in week 12. The repair of cementum was 59.6% by week 4 and 73.1% by week 12. The periodontal ligament thickness increased gradually from week 4 to week 8 and decreased by week 12.

Evidence Interpretation

The root-MIs contact is a potential risk during MIs insertion. The healing process of the roots starts after removing the MIs. More than 50% of root healing can be observed by the first 8 weeks after injury, and more than 70% of root repair occurs by the end of week 12. So, if the clinician has a root-MIs contact, he should remove the MIs and give a rest period of 12 weeks for the repair to occur. Also, the reinsertion of the MIs should be avoided at the same place and location.

Viewpoint

Ahmed study [42] was a well-conducted study. This study has a limited validity as most of the patients are adolescents with an age range from 13.5 to 21.6 years. As such, the present evidence cannot be applied to older patients with the same confidence. The sample size was small, and the healing observation period was short. The confidence interval was inconsistent with the p value regarding the healing difference between week 8 and week 12. So, a larger study with a longer observation period is recommended to have more confidence in the estimate of the injury healing.

Clinical Question 14: What Is the Incidence of Maxillary Sinus Penetration by Infrazygomatic Crest MIs?

Evidence

Retrospective Study
Jia/2018 [43]

In this study, the authors collected the data of 60 MIs which were inserted in the infrazygomatic crest in 32 patients (mean age 28 ± 6 years). The length of the MIs was 14 mm, and the diameter was 2 mm. The MIs were inserted after examining CBCT scans with an insertion angle of 29.6°. A force of 400–500 g was applied to MIs after 1 month of insertion. The researchers found that 47 out of 60 (78.3%) MIs penetrated the maxillary sinus without clinical symptoms. Two penetrated MIs failed, leading to a success rate of 95.7% for penetrated MIs compared with non-penetrated

MIs (100%) without a significant difference. The mean depth of penetration was 2.6 mm in 22 MIs. After penetration, the sinus membrane thickness increased statistically by 0.6 mm ($P = 0.001$) with a statistically significant decrease of the buccal (above the MIs) and palatal (below the MIs) bone by 0.1 and 0.4 mm, respectively ($P = 0.019$; $P = 0.002$). The incidence of membrane thickening was statistically higher with more than 1 mm penetration (88.2%) when compared with less than 1 mm penetration (37.5%) ($P = 0.017$). Also, the thickening of the sinus membrane was statistically greater by 0.8 mm with more than 1 mm penetration ($P = 0.03$).

Evidence Summary

Looking into the evidence, there is low evidence suggesting that the incidence of sinus penetration by infrazygomatic crest MIs is very high (47/60; 78.3%) with a small impact on the MIs success rate. The average depth of the penetration was 2.6 mm. The thickness of the sinus membrane statistically increased by 0.6 mm after penetration with associated bone resorption from buccal and palatal aspects. The higher incidence of membrane thickening (88.2%) was correlated with penetration of more than 1 mm when compared with penetration of less than 1 mm (37.5%) ($P = 0.017$).

Evidence Interpretation

In infrazygomatic crest MIs, the incidence of sinus penetration is 78.3%. Sinus penetration is not related to MIs success, and the common outcomes are increased sinus membrane thickening and decreased buccal and palatal bone thickening. The sinus penetration may be problematic for patients and may result in chronic sinusitis.

Viewpoint

It was a good study that addressed a relevant clinical question [43]. As it was a retrospective study, that means it is more prone to selection bias, and only the successful MIs will be followed up for a longer period with a CBCT observation. So, the failed cases would be removed if the final CBCT did not exist. Also, the sinus configuration may vary according to ethnicity and jaw geometry. As such, the generalizability is limited to Chinese ethnicity. Furthermore, this was low-quality evidence and further research with a better design and a larger sample size is required to be certain about this iatrogenic effect.

Authors' Recommendations

- Temporary skeletal anchorage devices are effective means of providing anchorage, and are more efficient than conventional anchorage appliances. Depending upon biomechanics, TSADs can provide absolute anchorage or may be associated with minimal anchorage loss. In some clinical situations, TSADs can even provide some space gain while also acting as an anchorage appliance.
- TSADs provide greater incisor retraction, less molar tipping, greater soft tissue effects, decreased number of visits and treatment duration than conventional anchorage.

- TSADs success rate is 86.5%. Buccal MIs are more effective than palatal MIs in providing anchorage, but palatal MIs have a greater success rate. The ideal site for buccal MIs placement is between the second premolar and the first molar in both jaws or between the first premolar and canine in the mandible. In the palate, the area 3–4 mm behind the incisive foramen and 3–9 mm lateral to the midpalatal suture is the best area for MIs placement. MIs placed in the zygomatic buttress area and distal to upper molars have increased failure rate. Also, infrazygomatic MIs are associated with sinus perforation though it does not affect its success rate.

- If a MI shows a lack of stability, it should be removed, and a new MI should be placed at a different location, or the anchorage requirement and the biomechanics should be reevaluated. Reinserting the MIs in the same location, even with a change of position and a pause period of 1–2 months, can result in an increased failure rate.

- The primary stability of MIs depends upon bone density, cortical bone thickness, and insertion torque. Most loading of the MIs is done immediately, especially in adult patients. The loading force usually ranges from 150 to 500 g.

- MIs are more effective than conventional mechanics for incisor and molar intrusion with no associated reactionary forces on anchoring/neighboring teeth. The best design of MIs is a small pitch with flutes. Ideally, root contact should be avoided. But if there is root contact, MIs should be removed immediately, and a pause period of up to 12 weeks should be given for cementum repair.

References

1. Kanomi R. Mini-implant for orthodontic anchorage. J Clin Orthod. 1997;31(11):763–7.
2. Alharbi F, Almuzian M, Bearn D. Anchorage effectiveness of orthodontic miniscrews compared to headgear and transpalatal arches: a systematic review and meta-analysis. Acta Odontol Scand. 2019;77(2):88–98. https://doi.org/10.1080/00016357.2018.1508742.
3. Sosly R, Mohammed H, Rizk MZ, Jamous E, Qaisi AG, Bearn DR. Effectiveness of miniscrew-supported maxillary incisor intrusion in deep-bite correction: a systematic review and meta-analysis. Angle Orthod. 2020;90(2):291–304. https://doi.org/10.2319/061119-400.1.
4. Rodriguez de Guzman-Barrera J, Saez Martinez C, Boronat-Catala M, Montiel-Company JM, Paredes-Gallardo V, Gandia-Franco JL, et al. Effectiveness of interceptive treatment of class III malocclusions with skeletal anchorage: a systematic review and meta-analysis. PLoS One. 2017;12(3):e0173875. https://doi.org/10.1371/journal.pone.0173875.
5. Sandler J, Murray A, Thiruvenkatachari B, Gutierrez R, Speight P, O'Brien K. Effectiveness of 3 methods of anchorage reinforcement for maximum anchorage in adolescents: a 3-arm multicenter randomized clinical trial. Am J Orthod Dentofac Orthop. 2014;146(1):10–20. https://doi.org/10.1016/j.ajodo.2014.03.020.
6. Upadhyay M, Yadav S, Nagaraj K, Patil S. Treatment effects of mini-implants for en-masse retraction of anterior teeth in bialveolar dental protrusion patients: a randomized controlled trial. Am J Orthod Dentofac Orthop. 2008;134(1):18–29.e1. https://doi.org/10.1016/j.ajodo.2007.03.025.
7. Sharma M, Sharma V, Khanna B. Mini-screw implant or transpalatal arch-mediated anchorage reinforcement during canine retraction: a randomized clinical trial. J Orthod. 2012;39(2):102–10. https://doi.org/10.1179/14653121226878.

8. Basha AG, Shantaraj R, Mogegowda SB. Comparative study between conventional en-masse retraction (sliding mechanics) and en-masse retraction using orthodontic micro implant. Implant Dent. 2010;19(2):128–36. https://doi.org/10.1097/ID.0b013e3181cc4aa5.

9. Al-Sibaie S, Hajeer MY. Assessment of changes following en-masse retraction with mini-implants anchorage compared to two-step retraction with conventional anchorage in patients with class II division 1 malocclusion: a randomized controlled trial. Eur J Orthod. 2014;36(3):275–83. https://doi.org/10.1093/ejo/cjt046.

10. Liu YH, Ding WH, Liu J, Li Q. Comparison of the differences in cephalometric parameters after active orthodontic treatment applying mini-screw implants or transpalatal arches in adult patients with bialveolar dental protrusion. J Oral Rehabil. 2009;36(9):687–95. https://doi.org/10.1111/j.1365-2842.2009.01976.x.

11. Ganzer N, Feldmann I, Bondemark L. Anchorage reinforcement with miniscrews and molar blocks in adolescents: a randomized controlled trial. Am J Orthod Dentofac Orthop. 2018;154(6):758–67. https://doi.org/10.1016/j.ajodo.2018.07.011.

12. Papadopoulos MA, Papageorgiou SN, Zogakis IP. Clinical effectiveness of orthodontic miniscrew implants: a meta-analysis. J Dent Res. 2011;90(8):969–76. https://doi.org/10.1177/0022034511409236.

13. Antoszewska-Smith J, Sarul M, Lyczek J, Konopka T, Kawala B. Effectiveness of orthodontic miniscrew implants in anchorage reinforcement during en-masse retraction: a systematic review and meta-analysis. Am J Orthod Dentofac Orthop. 2017;151(3):440–55. https://doi.org/10.1016/j.ajodo.2016.08.029.

14. Papageorgiou SN, Zogakis IP, Papadopoulos MA. Failure rates and associated risk factors of orthodontic miniscrew implants: a meta-analysis. Am J Orthod Dentofac Orthop. 2012;142(5):577–595 e7. https://doi.org/10.1016/j.ajodo.2012.05.016.

15. Alharbi F, Almuzian M, Bearn D. Miniscrews failure rate in orthodontics: systematic review and meta-analysis. Eur J Orthod. 2018;40(5):519–30. https://doi.org/10.1093/ejo/cjx093.

16. Cunha AC, da Veiga AMA, Masterson D, Mattos CT, Nojima LI, Nojima MCG, et al. How do geometry-related parameters influence the clinical performance of orthodontic mini-implants? A systematic review and meta-analysis. Int J Oral Maxillofac Surg. 2017;46(12):1539–51. https://doi.org/10.1016/j.ijom.2017.06.010.

17. Tsui WK, Chua HD, Cheung LK. Bone anchor systems for orthodontic application: a systematic review. Int J Oral Maxillofac Surg. 2012;41(11):1427–38. https://doi.org/10.1016/j.ijom.2012.05.011.

18. Kakali L, Alharbi M, Pandis N, Gkantidis N, Kloukos D. Success of palatal implants or mini-screws placed median or paramedian for the reinforcement of anchorage during orthodontic treatment: a systematic review. Eur J Orthod. 2019;41(1):9–20. https://doi.org/10.1093/ejo/cjy015.

19. Mecenas P, Espinosa DG, Cardoso PC, Normando D. Stainless steel or titanium mini-implants? A systematic review. Angle Orthod. 2020;90(4):587–97. https://doi.org/10.2319/081619-536.1.

20. Uesugi S, Kokai S, Kanno Z, Ono T. Prognosis of primary and secondary insertions of orthodontic miniscrews: what we have learned from 500 implants. Am J Orthod Dentofac Orthop. 2017;152(2):224–31. https://doi.org/10.1016/j.ajodo.2016.12.021.

21. Uesugi S, Kokai S, Kanno Z, Ono T. Stability of secondarily inserted orthodontic miniscrews after failure of the primary insertion for maxillary anchorage: maxillary buccal area vs midpalatal suture area. Am J Orthod Dentofac Orthop. 2018;153(1):54–60. https://doi.org/10.1016/j.ajodo.2017.05.024.

22. Mohammed H, Wafaie K, Rizk MZ, Almuzian M, Sosly R, Bearn DR. Role of anatomical sites and correlated risk factors on the survival of orthodontic miniscrew implants: a systematic review and meta-analysis. Prog Orthod. 2018;19(1):36. https://doi.org/10.1186/s40510-018-0225-1.

23. Winsauer H, Vlachojannis C, Bumann A, Vlachojannis J, Chrubasik S. Paramedian vertical palatal bone height for mini-implant insertion: a systematic review. Eur J Orthod. 2014;36(5):541–9. https://doi.org/10.1093/ejo/cjs068.

24. Sarul M, Minch L, Park HS, Antoszewska-Smith J. Effect of the length of orthodontic mini-screw implants on their long-term stability: a prospective study. Angle Orthod. 2015;85(1):33–8. https://doi.org/10.2319/112113-857.1.
25. Marquezan M, Mattos CT, Sant'Anna EF, de Souza MM, Maia LC. Does cortical thickness influence the primary stability of miniscrews?: a systematic review and meta-analysis. Angle Orthod. 2014;84(6):1093–103. https://doi.org/10.2319/093013-716.1.
26. Meursinge Reynders RA, Ronchi L, Ladu L, van Etten-Jamaludin F, Bipat S. Insertion torque and success of orthodontic mini-implants: a systematic review. Am J Orthod Dentofac Orthop. 2012;142(5):596–614.e5. https://doi.org/10.1016/j.ajodo.2012.06.013.
27. Meursinge Reynders R, Ronchi L, Ladu L, Van Etten-Jamaludin F, Bipat S. Insertion torque and orthodontic mini-implants: a systematic review of the artificial bone literature. Proc Inst Mech Eng H. 2013;227(11):1181–202. https://doi.org/10.1177/0954411913495986.
28. Ohashi E, Pecho OE, Moron M, Lagravere MO. Implant vs screw loading protocols in orthodontics: a systematic review. Angle Orthod. 2006;76(4):721–7.
29. Motoyoshi M, Matsuoka M, Shimizu N. Application of orthodontic mini-implants in adolescents. Int J Oral Maxillofac Surg. 2007;36(8):695–9. https://doi.org/10.1016/j.ijom.2007.03.009.
30. Brinley CL, Behrents R, Kim KB, Condoor S, Kyung HM, Buschang PH. Pitch and longitudinal fluting effects on the primary stability of miniscrew implants. Angle Orthod. 2009;79(6):1156–61. https://doi.org/10.2319/103108-554r.1.
31. Chang JZ, Chen YJ, Tung YY, Chiang YY, Lai EH, Chen WP, et al. Effects of thread depth, taper shape, and taper length on the mechanical properties of mini-implants. Am J Orthod Dentofac Orthop. 2012;141(3):279–88. https://doi.org/10.1016/j.ajodo.2011.09.008.
32. Gracco A, Giagnorio C, Incerti Parenti S, Alessandri Bonetti G, Siciliani G. Effects of thread shape on the pullout strength of miniscrews. Am J Orthod Dentofac Orthop. 2012;142(2):186–90. https://doi.org/10.1016/j.ajodo.2012.03.023.
33. Li F, Hu HK, Chen JW, Liu ZP, Li GF, He SS, et al. Comparison of anchorage capacity between implant and headgear during anterior segment retraction. Angle Orthod. 2011;81(5):915–22. https://doi.org/10.2319/101410-603.1.
34. Jain RK, Kumar SP, Manjula WS. Comparison of intrusion effects on maxillary incisors among mini implant anchorage, j-hook headgear and utility arch. J Clin Diagn Res. 2014;8(7):ZC21–4. https://doi.org/10.7860/JCDR/2014/8339.4554.
35. Atalla AI, AboulFotouh MH, Fahim FH, Foda MY. Effectiveness of orthodontic mini-screw implants in adult deep bite patients during incisor intrusion: a systematic review. Contemp Clin Dent. 2019;10(2):372–81. https://doi.org/10.4103/ccd.ccd_618_18.
36. Alsafadi AS, Alabdullah MM, Saltaji H, Abdo A, Youssef M. Effect of molar intrusion with temporary anchorage devices in patients with anterior open bite: a systematic review. Prog Orthod. 2016;17:9. https://doi.org/10.1186/s40510-016-0122-4.
37. Sugawara J, Baik UB, Umemori M, Takahashi I, Nagasaka H, Kawamura H, et al. Treatment and posttreatment dentoalveolar changes following intrusion of mandibular molars with application of a skeletal anchorage system (SAS) for open bite correction. Int J Adult Orthodon Orthognath Surg. 2002;17(4):243–53.
38. Han-ah L, Dds M, Young-chel P, Dds M, et al. Treatment and posttreatment changes following intrusion of maxillary posterior teeth with miniscrew implants for open bite correction. Korean J Orthod. 2008;38(1):31–40. https://doi.org/10.4041/kjod.2008.38.1.31.
39. Marzouk ES, Kassem HE. Evaluation of long-term stability of skeletal anterior open bite correction in adults treated with maxillary posterior segment intrusion using zygomatic miniplates. Am J Orthod Dentofac Orthop. 2016;150(1):78–88. https://doi.org/10.1016/j.ajodo.2015.12.014.
40. Liu Y, Yang ZJ, Zhou J, Xiong P, Wang Q, Yang Y, et al. Soft tissue changes in patients with dentoalveolar protrusion treated with maximum anchorage: a systematic review and meta-analysis. J Evid Based Dent Pract. 2019;19(4):101310. https://doi.org/10.1016/j.jebdp.2019.01.006.

41. Motoyoshi M, Uchida Y, Inaba M, Ejima K, Honda K, Shimizu N. Are assessments of damping capacity and placement torque useful in estimating root proximity of orthodontic anchor screws? Am J Orthod Dentofac Orthop. 2016;150(1):124–9. https://doi.org/10.1016/j.ajodo.2015.12.018.
42. Ahmed VK, Rooban T, Krishnaswamy NR, Mani K, Kalladka G. Root damage and repair in patients with temporary skeletal anchorage devices. Am J Orthod Dentofac Orthop. 2012;141(5):547–55. https://doi.org/10.1016/j.ajodo.2011.11.014.
43. Jia X, Chen X, Huang X. Influence of orthodontic mini-implant penetration of the maxillary sinus in the infrazygomatic crest region. Am J Orthod Dentofac Orthop. 2018;153(5):656–61. https://doi.org/10.1016/j.ajodo.2017.08.021.

Impacted Maxillary Canines

7

Contents

© The Author(s), under exclusive license to Springer Nature Switzerland AG 2023   171
S. Mheissen, H. Khan, *Orthodontic Evidence*,
https://doi.org/10.1007/978-3-031-24422-3_7

Abbreviations

CG   Control group
CRT   Conventional radiographic techniques
DCE   Deciduous canine extraction
EMC   Ectopic maxillary canines
HP   Horizontal parallax
OIIRR   Orthodontic-induced inflammatory root resorption
OPG   Orthopantomograph
PDC   Palatally displaced canine
SIRR   Severe incisor root resorption
SLOB   Same lingual opposite buccal
VP   The vertical parallax

Introduction

Maxillary canines are considered as the cornerstone of the mouth and are part of anterior dentition, which is known as the "Esthetic Zone." Maxillary canines are frequently impacted, with a prevalence of 1.7–2% [1, 2] in the general population, and up to 5% in orthodontic patients [3]. There is more predisposition of impaction in females, unilateral and in Class II division 2 malocclusion, with palatal impacted canines being more prevalent than buccal impacted canines [4, 5]. The etiology of maxillary impaction is multifactorial, with both genetic and environmental factors involved. The etiology of buccally impacted canines is mostly considered environmental, and for palatally impacted canines, it is thought to be genetic [6]. Two theories have been proposed for the etiology of palatally impacted canines; the guidance theory [7] and genetic theory [8].

Maxillary canines are palpable from the buccal aspect by 8–9 years of age. If the canines are not palpable after 10–11 years of age, clinical and radiographic investigations are undertaken to rule out any palatal displacement of the canines. Maxillary canine eruption is considered delayed if they do not erupt by 12.3 years in girls and 13.1 years in boys [9]. If the canine does not erupt by 13 years of age, its root apex is fused, or the patient has reached CVM stage 5, the canines are considered impacted [10].

Clinical examination of palatally displaced or impacted canines include visual inspection for the canine bulge, presence of retained deciduous teeth or lack of space, mobility of deciduous canines and marked change in angulation or direction of lateral incisors. In addition to that, impacted or displaced canines are many times associated with peg-shaped lateral incisors or other anomalies such as transpositions. After visual inspection, palpation of the buccal and palatal surfaces should be done. If the canine presence or position is not diagnosed through clinical examination a radiographic examination should be undertaken.

Radiographic evaluation to localize the presence and the buccolingual position of the canine includes using a single X-ray and measuring the canine to canine index or canine to incisor index [11]. In plain radiographs, mostly two radiographs taken at different angles are used to locate the position of the canine in so-called parallax techniques. These parallax techniques of radiograph, which can be vertical parallax (VP) or horizontal parallax (HP), use the same lingual opposite buccal (SLOB) rule. The HP depends on tube shifting in a horizontal direction mostly on periapical films while the vertical parallax depends on tube shifting in vertical direction, such as using a panoramic radiograph (7 degrees) and occlusal radiograph (60–65 degrees) together.

More recently, cone beam tomography images have been used to establish the canine position. Once the buccolingual position of the canine is established, different classifications are used to determine the severity of canine impaction. These classifications depend on sector classification, alpha (α) angle, beta(β) angle, Gamma (γ) angle and distance (d).

Classification Parameters of the Canine Impaction

Sector Classification

Ericson and Kurol [1, 12] in 1988 introduced five sector classification. In one study [12] by same authors the sector 1 was the most mesial sector that was over the central incisor, while in the second study [1] sector 1 was the most distal sector that was over the canine area at the corner of the mouth. The classification by Ericson and Kurol [1] is the most widely used (Fig. 7.1). In this classification, the most unfavorable sector is sector 5 and the most favorable is Sector 1. A modification of the

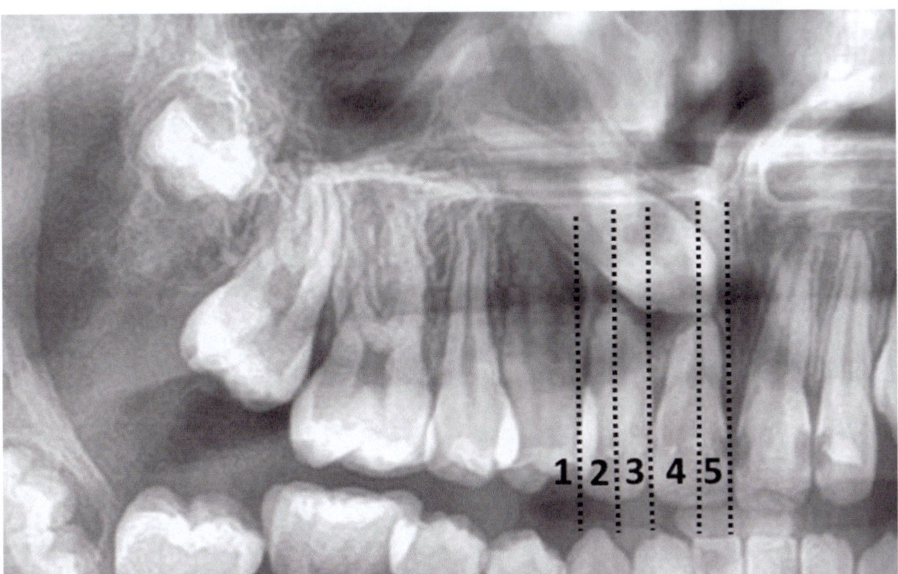

Fig. 7.1 The five-sectors classification introduced by Ericson and Kurol

five-sectors classification was the four sectors classification of Lindauer et al. [13] in which the authors combined sectors 4 and 5 of Ericson and Kurol [1] into one sector called sector 4 which was the most mesial and unfavorable sector. Crescini et al. [14] introduced three sectors classification, in which sector 1 was the most mesial and unfavorable sector while the sector 3 was the most distal and favorable sector.

Alpha (α) Angle

This angle was given by Ericson and Kurol [1, 12] to judge to mesial inclination of impacted canines. This is the angulation of the long axis of the canine to the upper midline (Fig. 7.2). α Angle is graded into three grades: Grade 1: 0°–15°, Grade 2: 16°–30° and Grade 3: ≥ 31°.

Beta (β) Angle

This angle was also proposed by Ericson and Kurol [12] and it is the angle between the maxillary canine long axis and adjacent lateral incisors' long axis (Fig. 7.2).

Gamma (γ) Angle

This angle indicates the canine angulation to the occlusal plane [15] (Fig. 7.2).

Distance (d)

It is the perpendicular distance from the canine tip to the occlusal plane (Fig. 7.2). Vermette [16] classified the severity of impaction according to the distance d as follows:

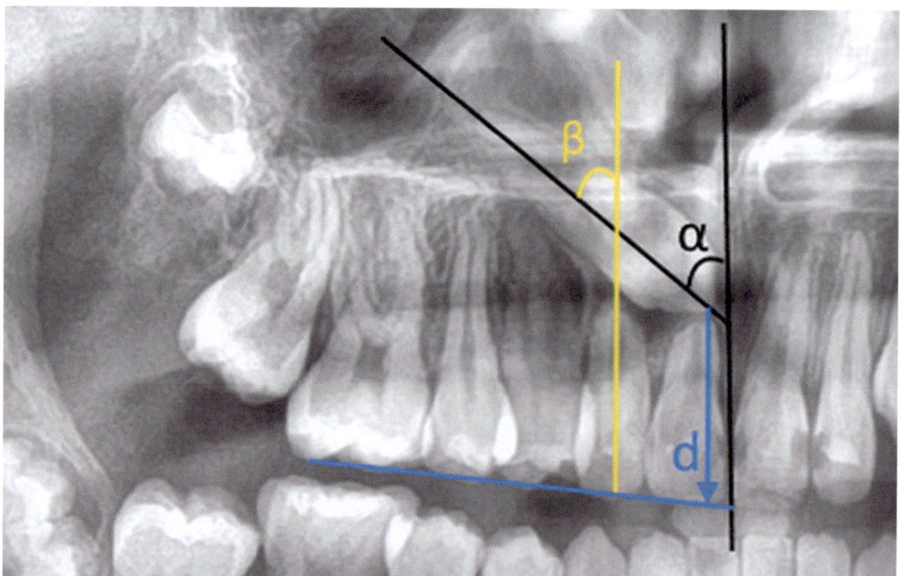

Fig. 7.2 Alpha, beta and gamma angles and distance d

- Mild impaction: Less than 12 mm distance to the occlusal plane.
- Moderate impaction: Between 12 and 15 mm distance.
- Severe impaction: Greater than 15 mm distance.

Once the position and severity of impacted canine are finalized, the clinician can use the evidence and the guidelines [17, 18] for managing displaced or impacted canines.

Clinical Diagnosis

Clinical Question 1: When the Maxillary Canine Bulge Should Be Palpable in Children?

Evidence

Longitudinal Study
Ericson and Kurol/1986 [19]
The researchers have randomly chosen 505 school children from the age range 8–12 years. The children were examined on two occasions at 2.5–3 years intervals. Four hundred ninety-two children attended the second examination. The researchers palpated the maxillary canine region palatally and buccally to detect the canine bulge. They found that the canine was palpable in 27% of 8 years old children, while in 73% of them, it was not palpable. In 10-year-old children, the canine was not palpable in 29% unilaterally or bilaterally, with a late occlusal development in 16%. At the age of 10–11 years, the number of unerupted or unpalpable canines decreased to 5%. In the second round of examination, most of the unpalpable canines erupted normally. The number of unerupted or unpalpable canines decreased to 3% in children of age 11–15 years. In children aged between 8 and 12 years, the radiographic examination was indicated in only 7.1%.

Evidence Summary
The best available evidence indicates that the canines become more palpable buccally in children over time. The unpalpable/unerupted canine decreased from 73% at the age of 8 to 29% at 10 years in school children. At the age of 10–11 years the unpalpable canine bulge decreased to 5% and in children between 11 and 15 years of age, this percentage decreased to 3%.

Evidence Interpretation
Maxillary canine bulge is palpable in the majority of children by the age of 10 years and before this age the detection of canine bulge is not recommended. If this bulge is not palpable clinically above 10 years of age, other diagnostic tools should be used.

Viewpoint
Ericson and Kurol study [19] provided us with good information relevant to our orthodontic practice. However, there are some limitations in this study. The

method of measurement was subjective without standard evaluation of the canine bulge or the indicators of palpable canine. The sample was Swedish and it is an established fact that the prevalence of impaction and the signs of impaction are different between ethnicities and races, so the generalizability of the findings is limited. Also, the observational studies rarely provide adequately robust evidence to recommend changes to clinical practice or health policy decision-making.

Radiographic and Impacted Canines

Clinical Question 2: When Is Radiographic Examination Indicated for Localization of Canine Impaction in Children?

Evidence

Longitudinal Study
Ericson and Kurol/1986 [19]
The researchers examined 505 school children on two occasions at 2.5–3 years intervals to detect displaced maxillary canines' signs. Out of 505 children, 315 were aged 10–13 years and the rest were at 8–10 years of age. They found that the need for radiographic examination in the primary examination, was 6.7% (21/315) in children at 10–13 years of age. In the second examination after 2.5–3 years interval, the total need for radiographic examination was 8% (41/505) in children over the age of 10 years. In children older than 10 years, the most common reason for radiographic examination was the asymmetric development with only palpable canines on one side. The inability to palpate the canine at this age was the second reason for radiographic examination.

Evidence Summary
The best available evidence indicates that the need for radiographic examination is approximately 8% in children above 10 years of age. Over age of 10 years, the asymmetrical development or lack of the canine bulge are predictor variables for ectopic canine eruption.

Evidence Interpretation
Radiographic examination can be done in children above 10 years of age if the canine is not palpable or palpable unilaterally.

Viewpoint
This study has been discussed before.

Clinical Question 3: Which Radiographic Method (Horizontal Parallax, Vertical Parallax or CBCT) Is More Accurate for the Detection of Impacted Canines?

Evidence

Systematic Reviews
Eslami/2017 [20]

This review included 8 studies that assessed the accuracy and the intra-modalities agreement of the CBCT and the conventional radiographical techniques (CRT) regarding the localization of the impacted canines. Two included studies compared the accuracy between the two methods. The authors found that the accuracy of CBCT ranged from 50% to 95%, and the accuracy of CRT ranged from 39% to 85% indicating a higher accuracy in the CBCT. Six included studies evaluated the inter-modalities (between different imaging) agreement in canine localization and found a significant difference with a wide range of agreement (kappa: 0.20 to 0.82, observed agreement: 64% to 84%) in canine localization. The treatment planning has a wide agreement of 0.36 to 0.72, as well. The review found a lack of robust evidence.

De Grauwe/2019 [21]

In this review, the authors included nine radiographic studies investigating impacted canine and root resorption. The review concluded that periapical radiograph is considered the most specific technique of the conventional X-rays to predict the buccolingual position of the impacted canine [22].

Cohort Studies
Ericson and Kurol/1987 [23]

In this trial the researchers recruited 84 children with 125 ectopic maxillary canines that they derived from clinical examinations of almost 3000 children. The sample age varied from 10 to 15 years. The authors used 2–3 periapical radiographs to investigate the suspected impaction. In cases with misplaced canines, they used supplemented vertex axial projection with a parallel X-ray to the root of the incisor. Further orthopantomographs (OPG) and lateral cephalometry were used for more details. For more information about root resorption, they used sagittal or frontal polytomography with hypocycloid movements.

The researchers found that most of those canines (70%) had abnormal positions, with 1.5% incidence of impacted canines in 3000 children. However, none of the radiographic methods gave the correct position of the canine for all cases. A conventional periapical radiograph was accurate in 92% of the patients, and the interpretation was difficult when the lateral incisor was tipped or proclined. Axial films or

OPG showed a less clear relationship between the canine and lateral incisor. The vertex axial projection was better in assessing the canine position in the dental arch compared to the conventional periapical technique and OPG.

Walker/2005 [24]

CBCT images were collected for 19 patients with ages 13.3 ± 2.98 years (range: 8–20 years). A total of 27 impacted or ectopically displaced canines were investigated; 8 patients were having bilaterally impacted/ectopic maxillary canines, and 11 were having unilateral-impacted canines. The researchers found that CBCT imaging of impacted canines can display the presence or absence of the canine, inclination of the tooth long axis, relative position; buccal and palatal, size of the follicle, thickness of the bone on the tooth, 3D proximity and roots resorption of adjacent teeth, other anatomic considerations and the overall dental development stage. In short, 3D imaging was helpful in managing impacted canines.

Retrospective Studies

Armstrong/2003 [25]

The authors collected data for 43 ectopic maxillary canines (EMC); 34 palatally EMC, and 9 buccally EMC. The mean age was 14 years and 11 months with a range of 12 years and 1 month to 28 years and 2 months. They compared the horizontal parallax (HP) technique and the vertical parallax (VP) radiography for localizing EMC. The correct diagnosis was higher in the HP technique (83%) than VP technique (68%) with a statistically significant difference. The mean diagnostic sensitivity was higher in HP technique (88%) than in the VP technique (69%). There were significantly more "unsure" diagnoses reported by the examiners with VP than with HP: 12% and 5%, respectively.

Mason/2001 [26]

In this study, the researchers collected data from 100 patients with 133 impacted canines; 87 (65%) were located palatally, 38 (28%) buccally, and 8 (6%) in the line of the arch. The researchers sent data to six examiners to predict the canine position using the parallax technique and magnification technique (panoramic radiography). They found that kappa statistics for the parallax technique ranged from 0.13 to 0.46 between the six examiners and ranged from 0.06 to 0.26 in the magnification technique. As such, the magnification technique was less accurate than vertical parallax for most examiners. Both methods were less sensitive in detecting buccally displaced canines, especially the magnification method.

Evidence Summary

The best available evidence suggests that the CBCT accuracy in localizing the impacted canine ranged between 50% and 95% while the accuracy of conventional radiograph techniques (CRT) ranged between 39% and 85%, which indicates that the accuracy of CBCT is higher than CRT. There is a wide range of agreement between observers (64%–84%) and modalities (0.2–0.82) in canine localization, which may result from the clinical and methodological differences between studies. On the other hand, low-level evidence [23] suggested that the conventional periapical radiograph is accurate in 92% of the examined cases with a clear difficulty when the lateral incisor is proclined or tipped. A less clear relation between canine and lateral incisor was observed in axial films or OPG. The correct diagnosis was higher in HP technique (83%) rather than VP technique (68%) with a statistically significant difference. The parallax technique was more accurate than the magnification technique in predicting the canine position.

Evidence Interpretation

Conventional radiographs provide sufficient information regarding ectopic/impacted maxillary canines in most cases. In CRT, the horizontal parallax technique is better than the vertical parallax and magnification technique (OPG).

CBCT is more accurate than conventional radiographs in localizing the impacted canines. But due to the high radiation dose of CBCT, it is recommended when conventional radiographs fail to provide sufficient information about the position of impaction or its associated pathology.

Viewpoint

The most interesting issue in diagnostic studies is the subjects' selection. In Eslami review [20] the patients' selection was at high risk of bias that limits the evidence. Also, there were methodological shortcomings due to the design of the studies and the inherent risk of bias, as well.

Ericson & Kurol trial [23] was an ambitious study with good information, but the study design is more prone to selection bias with no standard method in the measurements for determining the canine position. There was no information regarding the three-dimensional canine position and the angulation as well. The wide range of age suggests a longer follow-up duration rather than one year.

Walker trial [24] was a CBCT study, but the low number of participants and their charchterstics may reduce the quality of the evidence.

Mason study [26] is a retrospective study, which is more prone to selection bias. The number of cases were good, but there was no information about the severity or precise position of the impacted canines that play a role in detecting the canine position. The examiners were from different dental specialties and with different experiences, which may lead to different kappa values. Interestingly, the examiners familiarity and experience with the technique play a fundamental role in his decision.

Albeit De Grauwe review [21] provides useful information but there was no information about the included studies' design and their quality which may reduce the quality of the evidence.

Clinical Question 4: What Is the Best Radiographic Technique for the Detection of Impaction-Related Root Resorption?

Evidence

Systematic Review
De Grauwe/2019 [21]
This review included nine studies that investigated root resorption associated with teeth impaction. One included trial [27] found that CBCT has a better detection rate (63%) of impaction-related root resorption when compared to plain film. Another

trial [28] revealed that CBCT was superior to intraoral radiography regarding the diagnosis of internal and external cervical root resorptions. Also, a higher incidence of dilaceration and root resorption was observed in CBCT than in 2D radiography [29–31]. The periapical and occlusal radiographs have a higher specificity (diagnosis of no root resorption when there is no root resorption) between the CRTs to predict root resorption. In contrast, panoramic radiograph has a higher sensitivity (diagnosis of root resorption when there is root resorption) in predicting root resorption.

Evidence Summary

The best available evidence suggests that CBCT is the best radiographic tool to detect root resorption associated with canine impaction. In CRTs, if there is a true root resorption, the panoramic radiograph is the best 2D technique to detect this root resorption. In contrast, the periapical and occlusal radiographs are the most specific technique if there is no true root resorption.

Evidence Interpretation

For impaction-related root resorption, a CBCT radiograph is the best technique for detecting this problem. However, if only the 2D radiographs are available, the panoramic radiograph is superior to other 2D techniques in detecting impaction-related root resorption.

Viewpoint

The review has already been discussed.

Surgical Techniques

Clinical Question 5: What Is the Best Flap Technique (Closed Versus Open) for Palatal Impacted Canine?

Evidence

Systematic Reviews and Meta-Analyses
Parkin/2017 [32]
In this Cochrane review, the authors included three RCTs to answer the aforementioned question. They found that there is no statistically significant difference in treatment success between the two techniques (risk ratio: RR;0.99, 95% CI: 0.93 to 1.06, P = 0.79, three studies, 141 participants, low-quality evidence). There were three failures in the open technique out of 69, and two failures in the closed technique out of 72 participants. One failure was due to the detachment of the gold chain in the closed group. One included study reported post-surgical infection in one case and pain during traction in another case because of that the chain perforated the palatal mucosa in the closed technique [33]. Two included studies reported no

difference between the two methods regarding the midpalatal (RR; 1.32, 95% CI: 0.63 to 2.77, P = 0.47) or mid-buccal gingival rescission (MD; −0.02 mm, 95% CI: −0.21 to 0.16, P = 0.81) [33, 34]. Likewise, there was no evidence of differences between the two methods regarding the length of the surgical time (MD; −3.30 minutes, 95% CI: −9.97 to 3.36, P = 0.33) or the gingival indexes.

Cassina/2017 [35]

This systematic review included eight trials; 4 were randomized controlled trials, and 4 were non-randomized trials. The authors compared open versus closed surgical techniques regarding the treatment duration and adverse effects. The pooled estimate of three studies in meta-analysis resulted in a statistically significant reduction of 2.14 months (MD;-2.14, 95% CI: −0.05 to −4.23, P < 0.05) in the initial alignment of the impacted canine to the dental arch in the open exposure group when compared with closed exposure group. In this respect, one study suggested that the overall treatment duration was less but not statistically significant in open technique (MD: −3.78 months; 95% CI: −9.21 to 1.65 months; P > 0.05). The open exposure technique was associated with lower odds of ankylosis (OR = 0.15; 95% CI 0.03–0.83; P < 0.05, one trial) [36]. However, there was no statistically significant difference between the two techniques regarding the re-exposure need, post-operative pain, difficulty in speech and eating, canine discoloration, and canine esthetics. The authors graded the evidence as low to very low quality.

Systematic Review
Sampaziotis/2018 [37]

This review included nine studies; 3 RCTs, 3 quasi-RCTs, and 3 non-RCTs. The authors investigated the differences between the open versus closed technique in the impacted palatal canines. No difference was found between closed versus open techniques regarding the periodontal status in the three studies. On the other hand, one included retrospective study [38] reported that the closed technique has a better periodontal outcome as the attachment loss was greater in the open technique from the palatal aspect. The included studies reported conflicting results regarding the treatment duration without conclusive evidence, as well. There was no difference between the two techniques regarding the relocation of the impacted canine in one study [39]. In contrast in another included study [34], the relocation of the impacted canine was quicker in the open technique. There was no difference between the two techniques regarding the esthetic results and the pain perception, while there was contradictory data regarding the failure rate and the re-exposure.

Evidence Summary

The best available evidence suggests that there is no difference between the closed and the open flap techniques for managing palatally impacted canines. There was no statistically significant difference in the success rate between the two techniques

(RR 0.99, 95% CI; 0.93–1.06). Likewise, there was no evidence of the differences between the two techniques regarding the gingival recession or the length of treatment time. Only one review with very low evidence [38], reported that the closed technique has a better periodontal outcome as there was greater attachment loss in the open technique from the palatal aspect. Furthermore, there was no difference between the two techniques regarding the secondary outcomes; the re-exposure need, post-operative pain, difficulty in eating, difficulty in speech, canine discoloration, and canine esthetics. On the other hand, the canine alignment time was statistically shorter in the open technique by 2.14 months (MD;-2.14, 95% CI: −0.05 to-4.23; P < 0.05) compared to the closed technique. Finally, the open technique showed a lower likelihood of canine ankylosis by 85% when compared to the closed technique.

Evidence Interpretation

There are no major differences between the two techniques for managing palatal-impacted canines. The clinician can use either of them in accordance with the surgeon's skills, patients' oral hygiene, and the severity of the impaction. The open technique can be used in cases with high chances of bond failure and ankylosis.

Bond failure mostly occurs if the optimum bonding surface is not available such as in the case of rotated canines. The chances of ankylosis are more common in adult' patients or in patients with a previous history of trauma. If the patient is unwilling to undergo a second surgery, open procedure should be used for canine traction. But there are also some practical limitations of using open procedures, such as deeply impacted canines that are close to adjacent roots or sinuses. In such cases, it is difficult to maintain good oral hygiene, and there is a possibility of iatrogenic damage so such cases should be managed according to their merits.

Viewpoint

Parkin review [32] was a well-conducted Cochrane review. The main shortcomings were the high risk of bias in two of the included studies with a small sample size that reduced the quality of the evidence and increased the uncertainty. There was no investigation of the severity of the canine impaction on the technique, which may be a confounding factor. Finally, there were only a few studies included.

Cassina review [35] was a well-conducted review with some limitations. There were a limited number of available trials with moderate to high risk of bias. Including non-randomized controlled trials may influence the results of meta-analysis, but the authors removed them in the sensitivity analysis to get robust results. Also, there was not enough information regarding the individual patient data, but the authors tried to remove confounding by re-analysis.

Sampaziotis review [37] was a systematic qualitative review without meta-analysis, which may lead to inaccurate results. The different designs with a serious risk of bias in the non-RCTs may reduce the quality of the evidence.

Interceptive Treatment

Clinical Question 6: Is Interceptive Treatment Effective in Managing Palatally Displaced Canines (PDCs)?

Evidence

Systematic Reviews and Meta-Analyses
Benson/2021 [40]

This Cochrane review included four RCTs that investigated interceptive procedures to promote the eruption of palatally displaced canines (PDCs). In one RCT, the deciduous canine extraction (DCE) promoted a successful eruption of the PDCs (RR; 2.78, 95% CI: 0.90–9.23, 45 patients) when compared to the non-extraction group at 12 months, but this was not statistically significant. Likewise in three RCTs, there was no statistically significant difference between primary canine and first molar extraction group and non-extraction group regarding the eruption of PDCs (RR;0.68,95%CI: 0.35–1.31, 119 patients) at 12 months and (RR; 0.61, 95% CI: 0.29–1.25) at 24 months. Furthermore, there was no statistically significant difference between extraction and non-extraction groups regarding the root resorption of the adjacent teeth (RR; 0.60, 95% CI: 0.28–1.31, 96 patients). The evidence for the present findings was very low.

Alyammahi/2018 [41]

The authors included five RCTs in this review, which investigated the effectiveness of interceptive treatment on PDC, with 214 individuals having a follow-up period of 48 months. The authors concluded that DCE did not significantly stimulate the PDC eruption in 12 months follow-up (RR: 1.537, 95% CI: 0.66–3.60, P = 0.32; n = 67 participants). In contrast, DCE had a statistically significant effect on the eruption of PDC in a follow-up period of more than 12 months (RR: 1.78, 95% CI: 1.38–2.31, P < 0.001; 5 studies, 214 participants). Furthermore, the mean eruption time was 15.6 ± 5.6 months in the extraction group, while it was 18.8 ± 5.8 months in the control group. The authors graded the evidence as moderate quality.

Randomized Controlled Trials
Baccetti/2011 [42]

This trial was included in the aforementioned review [41]. The author recruited 120 participants with an age of 9.5–13 years in this trial. They allocated the subjects into four groups; 40 participants in RME followed by transpalatal arch TPA with deciduous canine extraction (RME/TPA/DCE group), 25 participants in TPA plus deciduous canine extraction (TPA/DCE group), 25 participants in the deciduous canine extraction group (DCE group), and 30 subjects as a control group without treatment. The rate of successful eruption was 80% (32/40 subjects) in RME/TPA/DCE group, 79.2% (19/24 subjects) in TPA/DCE group, 62.5% in the DCE group, and 27.6% in the control group with statistically significant differences between all the groups.

Baccetti/2009 [43]

This trial also was included in the aforementioned review [41]. The authors randomly allocated 60 children aged 7.6–9.6 years into two groups; 35 subjects in the RME group and 25 subjects in the non-treated control group. Regarding the dropout, the final sample consisted of 32 subjects in the RME group and 22 subjects in the control group. The authors concluded that the successful eruption rate was 65.7% in the RME group and 13.6% in the control group after a mean observation period of 4.11 years. The differences were statistically significant.

Naoumova/2018 [44]

The authors recruited 67 patients (40 females and 27 males) with an age of 11.35 ± 1 years and randomly allocated them to primary canine extraction and non-extraction groups. The patients were examined clinically and radiographically by OPG at baseline, after 6 months, and 12 months. They measured the Alpha (α) angle, sector of canine, and the distance of the canine cusp tip to the occlusal plane. The authors found that PDCs that erupted spontaneously in the non-extraction group had a significantly smaller α angle and were positioned in a "lower sector" when compared with spontaneously erupted PDCs in the extraction group. The PDCs that showed no eruption in both extraction and non-extraction groups were positioned significantly more horizontally with a larger α angle, in a higher sector, and root development was more advanced. In addition to that, the children who showed no spontaneous eruption were older. PDCs that spontaneously erupted had 20° of α angle and were in sector 2. PDCs with 30° α angle did not erupt spontaneously. Interestingly, the PDCs located in sector 4 did not erupt despite deciduous canine extraction.

Naoumova/2015 [45]

This trial was included in both reviews [40, 41]. In this study, 67 patients (40 girls and 27 boys) with age of 11.4 ± 1.0 years were included. There were 45 unilateral and 22 bilateral PDCs. The children were randomly allocated to the extraction group (DCE) or non-extraction control group (CG). In the extraction group, the clinician extracted the deciduous canines. The researchers found that the extraction group had more spontaneous eruptions of the PDCs, and this was statistically significant, 69% and 39%, in EG and CG, respectively.

Armi/2011 [46]

This RCT comprised of 64 subjects with PDCs and divided them into three groups: cervical pull headgear (HG) for one year and 12–14 hour/day, rapid maxillary expansion (7 mm) and cervical pull headgear (RME/HG), or untreated control group (CG). The authors found that the successful eruption was 85.7% in the RME/HG group and 82.3% in the HG group. Both treatment groups have a significantly greater successful eruption rate than the success rate in untreated control subjects (36%).

Leonardi/2004 [47]

This trial was included in Alyammahi review [41]. In this longitudinal study, the researchers randomly assigned 46 subjects with PDCs (62 maxillary canines) into three groups; extraction of deciduous canines (DCE), extraction of deciduous canines with cervical headgear (DCE/HG), and non-treated group (CG). They found that the eruption rate was similar in DCE group (50%) and CG, however, the eruption rate was significantly higher (80%) in DCE/HG group after 18 months. There was no difference between the DCE group and DCE/HG in terms of the duration of successful eruption.

Evidence Summary

The best available evidence suggests that the interceptive treatment by deciduous canine extraction stimulated the PDC eruption by 178%, but this was not statistically significant due to the wide confidence range, which included the value of no effect in one review [40]. On the other hand, DCE promoted PDC eruption by 1.78 times more than the non-extraction group [41]. Moreover, the PDC eruption takes more than 1 year after primary canine extraction, with an average time of 15.6 ± 5.6 months in the extraction group and 18.8 ± 5.8 months in the non-extraction group. The deciduous canine extraction has limited or no benefit when the α angle becomes 30° or more (more horizontal location), and the PDC is located in sector 4 or above. The eruption is easier and spontaneous when the PDC is in Sector 2 with an α angle of 20°. In one trial [42], there was a statistically significant higher successful eruption in the TPA group with or without RME (79.2–80%) and DCE than in the DCE alone group or control, 62.5%, and 27.6%, respectively. Likewise, RME had a higher successful canine eruption rate of 65.7% compared to 13.6% in control [43].

Evidence Interpretation

In children aged 10–13 with PDCs, there is a good chance of spontaneous eruption of permanent canine after primary canine extraction, but it takes more than a year.

The factors which may increase the chance of eruption are low α angle and lower sector. There is no benefit of interceptive orthodontics if the α angle is greater than 30° and the palatally displaced canine is in sector four or higher. RME, along with canine extraction, is beneficial if there is a maxillary transverse discrepancy. After RME, a TPA should be used to maintain the transverse dimension. Also, giving a TPA is more beneficial after primary canine extraction as it helps in the maintenance of transverse dimension and provides some limited anteroposterior anchorage.

Viewpoint

Benson et al. [40] review included a low number of studies; only 4 RCTs. The authors assessed two RCTs at high risk of bias due to the younger patients (8 years) recruited in those studies, the very high number of patients who were judged to have bilateral PDCs, and the uncertainty in the diagnosis of the PDCs as sector 1 has no overlap with the root of upper lateral which is considered normal before the full development of the lateral incisor root.

Alyammahi review [41] appraised three studies as having a high risk of bias, while two studies were at low risk of bias. The authors reported a risk difference (RD) of 0.287 that lead to the number needed to treat (NNT) of 3.48, which means the clinician needs to extract 4 primary canines to prevent one impaction.

There was not enough information regarding the randomization and blinding in Baccetti trial [42], which may reduce its quality and increase the selection bias. The alpha angle was 15° in the eligibility criteria, which means only mild cases of PDC were selected. There was no information about the transverse problems and/or crowding in the maxilla that restricted the need for the maxillary expansion. On the other hand, another RCT by Baccetti [43] has limitations related to randomization and blinding. Also, there was insufficient information regarding the malocclusion in the transverse plane and crowding. The prediction of the impaction was based on the postero-anterior (PA) radiographs, which may confuse the examiner. Furthermore, the dropout may lead to bias.

Naoumova trials [44, 45] excluded cases having more than 2 mm of crowding in the maxilla and root resorption of the Grades 3 and 4 of adjacent roots, which led to restricting the results of this study to uncrowded cases and the cases with limited root resorption of the adjacent teeth. The results of this study can only be generalized to the Caucasian population aged 10–13 years with PDCs located in sectors 2–4 with mild space deficiency in the maxilla.

Amri and Leonardi trials [46, 47] did not have sample size calculations, that might lead to underpowered study. The researchers reported that the severity of canine displacement was similar in the three groups at T1, but they did not provide enough information regarding the canine position, angulation, and sectors. So, confounders may affect the study findings of these trials, which leads to misinterpretation of the results.

Clinical Question 7: Are There Any Adverse Effects of Interceptive Treatment of Palatally Displaced Canines?

Evidence

Systematic Review
Alyammahi/2018 [41]
In this systematic review, one included RCT [45] reported that there was no statistically significant effect of extraction on the root resorption of the adjacent teeth (RR: 0.60, 95% CI: 0.28–1.30, P = 0.2; n = 67 participants). In addition to that, one included RCT [48] reported a decrease in the length of the primary canine region post-extraction without midline shift.

Randomized Controlled Trial
Naoumova/2018 [44]
The authors randomly allocated 67 patients to extraction and non-extraction groups. The side effect of primary canines extraction was reported. Midline shift of

0.5–1.5 mm on the extraction side was noticed in 6 of the 35 patients after 1 year. After 6 months, unwanted movement in 37% of the patients was seen; rotation in 6 premolars and movement of 4 premolars and 4 laterals into the extraction sites.

Evidence Summary

The best available evidence suggests that interceptive treatment by extraction of primary/deciduous canine is associated with some iatrogenic effects. These iatrogenic effects include drifting of neighboring teeth into the extraction space, midline shift, rotation of other teeth, and lack of space. There was no evidence for other effects of DCE, such as the adjacent root resorption.

Evidence Interpretation

Interceptive treatment for palatally displaced maxillary canines is associated with side effects such as midline deviation, decrease in arch length, tipping of teeth into extraction space and rotation of teeth. So, some mechanotherapy is always required post-interceptive treatment to correct these problems.

Viewpoint

The included review and the RCT have already been discussed.

Treatment Duration

Clinical Question 8: What Is the Duration of Active Traction and Total Treatment of Palatally Displaced Maxillary Impacted Canines?

Evidence

A Prospective Study
Crescini/2007 [14]

This study recruited 168 participants (40 males and 128 females) with impacted canines and an age range of 12.8–52 years. The researchers evaluated the position of the canine by α angle, d-distance from the canine tip to the occlusal plane, and the three sectors. They found that the overall treatment duration was 22 ± 4.8 months with a traction phase of 8 ± 2.3 months (range 4–13). Interestingly, the authors found that 1 more week of active orthodontic traction was required for either every $5°$ of α-angle or 1 mm increase of distance d. The sector 1 which was the most mesial sector, probably increases the traction time by 6 weeks when compared to sector 3.

A Retrospective Studies
Stewart/2001 [49]

The authors collected the data from three private clinics for 47 adolescent participants who underwent orthodontic treatment for impacted canines; 29 children with unilateral impactions and 18 children with bilateral impactions. They compared them with participants without impaction as treated control for treatment duration. They found that the treatment duration was 25.8 months for the unilateral-impacted group, 32.3 months for the bilateral-impacted canines, and 22.4 months for the control group.

Arriola-Guillen/2019 [50]

The authors included 30 patients (11 males and 19 females; age of 18.16 ± 7.32 years) with 45 impacted canines who were treated in a private clinic. The authors found that the duration of active orthodontic traction was 8.40 ± 3.26 months with a range of (4–16 months). The sex had a statistically significant effect on the traction duration as the traction duration was higher by 2.049 months in females than males. The duration increased statistically by 2.74 months in bilateral cases when compared with unilateral impactions. The traction time of the impacted canines increased by 2.35 months (P = 0.046) in the higher sectors 4 or 5 when compared to the lower sectors. The traction time increased statistically in bicortical (in the middle of the two cortical plates) centered canine traction by 2.85 months (P = 0.001) and by 0.055 months (P = 0.009) for each degree increase in β angle.

Evidence Summary

The best available evidence suggests that the total time duration for traction of impacted canine to the occlusal plane is 8.40 ± 3.26 months, with a range of 4–16 months. Canine traction can take more time in females than males by 2.049 months. Bilateral traction takes more time than unilateral traction by 2.74 months. Likewise, total treatment duration increased by 3.4 and 9.9 months in unilateral and bilateral impaction, respectively.

Higher sector (mesial position) of 4 or 5 is associated with an extra traction duration of 2.35 months than the lower sectors. A 5° of α-angulation opening or 1 mm extra d-distance may increase the traction time by 1 week. The bicortical impaction and higher β angle may increase the traction duration, as well.

Evidence Interpretation

In impacted canines, the duration of active traction is approximately 8 months, meaning impacted canine cases take slightly more treatment time than conventional cases of comprehensive orthodontic treatment. Factors that increase traction time to occlusal plane and treatment duration are gender, higher sectors, higher α, β angle, bilateral and bicortical impaction.

Viewpoint

Crescini study [14] provided us with good information. The lack of randomization and blinding might reduce the quality of the evidence. It is worth noticing that the age range in this study was wide, 12.5–52 years, which might confound the results.

Stewart study [49] design is retrospective which is more prone to selection bias. There were gender differences between the control and the impaction group, which may confound the findings. The records were collected from three clinics, which may enhance the applicability of the results.

Arriola-Guillen study [50] was done in a private practice setting by an orthodontist with 20 years of experience. The design of the study has shortcomings, as it was a retrospective design without a control group which is similar to the case series. The long experience years of the orthodontist may play a role in the treatment duration and may also restrict the external validity of the findings.

Failure of the Treatment

Clinical Question 9: What Factors Influence the Successful Traction of Impacted Canines?

Evidence

Cases Series
Becker/2010 [51]
The authors analyzed data of failed treatment for 28 referred patients (18 females, 10 males; age: 17.4 ± 4.3 years) with 37 impacted canines. Of those, 26 impactions were palatal, 9 were buccal, and 2 were in the mid-alveolus. Most of the patients (26/28; 92.9%) were referred after performing the surgery. The mean duration of the treatment failure, from start to realization of failure, was 26.2 ± 17.2 months. The major reasons for failure were inadequate anchorage 18/37 (48.6%), mistaken location and directional traction 15/37 (40.5%) and ankylosis 12/37 (32.4%). The success rate of the revised treatments was 71.4%, with a mean duration of 14.4 ± 7.2 months. Surgical luxation and subsequent traction were used for treating 7 ankylosed teeth but only three of them succeeded. Repeat surgery was needed for 62.9% of the canines mostly to redirect the ligature wires.

Evidence Summary
The best available evidence suggests that the reasons for failure in impacted canines' traction are mainly poor anchorage (48.6%), poor diagnosis (40.5%) for the impaction location and the elastic traction to the archwire, and ankylosis (32.4%). The success rate of re-treatment of the failed cases was 71.4%, with a mean duration of 14.4 ± 7.2 months. The need for another surgery was 62.9%.

Evidence Interpretation
Factors that may influence the success of treating impacted canines are:

- Precise diagnosis for the canine location.
- Early diagnosis of ankylosis and surgical luxation of the ankylosed teeth.
- Appropriate traction mechanics and direction.
- Suitable plan for the anchorage requirements.

Viewpoint

Becker study [51] was of very low evidence but it provided the clinician with useful information regarding clinical causes of impacted teeth, traction failure and the success rate of re-treatment.

Adverse Effects

Clinical Question 10: What Is the Prevalence of Root Resorption (RR) in Adjacent Teeth To Impacted Canines and the Related Factors?

Evidence

Systematic Review
Schroder/2018 [52]

The authors included 18 studies to investigate root resorption in the adjacent teeth to impacted canines. These canines' were mostly palatal (56.99%), followed by buccal (29.35%) and the least common were in the arch (19.59%) canines. They found different prevalence values for RR in central incisors, with a range of 1.19%–35.06%. Different RR values in lateral incisors ranged from 8.20% to 89.61%, while RR in premolars ranged from 4.48% to 11.72% in five included studies. There was a significant difference in the RR values between group A with a contact between the impacted canine and the neighboring teeth and group B without contact. The RR of the lateral incisors was 44.50% in group A and 7.35% in group B.

There were differences in the location of RR; the apical third RR was 56.87%, and the cervical third RR was 6.10%. RR severity prevalence was 43.20% and 30.90%, from slight to severe, respectively.

Cohort Studies
Ericson and Kurol/1987 [23]

This trial comprised 84 children with 125 ectopic erupted maxillary canines. The age varied from 10 to 15 years. The researchers used sagittal or frontal polytomography with hypocycloid movements for detection of root resorption. They found that 12 lateral incisors and one central incisor have root resorption. 12.5% of adjacent teeth to impacted canines showed a degree of root resorption. Females have more root resorption on laterals than males by 12:1.

Ericson and Kurol/1988 [12]

This study comprised two groups; a resorption group of 40 lateral incisors with root resorption caused by the ectopic eruption (age 10–15 years) and a control group of 118 ectopic eruptions without lateral incisor resorption (age 10.1–14.9 years). The authors found that the risk of root resorption of the lateral incisor increases by 50% if the α angle was greater than 25°. Also, the mesial inclination of the canine to the midline, in the axial-vertex occlusal film, was significantly higher in the resorption group (34.5°) than in the control group (16.4°). OPG showed that 65% and 28% of canines were in the most medial sectors in the resorption and control groups, respectively. Interestingly, when the canine cusp was positioned mesially to the lateral incisor, the risk increased three times, and the lateral incisor' root was resorbed.

Retrospective Studies
Guarnieri/ [53]
The researchers recruited 50 patients (22 male and 28 female) with 69 impacted maxillary canines. Their age ranged from 9 to 15 years (mean age: 11.7 years). Five patients were in early mixed dentition, 20 patients had late mixed dentition, and 24 patients had permanent dentition. Fifty impacted canines (72%) were palatal, 13 canines (19%) were buccal, and 6 canines (9%) were in the mid-alveolus. The authors assessed the effect of the impacted canine on the adjacent root resorption on CT scans. The prevalence of root resorption of the adjacent teeth was 34% of the impacted cases. Twenty resorption cases (92%) showed that the lateral incisors were resorbed, while central incisors were resorbed in one case, and both central and lateral incisors were resorbed in one case. Twelve cases (52%) showed resorption in apical third, while 11 cases (48%) showed resorption in the middle third. In the vast majority of the cases (70%) resorption was mild, in 26% it was moderate, while in one case (4%) there was severe resorption.

The authors found that the predictive value of β angle is equal to 76% while α and γ angles do not seem to be statistically significant. Thus:

- If β angle >54° the likelihood of root resorption is greater than 61% irrespective of the evaluation of the analysis of Lindauer [13].
- If β angle <18° and Lindauer [13] sector, is I, the likelihood of root resorption is 0.06%.

Walker/2005 [24]
CBCT images were collected for 19 patients with age ranging from 8 to 20 years (13.3 ± 2.98). There were 27 ectopically erupted or impacted maxillary canines, including 16 bilateral impactions and 11 unilateral impactions. Researchers found that resorption of adjacent teeth to the impacted canine was present in 66.7% (18) of the lateral incisors and 11.1% (3) of the central incisors. The proximity of the impacted canine to the incisors was correlated with their resorption. All central incisor resorption cases also had lateral resorption. In one case, there was resorption on the first premolar. In 63.0% of the 27 cases, the impacted canine was in contact (distance less than 0.5 mm) with the lateral incisor, and the impacted canine was in contact with the central incisor in 18.5% of the 27 cases. The average distances of the impacted canine to the lateral and central incisors were 1.4 ± 2.15 mm and 3.5 ± 2.90 mm, respectively.

Chaushu/2015 [54]

In this study, researchers collected data from two groups: Severe incisor root resorption (SIRR) group that comprised 55 consecutive patients (77 impacted canines) with SIRR of 96 incisors (more than root third is affected) and the control group that comprised 57 consecutive control subjects (72 canines). The researchers found that there is a statistically significant higher ratio (2.5:1) of lateral resorption than centrals (69 lateral and 27 central). The risk of females having SIRR was higher than males by 4.2 times. The risk of SIRR for canines positioned in sector 5 was higher than for canines positioned in sectors 2 and 3 by 5.5 and 3.5 times, respectively. Similarly, the risk of SIRR associated with a canine in sector 3 was higher than the risk of SIRR with canines in sectors 1 and 2 by 3 times. The pattern of impacted maxillary canines associated SIRR was mostly oblique rather than horizontal.

Evidence Summary

The best available evidence suggests that the contact between impacted canines with adjacent teeth may be associated with root resorption. The root resorption of the centrals ranged between 1.19% and 35.06%. RR of the lateral incisors ranged between 8.20% and 89.61%. RR of the premolars ranged from 4.48% to 11.72%. Even if there was no contact, there was incidence of root resorption, the root resorption in the lateral incisors without clear contact was 7.35%, while it was 44.50% in the contact group. All central incisor resorption cases were also having lateral resorption. There was a statistically significant higher ratio (2.5:1) of lateral incisors root resorption than central incisors. Risk of root resorption of the lateral incisor increases by 50% if the α angle was greater than 25°. If β angle was higher than 54°, the probability of having root resorption was greater than 61%. Risk of SIRR when canine positioned in sector 5 was higher than canines positioned in sectors 2 and 3 by 5.5 and 3.5 times, respectively. More RR was reported in apical third (56.87%) than in the cervical third (6.10%).

Evidence Interpretation

Different factors contribute to root resorption of adjacent teeth to impacted canines. Greater the physical proximity of the impacted canine crown to the root of adjacent teeth (increase β angle, mesial sector), the more would be the chances of root resorption. The lateral incisor has more chances of root resorption than the central incisors. Apical third of these teeth showed more resorption than cervical third. The clinician should consider the root resorption of adjacent teeth if the aforementioned factors raise red flags.

More root resorption is diagnosed using CBCT as compared to conventional radiographs. So, if the plain radiographic findings are doubtful, the clinician should opt for CBCT.

Viewpoint

Schroder review [52] provided us with a good information that add to the knowledge regarding the prevalence of RR in different races and origins. The included studies have shortcomings related to high or unclear risk of bias resulting from no sufficient description of the eligibility criteria or the compared groups.

In Ericson and Kurol [12], there was a lack of blinding and randomization that would decline the quality of the evidence. There was not enough reporting on the differences between canine locations to the arch (buccal, lingual, or medial).

Chaushu study [54] was an observational study with the involvement of two different geographic areas with selected cases that may limit the generalizability of the results. The sample size was low, and a larger sample size is recommended. The confounding factors of canine positions, bilateral versus unilateral impaction and differences in age between groups may reduce the certainty of the evidence.

Clinical Question 11: What Is the Effect of Impacted Canine Treatment on Orthodontic Induced Inflammatory Root Resorption?

Evidence

Retrospective Studies
Arriola-Guillen/2019 [55]

In this study, the authors included 45 patients treated in private practice and divided them according to the complexity of impacted canines' traction into two groups; 20 patients in the low complex treatment group (the canine is located in sectors 1 and 2), and 25 patients in the highly complex treatment group (the canine is located in sectors 3, 4, and 5). The authors assessed the root resorption of the upper four incisors before and after the treatment on CBCT scans. They found that there were no statistically significant differences between the two groups regarding root resorption after the treatment. The resorption in root length ranged from 1 to 1.5 mm in the four incisors; (MD; −0.01, −0.11 mm in the lateral and central incisors, respectively). The area of resorption ranged from 3 to 4 mm^2 (MD; −0.22, 0.17 mm^3 in the lateral and central incisors, respectively). There was no effect of the complexity of the treatment on root resorption.

Brusveen/2012 [56]

The authors collected the data of 66 patients: 32 patients (20 females, 12 males) had a unilateral impaction with a mean age of 13.9 years (range, 10.0–33.4 years), and 33 patients (21 females, 13 males) as a non-impacted canine group with a mean age of 13.4 years (range, 9.8–35.0 years) for comparison. They assessed the orthodontic-induced root resorption using intraoral periapical films by measuring the lengths of the maxillary incisors. There was no difference between the two groups regarding tooth shortening, with a mean value of incisors shortening ranged between 0.26 and 0.72 mm for the two groups.

Evidence Summary

In the absence of high-quality evidence, the best available evidence suggests that the treatment of impacted canines did not have an impact on the OIIRR of the central and lateral incisors. The root resorption of the incisors ranged between 0.26 and 0.72 mm in one study [56] and 1 and 1.5 mm in another study [55] due to differences in the radiographic methods and other variables.

Evidence Interpretation

According to the existing evidence, the impacted canine treatment does not influence the OIIRR of the upper incisors.

Viewpoint

Notwithstanding the fact that Arriola-Guillens study [55] was a retrospective study, the authors considered the severity of the impaction for assessing the root resorption. The main shortcoming in this study is that the height of the canine crown from the occlusal plane (d-distance) in the two groups was 11 mm, which suggests that the two groups impaction was mild. Also, there was a lack of information regarding unilateral and bilateral impaction in this study.

Brusveen study [56] was a retrospective study. The impaction characteristics suggest that most of the impacted canines were located in sectors 1, 2, and 3 (56%), and only 44% were located in sectors 4 and 5, which may affect the root resorption of the incisors. Also, only 21.9% of impacted canines crowns were located in the apical third of the incisors' root, while 0% were located above the apex that may be considered as a non-apical resorption factor. Finally, the follicle tooth ratio was 1.5 and not significantly correlated to the RR.

Different mechanics, canine position, and length of treatment may be considered as factors for root resorption. These factors should be taken into account in future RCTs to be certain about the OIIRR due to canine impactions.

Authors' Recommendations

- The canine bulge is palpable in most children after 10 years of age. So radiographic examination is justified if the canine is not palpable after this age, or there is asymmetrical eruption.
- Traditionally 2-D radiographs are used for localization of impacted canines. Mostly two radiographs with cone shift techniques are used. In conventional radiographs, horizontal parallax has better accuracy than vertical parallax, with parallax technique better than magnification technique. For detection of root resorption panoramic X-rays are better than periapical and occlusal X-rays.
- CBCT is the best imaging technique for localization of impacted canine position and detection of root resorption of neighboring teeth. But it should only be used if the clinician believes that conventional radiographic techniques would fail to provide the required information.
- Chances of root resorption of a neighboring teeth increase as its physical proximity with impacted canine crown increases. Increase in mesial sector and angulation of canine increase the chances of adjacent teeth-root resorption. There are more chances of root resorption on lateral incisors and at the apical thirds of the roots of adjacent anterior teeth. Orthodontic treatment of impacted teeth does not induce extra root resorption of anterior teeth.

- There are no major differences between open versus closed eruption exposure techniques for palatal impacted canines. The open technique can be more beneficial in cases with high chances of ankylosis, and in patients who are unwilling to undergo a second episode of surgery in case of bond or attachment failure.
- Interceptive orthodontics for PDCs can be successfuly carried out after 10 years of age in patients with an alpha angle less than 20° and a lower sector of canine crown (sectors 1 and 2). Interceptive orthodontics can be done by extraction of deciduous canine and use of RME, headgear, and TPA. It mostly takes more than a year for spontaneous eruption of PDC if optimum space is provided for it. Interceptive orthodontic treatment for PDCs is also associated with iatrogenic effects such as neighboring tooth migration and rotation into the extraction space.
- Treatment duration of impacted canine cases is longer than conventional cases of comprehensive orthodontic treatment. Factors that increase traction to occlusal plane and treatment duration are gender, higher sectors, higher α and β angle, bilateral impaction, and bicortical impaction. Successful treatment depends upon precise diagnosis and biomechanics.
- If an impacted canine is ankylosed, traction should always be done after surgical luxation of the canine.

References

1. Ericson S, Kurol J. Early treatment of palatally erupting maxillary canines by extraction of the primary canines. Eur J Orthod. 1988;10(4):283–95.
2. Ericson S, Kurol J. Radiographic assessment of maxillary canine eruption in children with clinical signs of eruption disturbance. Eur J Orthod. 1986;8(3):133–40.
3. Celikoglu M, Kamak H, Oktay H. Investigation of transmigrated and impacted maxillary and mandibular canine teeth in an orthodontic patient population. J Oral Maxillofac Surg. 2010;68(5):1001–6. https://doi.org/10.1016/j.joms.2009.09.006.
4. Stivaros N, Mandall NA. Radiographic factors affecting the management of impacted upper permanent canines. J Orthod. 2000;27(2):169–73. https://doi.org/10.1093/ortho/27.2.169.
5. Mossey PA, Campbell HM, Luffingham JK. The palatal canine and the adjacent lateral incisor: a study of a west of Scotland population. Br J Orthod. 1994;21(2):169–74.
6. Kokich VG. Surgical and orthodontic management of impacted maxillary canine. Am J Orthod Dentofac Orthop. 2004;126(3):278–83.
7. Becker A, Smith P, Behar R. The incidence of anomalous maxillary lateral incisors in relation to palatally-displaced cuspids. Angle Orthod. 1981;51(1):24–9. https://doi.org/10.1043/0003-3219(1981)051<0024:tioaml>2.0.co;2.
8. Peck S, Peck L, Kataja M. The palatally displaced canine as a dental anomaly of genetic origin. Angle Orthod. 1994;64(4):249–56. https://doi.org/10.1043/0003-3219(1994)064<0249:wnid>2.0.co;2.
9. Hurme VO. Ranges of normalcy in the eruption of permanent teeth. J Dent Child. 1949;16(2):11.
10. Baccetti T, Franchi L, De Lisa S, Giuntini V. Eruption of the maxillary canines in relation to skeletal maturity. Am J Orthod Dentofacial Orthop. 2008;133(5):748–51. https://doi.org/10.1016/j.ajodo.2007.10.031.

11. Chaushu S, Becker A, Zeltser R, Branski S, Vasker N, Chaushu G. Patients perception of recovery after exposure of impacted teeth: a comparison of closed- versus open-eruption techniques. J Oral Maxillofac Surg. 2005;63(3):323–9. https://doi.org/10.1016/j.joms.2004.11.007.
12. Ericson S, Kurol J. Resorption of maxillary lateral incisors caused by ectopic eruption of the canines. A clinical and radiographic analysis of predisposing factors. Am J Orthod Dentofacial Orthop. 1988;94(6):503–13.
13. Lindauer SJ, Rubenstein LK, Hang WM, Andersen WC, Isaacson RJ. Canine impaction identified early with panoramic radiographs. J Am Dent Assoc. 1992;123(3):91–2. 5–7
14. Crescini A, Nieri M, Buti J, Baccetti T, Pini Prato GP. Orthodontic and periodontal outcomes of treated impacted maxillary canines. Angle Orthod. 2007;77(4):571–7. https://doi.org/1 0.2319/080406-318.1.
15. Alqerban A, Jacobs R, Fieuws S, Willems G. Predictors of root resorption associated with maxillary canine impaction in panoramic images. Eur J Orthod. 2016;38(3):292–9. https://doi. org/10.1093/ejo/cjv047.
16. Vermette ME, Kokich VG, Kennedy DB. Uncovering labially impacted teeth: apically positioned flap and closed-eruption techniques. Angle Orthod. 1995;65(1):23–32.; discussion 3. https://doi.org/10.1043/0003-3219(1995)065<0023:Ulitap>2.0.Co;2.
17. Counihan K, Al-Awadhi EA, Butler J. Guidelines for the assessment of the impacted maxillary canine. Dent Update. 2013;40(9):770–2., 5–7. https://doi.org/10.12968/denu.2013.40.9.770.
18. Husain J, Burden D, McSherry P, Morris D, Allen M. National clinical guidelines for management of the palatally ectopic maxillary canine. Br Dent J. 2012;213(4):171–6. https://doi. org/10.1038/sj.bdj.2012.726.
19. Ericson S, Kurol J. Longitudinal study and analysis of clinical supervision of maxillary canine eruption. Community Dent Oral Epidemiol. 1986;14(3):172–6.
20. Eslami E, Barkhordar H, Abramovitch K, Kim J, Masoud MI. Cone-beam computed tomography vs conventional radiography in visualization of maxillary impacted-canine localization: a systematic review of comparative studies. Am J Orthod Dentofacial Orthop. 2017;151(2):248–58. https://doi.org/10.1016/j.ajodo.2016.07.018.
21. De Grauwe A, Ayaz I, Shujaat S, Dimitrov S, Gbadegbegnon L, Vande Vannet B, et al. CBCT in orthodontics: a systematic review on justification of CBCT in a paediatric population prior to orthodontic treatment. Eur J Orthod. 2019;41(4):381–9. https://doi.org/10.1093/ejo/cjy066.
22. Tsolakis AI, Kalavritinos M, Bitsanis E, Sanoudos M, Benetou V, Alexiou K, et al. Reliability of different radiographic methods for the localization of displaced maxillary canines. Am J Orthod Dentofac Orthop. 2018;153(2):308–14. https://doi.org/10.1016/j.ajodo.2017.06.026.
23. Ericson S, Kurol J. Radiographic examination of ectopically erupting maxillary canines. Am J Orthod Dentofacial Orthop. 1987;91(6):483–92.
24. Walker L, Enciso R, Mah J. Three-dimensional localization of maxillary canines with cone-beam computed tomography. Am J Orthod Dentofacial Orthop. 2005;128(4):418–23. https:// doi.org/10.1016/j.ajodo.2004.04.033.
25. Armstrong C, Johnston C, Burden D, Stevenson M. Localizing ectopic maxillary canines-horizontal or vertical parallax? Eur J Orthod. 2003;25(6):585–9.
26. Mason C, Papadakou P, Roberts GJ. The radiographic localization of impacted maxillary canines: a comparison of methods. Eur J Orthod. 2001;23(1):25–34. https://doi.org/10.1093/ejo/23.1.25.
27. Jawad Z, Carmichael F, Houghton N, Bates C. A review of cone beam computed tomography for the diagnosis of root resorption associated with impacted canines, introducing an innovative root resorption scale. Oral Surg Oral Med Oral Pathol Oral Radiol. 2016;122(6):765–71. https://doi.org/10.1016/j.oooo.2016.08.015.
28. Patel S, Dawood A, Wilson R, Horner K, Mannocci F. The detection and management of root resorption lesions using intraoral radiography and cone beam computed tomography - an in vivo investigation. Int Endod J. 2009;42(9):831–8. https://doi.org/10.1111/j.1365-2591 .2009.01592.x.
29. Durack C, Patel S, Davies J, Wilson R, Mannocci F. Diagnostic accuracy of small volume cone beam computed tomography and intraoral periapical radiography for the detection of

simulated external inflammatory root resorption. Int Endod J. 2011;44(2):136–47. https://doi.org/10.1111/j.1365-2591.2010.01819.x.
30. Ren H, Chen J, Deng F, Zheng L, Liu X, Dong Y. Comparison of cone-beam computed tomography and periapical radiography for detecting simulated apical root resorption. Angle Orthod. 2013;83(2):189–95. https://doi.org/10.2319/050512-372.1.
31. Sun H, Wang Y, Sun C, Ye Q, Dai W, Wang X, et al. Root morphology and development of labial inversely impacted maxillary central incisors in the mixed dentition: a retrospective cone-beam computed tomography study. Am J Orthod Dentofac Orthop. 2014;146(6):709–16. https://doi.org/10.1016/j.ajodo.2014.07.026.
32. Parkin N, Benson PE, Thind B, Shah A, Khalil I, Ghafoor S. Open versus closed surgical exposure of canine teeth that are displaced in the roof of the mouth. Cochrane Database Syst Rev. 2017;8:Cd006966. https://doi.org/10.1002/14651858.CD006966.pub3.
33. Parkin NA, Deery C, Smith AM, Tinsley D, Sandler J, Benson PE. No difference in surgical outcomes between open and closed exposure of palatally displaced maxillary canines. J Oral Maxillofac Surg. 2012;70(9):2026–34. https://doi.org/10.1016/j.joms.2012.02.028.
34. Smailiene D, Kavaliauskiene A, Pacauskiene I, Zasciurinskiene E, Bjerklin K. Palatally impacted maxillary canines: choice of surgical-orthodontic treatment method does not influence post-treatment periodontal status. A controlled prospective study. Eur J Orthod. 2013;35(6):803–10. https://doi.org/10.1093/ejo/cjs102.
35. Cassina C, Papageorgiou SN, Eliades T. Open versus closed surgical exposure for permanent impacted canines: a systematic review and meta-analyses. Eur J Orthod. 2018;40(1):1–10. https://doi.org/10.1093/ejo/cjx047.
36. Koutzoglou SI, Kostaki A. Effect of surgical exposure technique, age, and grade of impaction on ankylosis of an impacted canine, and the effect of rapid palatal expansion on eruption: a prospective clinical study. Am J Orthod Dentofac Orthop. 2013;143(3):342–52. https://doi.org/10.1016/j.ajodo.2012.10.017.
37. Sampaziotis D, Tsolakis IA, Bitsanis E, Tsolakis AI. Open versus closed surgical exposure of palatally impacted maxillary canines: comparison of the different treatment outcomes-a systematic review. Eur J Orthod. 2018;40(1):11–22. https://doi.org/10.1093/ejo/cjw077.
38. Wisth PJ, Norderval K, Booe OE. Comparison of two surgical methods in combined surgical-orthodontic correction of impacted maxillary canines. Acta Odontol Scand. 1976;34(1):53–7. https://doi.org/10.3109/00016357609026558.
39. Iramaneerat S, Cunningham SJ, Horrocks EN. The effect of two alternative methods of canine exposure upon subsequent duration of orthodontic treatment. Int J Paediatr Dent. 1998;8(2):123–9. https://doi.org/10.1046/j.1365-263x.1998.00075.x.
40. Benson PE, Atwal A, Bazargani F, Parkin N, Thind B. Interventions for promoting the eruption of palatally displaced permanent canine teeth, without the need for surgical exposure, in children aged 9 to 14 years. Cochrane Database Syst Rev. 2021;12:CD012851. https://doi.org/10.1002/14651858.CD012851.pub2.
41. Alyammahi AS, Kaklamanos EG, Athanasiou AE. Effectiveness of extraction of primary canines for interceptive management of palatally displaced permanent canines: a systematic review and meta-analysis. Eur J Orthod. 2018;40(2):149–56. https://doi.org/10.1093/ejo/cjx042.
42. Baccetti T, Sigler LM, McNamara JA Jr. An RCT on treatment of palatally displaced canines with RME and/or a transpalatal arch. Eur J Orthod. 2011;33(6):601–7. https://doi.org/10.1093/ejo/cjq139.
43. Baccetti T, Mucedero M, Leonardi M, Cozza P. Interceptive treatment of palatal impaction of maxillary canines with rapid maxillary expansion: a randomized clinical trial. Am J Orthod Dentofacial Orthop. 2009;136(5):657–61. https://doi.org/10.1016/j.ajodo.2008.03.019.
44. Naoumova J, Kjellberg H. The use of panoramic radiographs to decide when interceptive extraction is beneficial in children with palatally displaced canines based on a randomized clinical trial. Eur J Orthod. 2018;40(6):565–74. https://doi.org/10.1093/ejo/cjy002.

45. Naoumova J, Kurol J, Kjellberg H. Extraction of the deciduous canine as an interceptive treatment in children with palatal displaced canines - part I: shall we extract the deciduous canine or not? Eur J Orthod. 2015;37(2):209–18. https://doi.org/10.1093/ejo/cju040.

46. Armi P, Cozza P, Baccetti T. Effect of RME and headgear treatment on the eruption of palatally displaced canines: a randomized clinical study. Angle Orthod. 2011;81(3):370–4. https://doi.org/10.2319/062210-339.1.

47. Leonardi M, Armi P, Franchi L, Baccetti T. Two interceptive approaches to palatally displaced canines: a prospective longitudinal study. Angle Orthod. 2004;74(5):581–6. https://doi.org/10.1043/0003-3219(2004)074<0581:tiatpd>2.0.co;2.

48. Bazargani F, Magnuson A, Lennartsson B. Effect of interceptive extraction of deciduous canine on palatally displaced maxillary canine: a prospective randomized controlled study. Angle Orthod. 2014;84(1):3–10. https://doi.org/10.2319/031013-205.1.

49. Stewart JA, Heo G, Glover KE, Williamson PC, Lam EW, Major PW. Factors that relate to treatment duration for patients with palatally impacted maxillary canines. Am J Orthod Dentofacial Orthop. 2001;119(3):216–25. https://doi.org/10.1067/mod.2001.110989.

50. Arriola-Guillen LE, Aliaga-Del Castillo A, Ruiz-Mora GA, Rodriguez-Cardenas YA, Dias-Da Silveira HL. Influence of maxillary canine impaction characteristics and factors associated with orthodontic treatment on the duration of active orthodontic traction. Am J Orthod Dentofacial Orthop. 2019;156(3):391–400. https://doi.org/10.1016/j.ajodo.2018.10.018.

51. Becker A, Chaushu G, Chaushu S. Analysis of failure in the treatment of impacted maxillary canines. Am J Orthod Dentofacial Orthop. 2010;137(6):743–54. https://doi.org/10.1016/j.ajodo.2008.07.022.

52. Schroder AGD, Guariza-Filho O, de Araujo CM, Ruellas AC, Tanaka OM, Porporatti AL. To what extent are impacted canines associated with root resorption of the adjacent tooth?: a systematic review with meta-analysis. J Am Dent Assoc. 2018;149(9):765–77 e8. https://doi.org/10.1016/j.adaj.2018.05.012.

53. Guarnieri R, Cavallini C, Vernucci R, Vichi M, Leonardi R, Barbato E. Impacted maxillary canines and root resorption of adjacent teeth: a retrospective observational study. Med Oral Patol Oral Cir Bucal. 2016;21(6):e743–e50. https://doi.org/10.4317/medoral.21337.

54. Chaushu S, Kaczor-Urbanowicz K, Zadurska M, Becker A. Predisposing factors for severe incisor root resorption associated with impacted maxillary canines. Am J Orthod Dentofacial Orthop. 2015;147(1):52–60. https://doi.org/10.1016/j.ajodo.2014.09.012.

55. Arriola-Guillen LE, Ruiz-Mora GA, Rodriguez-Cardenas YA, Aliaga-Del Castillo A, Boessio-Vizzotto M, Dias-Da Silveira HL. Influence of impacted maxillary canine orthodontic traction complexity on root resorption of incisors: a retrospective longitudinal study. Am J Orthod Dentofacial Orthop. 2019;155(1):28–39. https://doi.org/10.1016/j.ajodo.2018.02.011.

56. Brusveen EM, Brudvik P, Boe OE, Mavragani M. Apical root resorption of incisors after orthodontic treatment of impacted maxillary canines: a radiographic study. Am J Orthod Dentofacial Orthop. 2012;141(4):427–35. https://doi.org/10.1016/j.ajodo.2011.10.022.

Orthodontic-Induced Inflammatory Root Resorption

8

Contents

Abbreviations

CAT	Clear aligners therapy
CB	Conventional brackets
ETT	Endodontically treated teeth
FA	Fixed appliance
LIPUS	Low-intensity pulsed ultrasound
LLLT	Low-level laser therapy
NSAIDs	Nonsteroidal anti-inflammatory drugs
OIIRR	Orthodontic-induced inflammatory root resorption
OVX	Ovariectomy
P	Pause
PGE	Prostaglandin
RR	Root resorption
SEM	Scanning electron microscopy
SLB	Self-ligating brackets
VT	Vital teeth
WP	Without pause

Introduction

One of the undesired iatrogenic effects of orthodontic treatment is root resorption [1]. Ottolengui in 1914 correlated root resorption to orthodontic treatment [2]. Ketcham was the first one who used radiographs to assess root resorption in 385 orthodontic-treated patients in his practice in 1926 [3]. Orthodontic induced inflammatory root resorption (OIIRR) results from the inflammatory process around the root, which is related to the orthodontic forces. Different factors may increase root resorption, which are divided into two categories: general factors and orthodontic factors. The general factors include systematic diseases, metabolism discords, hormonal conditions, medications [4], chemotherapy, radiotherapy, ethnicity [5], positive family history [6], type of malocclusions such as Class II division 2 [7], habits [8], tooth type [9], root form [5, 10], and previous history of trauma or previous root resorption [11]. The orthodontic-related factors comprise the characteristics of orthodontic forces, such as its magnitude, direction, and type. Treatment duration and different orthodontic appliances also fall in the orthodontic factors category. Root resorption is classified according to its severity. Mostly Levander and Malmgren classification [12] is used. The five grades of this classification are: Grade 0 having no root resorption, Grade 1 having irregular root outline, Grade 2 having <2 mm root resorption (minor), Grade 3 having >2 mm root resorption (severe), and Grade 4 having resorption >1/3 of root length (extreme).

OIIRR

Clinical Question 1: What Is the Average Amount of Orthodontic-Induced Inflammatory Root Resorption (OIIRR)?

Evidence

Systematic Review and Meta-Analysis
Samandara/2019 [13]

Seventeen studies that investigated the OIIRR were included in this review. It was found that the average linear OIIRR was 0.8 mm (95% CI: 0.5 to 1.0 mm) with fixed appliances using CBCT assessment. The total amount of OIIRR was significantly higher after treatment completion (1.1 mm) when compared with the initial stages of treatment (0.5 mm). Longer treatment duration was accompanied with higher root resorption by 0.36 mm/year. Furthermore, the volumetric OIIRR after fixed appliance treatment was 15.4 mm^3 (95% CI: -4.1 to 35.0 mm^3) in the three included studies. The authors assessed the level of the evidence as low.

Systematic Review
Weltman/2010 [11]

This review included 11 trials that compared orthodontically treated teeth with control teeth, which did not undergo orthodontic treatment. The study found that all teeth experiencing orthodontic movement had significantly higher RR than the control teeth.

Evidence Summary

The best available evidence suggests that orthodontic treatment is always accompanied by OIIRR. The average amount of linear root resorption is 0.8 mm in a comprehensive orthodontic treatment which increases at the rate of 0.36 mm/year for increased treatment duration. Volumetric OIIRR was 15.4 mm^3 after fixed orthodontic treatment.

Evidence Interpretation

There is always a small amount (0.8 mm) of root resorption associated with orthodontic treatment. This resorption is progressive and increases as the treatment duration increases. The patient and his parents should be informed about this iatrogenic effect before commencing the treatment.

Viewpoint

Samandara review [13] has low evidence regarding root resorption. The high risk of bias, the imprecision, and inclusion of non-randomized studies have reduced the quality of the evidence. Furthermore, the search for this review was done by 2015 and updated by 2017, which was 2 years before publishing and a further update was needed.

Weltman review [11] provided well-structured information. The authors in this review defined the inclusion criteria, but they included many comparison groups which do not meet their comparison group. Also, they used an uncommon tool for risk of bias without a reference for its validity that resulted in a moderate risk of bias in most included studies. The aforementioned issues might reduce the quality of the evidence.

Tooth and OIIRR

Clinical Question 2: Which Teeth Are Most Affected by Root Resorption?

Evidence

Systematic Review and Meta-Analysis
Samandara/2019 [13]

According to this review, the most affected teeth by OIIRR are the central incisors (0.8 mm, 95% CI; 0.4 to 1.3 mm), followed by lateral incisors (0.7 mm, 95% CI: 0.4 to 1.1 mm), then canines (0.4 mm, 95% CI; −0.3 to 1.0 mm). OIIRR in the anterior teeth (0.9, 95% CI: 0.6–1.1) was significantly greater than the OIIRR of the posterior teeth (OIIRR; 0.2 mm, 95% CI: −0.3 to 0.8 mm). The upper anterior teeth showed the largest amount of OIIRR (0.8 mm, 95% CI: 0.6–1.1 mm), followed by the lower anterior teeth (0.6 mm, 95% CI: −0.1 to 1.3 mm), the lower posterior teeth (OIIRR; 0.3 mm, 95% CI; −0.4 to 1.0 mm), and the upper posterior teeth (0.2 mm, 95% CI: −0.4 to 0.8 mm). The evidence was of low quality.

Retrospective Study
Fernandes/2019 [14]

The authors assessed OIIRR in 2173 maxillary incisors on periapical radiographs. The sample included 231 males and 333 females from three institutions. The authors found that laterals are more likely to have OIIRR than centrals (OR: 1.54, 95%CI: 1.25–1.83, p < 0.001). In other words, upper laterals have a higher risk of OIIRR than centrals by 54%.

Evidence Summary

The best available evidence suggests that the upper anterior teeth showed a greater amount of root resorption (MD; 0.8 mm, 95% CI: 0.6–1.1 mm) than lower anterior teeth (0.6 mm), lower posterior teeth (0.3 mm) and upper posterior teeth (0.2 mm).

Furthermore, low-level evidence suggests that laterals have a higher risk of root resorption than centrals by 54%.

Evidence Interpretation

In clinical orthodontics, the upper anterior teeth are the most affected teeth by root resorption, followed by lower anterior teeth. This might be due to different treatment modalities and movements of the anterior teeth done during the course of orthodontic treatment. Mostly on anterior teeth especially the upper anterior teeth, torque, and intrusive forces are given for ideal occlusal relationship. Both these types of forces are known to increase the chances of root resorption.

Viewpoint

The systematic review has already been discussed.

The retrospective design and use of periapical radiographs in Fernandes study [14] may be considered limitations of this study. Also, the majority of the sample was of White origin that may limit the generalizability. However, the large number of patients is a strong point of this study.

Teeth Morphology and OIIRR

Clinical Question 3: What Is the Effect of Root Morphology on Root Resorption?

Evidence

Ambidirectional Study
Brin/2003 [15]

The authors assessed the records of 138 Class II patients who completed the fixed appliance treatment phase. At the beginning of fixed appliance treatment, 35.5% of the maxillary incisors showed some kind of unusual root morphology. The authors found that a tooth with unusual root shape had slightly more risk of moderate to severe OIRR than a tooth with normal root shape.

Prospective Study
Smale/2005 [16]

The authors included 290 orthodontic patients; 191 females and 99 males aged 19.2 ± 10.6 years with a range of (10.1–57.1) years. The authors treated the patients with fixed appliances, either with 0.018 or 0.022-in slot and measured the length of four incisors on periapical radiographs before and after approximately 6 months (6.4 ± 0.9) of the active treatment. Univariate linear regression indicated that root form affects root resorption. Deviated and pointed roots of central incisors have a higher likelihood of root resorption by 0.14 and 0.16, respectively, and this was statistically significant. While normal roots were associated with less OIIRR (-0.21, $p < 0.001$).

Likewise, higher odds of root resorption were found in deviated and pointed lateral roots (0.22 and 0.21, respectively), and a lower likelihood of OIIRR was reported for normal lateral roots (−0.34, p < 0.001).

Retrospective Studies
Kook/2003 [17]

The authors collected data for 114 patients from four offices to compare OIIRR in normal and deformed maxillary laterals. Sixty-nine patients had 44 peg shape laterals and 25 small laterals, and 43 patients were in a control group. The average amount of RR was 1.06 mm in peg shape laterals and 1.30 mm in small laterals. There was no statistically significant difference between peg-shaped laterals and normal lateral incisors regarding OIIRR; 1.09 mm and 0.88 mm in peg-shaped and normal lateral incisors, respectively. In contrast, there was a statistically significant difference in OIIRR between small laterals (1.03 mm) and normal lateral incisors (1.62 mm).

Fernandes/2019 [14]

Authors collected data from three institutions to investigate factors that affect OIIRR in the maxillary incisors. The authors assessed data of 564 patients (231 males and 333 females) with 2173 maxillary incisors on periapical radiographs. They found the root shape has an impact on the OIIRR. A higher odd was found in the triangular root than in rhomboid root (OR:1.44, 95%CI: 0.98–2.09, p = 0.06). Likewise, dilacerated roots had a higher risk of OIIRR (OR; 2.26, 95%CI: 1.53 to 3.36, p < 0.001). Pipette root shape also had a higher risk of OIIRR than rhomboid roots (OR; 1.71, 95%CI: 0.99–2.49, p = 0.052).

Evidence Summary

Looking into the evidence collectively, the available evidence suggests that abnormal or deviated root morphology may be considered a risk factor for root resorption, as these deformed teeth have moderate to severe OIIRR more than teeth with normal root shape. In this respect, maxillary incisors having deviated and pointed roots have a higher risk of OIIRR. Dilacerated roots were at higher risk of OIRR than rhomboid roots by 126%. Likewise, teeth with triangular or pipette root shape have a higher risk of OIIRR than teeth with normal root shape by 44% and 71%, respectively.

Peg shaped laterals had a higher amount of OIIRR than normal incisors, but this was not statistically significant. In contrast, small laterals had a less OIIRR (1.03 mm) than incisors (1.62 mm).

Evidence Interpretation

Abnormal root morphology increases the chances of orthodontic-induced root resorption. Teeth with dilacerated, pointed, pipette, and triangular roots have more chances of root resorption than teeth with normal root shape. Peg-shaped lateral incisors may have more chances of root resorption.

In case of abnormal root morphology, the clinician should take detailed informed consent from the patient. Also, root resorption in susceptible teeth should be monitored periodically following the ALARP (as low as reasonably practicable) principle. If there is moderate to severe root resorption, a rest period should be given, and a revised realistic treatment plan should be adopted.

Viewpoint

Brin study [15] was of a retrospective design that followed up Class II patients' treatment. There was a lack of sample size calculation that may underpower the findings. The prevalence of traumatized teeth in the sample may confound the results. The authors found that the root morphology was repeatable in 89% of the sample using OPG, which may leave room for error.

Smale study [16] provides good information regarding OIIRR but the use of different treatment appliances with different sequences of archwires in both modalities may confound the findings. Other factors that may reduce the quality of the evidence are the wide age range, the difficulty in standardizing the periapical radiographs, and the lack of sample size calculation. Kook et al. study [17] was of a retrospective design and collected data from different clinics that may provide a better overall assessment of the OIRR. However, the extraction pattern, the experience of the clinician, the mechanotherapy used, the intrusion movement, and the uneven gender distribution may confound the findings. Interestingly, the findings are applicable to adolescent female patients with a Class I of malocclusion and non-extraction treatment.

Clinical Question 4: What Is the Effect of Root Length on OIIRR?

Evidence

Retrospective Studies
Fernandes/2019 [14]

The authors assessed the length of 2173 maxillary incisors on periapical radiographs. They found that root length has an impact on the OIIRR (OR:1.29, 95%CI: 1.2 to 1.37, P < 0.001). Thus, the risk of OIRR increases by 29% for each additional millimeter of root length.

Mirabella/1995 [18]

Authors collected 500 orthodontic patient records before and after treatment from four practices. After removing incomplete records, 343 records remained. The age range was 20 to 70.1 years, with an average treatment duration of 2 ± 0.7 years. The root resorption was assessed using periapical radiographs of maxillary anterior teeth. They found that increased tooth length was associated with greater root resorption.

Evidence Summary

The best available evidence suggests that there is a positive association between root length and root resorption. Longer roots have a higher likelihood of OIIRR; for every additional millimeter of root length, there is an increase in the risk to root resorption by 29%.

Evidence Interpretation

There are more chances of root resorption in teeth with long roots. This can be due to the higher moment-to-force ratio required to move these teeth.

Viewpoint

Mirabella study [18] had a large sample. However, the authors excluded 157 records from the study that may increase the selection bias. Other different factors may also confound the results. Interestingly, it would be better to assess the ratio of root resorption rather than the sole measurement; for instance, the ratio of 1 mm root resorption in 10 mm root is equal to 1.5 mm in 15 mm root.

Force Direction Effect

Clinical Question 5: Which Type of Tooth Movement Is Associated with OIIRR?

Evidence

Systematic Review and Meta-Analysis
Bellini-Pereira/2020 [19]

This systematic review included 14 studies: three were RCTs, six were prospective studies, and five were retrospective studies. The authors pooled seven studies in a meta-analysis to evaluate the OIIRR in upper anterior and posterior teeth after tooth intrusion. The maxillary incisors intrusion movement, with a range of (1.55–2.48 mm), yielded an OIIRR of 0.72 mm (95% CI: 0.16–1.28, $P < 0.01$, 4 studies). Likewise, the maxillary molars intrusion movement with a range of (2.79–3.40 mm) resulted in OIRR of 0.41 mm (95% CI: −0.24 to 1.07, $P = 0.22$, 3 studies), but this was not statistically significant. The evidence was graded as moderate for anterior intrusion and low for posterior intrusion.

Systematic Reviews
Roscoe/2015 [20]

In this review, four included studies found that root resorption in the bucco-cervical and lingual-apical regions were associated with buccal tipping. Also, OIIRR in buccal-apical and palatal-cervical regions was associated with buccal root torque. OIIRR in distal surfaces was associated with extrusion movement. The impact of intrusion movement on OIIRR was not clear in this study.

Weltman/2010 [11]

In this review, one RCT [21] compared intrusive and extrusive forces with a control group. The study found that there was no difference between extrusive force and the control group regarding RR. Intrusive force significantly increased the percentage of OIIRR area by fourfolds. The correlation between RR after intrusion and extrusion in the same patient was significantly strong r = 0.774 (P = 0.024). Another included RCT [22] reported that the volume of RR craters was correlated with the intrusive force magnitude.

Randomized Controlled Trial

Han/2005 [21]

This trial was included in the Weltman systematic review [11]. The intervention sample comprised of 18 upper first premolars in nine patients with a mean age of 15.3 years (12.7–20 years). A control group of 11 extracted premolars were randomly obtained before active treatment from six patients. The researchers randomly assigned one premolar to the intrusion group and the other to the extrusion group. The patients applied a force of 100 cN (100 g) on each premolar using an elastic band which was changed daily. After 8 weeks, the 18 teeth were extracted and examined using scanning electron microscopy (SEM). The average percentage of root resorption in control, extruded and intruded teeth were 0.52 ± 0.39%, 1.28 ± 0.43%, and 5.75 ± 1.38%, respectively. The OIRR was significantly higher in the intrusion group than in the extrusion group (P = 0.006).

Evidence Summary

Looking into the available evidence collectively, intrusion forces result in apical root resorption for maxillary incisors and maxillary molars by 0.72 mm and 0.41 mm, respectively [19]. Buccal tipping was associated with root resorption in the bucco-cervical and lingual-apical regions. Buccal root torque was associated with RR in buccal-apical and palatal-cervical regions, while extrusion movement was associated with RR in distal surface [20]. In contrast, another review [11] found no difference in RR between extrusive force and the control group. However, when extrusion was compared with intrusion tooth movement, an RCT [21] found that the RR was significantly higher in the intrusion group than in the extrusion group, 5.75 ± 1.38% and 1.28 ± 0.43%, respectively (P = 0.006). Moreover, the amount of root resorption caused by intrusion force [22] was associated with the magnitude of the force.

Evidence Interpretation

Low to moderate quality evidence indicates that incisor intrusion is associated with more root resorption than molar intrusion. Intrusive tooth movement is associated more with root resorption than extrusive tooth movement. As such, light forces can be given for intrusive movements under careful observation. Furthermore, according to the present evidence, tipping, torque, and extrusion are associated with root resorption and region of root resorption depends upon the type of tooth movement.

Viewpoint

The clinician should interpret the Bellini-Pereira review [19] results with caution due to the clinical heterogeneity and the different imaging methods between included studies. However, to some extent, the author undertook a sensitivity analysis to control these factors and found a minor impact of the imaging methods on the outcome measures.

The included studies, in Roscoe [20] review, were of different quality due to the absence of a control group, the lack of randomization, the selection criteria of patients, and methodological differences in measurement. In Han trial [21] there was a lack of sample size calculation which is a crucial point. The low sample size may underpower the study. The lack of information regarding allocation concealment and improper blinding may also reduce the certainty of the findings. It is worth mentioning that the force application was made by the patients themselves that may confound the results as the force application was not uniform.

The Influence of Force on OIRR

Clinical Question 6: What Is the Effect of Force Magnitude on Root Resorption?

Evidence

Systematic Review
Currell/2019 [23]
This systematic review synthesized qualitatively 25 studies for 24 RCTs. Eleven included trials evaluated the effect of heavy and low force on root resorption and found a positive association between OIIRR and the magnitude of force. However, the evidence was of very low to low quality.

Weltman/2010 [11]
In this review, four split-mouth studies compared heavy (225 g) versus light continuous force (25 g) and found that heavy continuous force produced significantly more root resorption than light continuous force. An included RCT [22] reported that the volume of RR craters was correlated with the intrusive force magnitude. The mean volume of the resorption craters was 3.49 and 11.59 times greater in the light and heavy orthodontic force group, respectively, than in the control group.

Roscoe/2015 [20]
This systematic review investigated OIRR and included 21 studies; 11 were RCTs, 8 were non-randomized controlled trials, and two were cohort studies. The review found a positive correlation between heavy forces and increased root resorption in 12 included studies.

Evidence Summary
Looking into the available evidence collectively, the best available evidence suggests that there is a positive association between the amount of root resorption and

the magnitude of the applied force. Both light and heavy continuous orthodontic forces cause greater volumetric resorption carters than the control group by 3.49 and 11.59 times, respectively.

Evidence Interpretation

The force magnitude has a positive correlation with the amount of root resorption. Both light and heavy forces are associated with root resorption, so some root resorption is inevitable even if the clinician uses light orthodontic forces.

From a clinical point of view, the clinician should apply low-level forces, and ideally light continuous forces should be preferred over heavy continuous forces. The prime examples of heavy continuous forces are those applied with a high stretch of power chains or NiTi coil springs. The clinician should also assess root resorption in cases where orthopedic forces are used as these forces are heavy and might be correlated with significant root resorption.

Viewpoint

Though Currell review [23] was a well-conducted study and included only the randomized controlled trials, there were some shortcomings in this review. The authors did not assess the root resorption quantitively, even for some trials out of the 24 included RCTs. Most of the included trials were having unclear to high risk of bias that may reduce the quality of the evidence.

The rest of the reviews have been discussed before.

Clinical Question 7: What Is the Effect of Force Regime (Continuous Versus Intermittent Versus Interrupted Forces) on Root Resorption?

Evidence

Systematic Review
Weltman/2010 [11]

In this review, one included trial [24] compared continuous versus discontinuous force and found that continuous force of 100 g for 24 hours/day by elastics produced significantly more RR than a discontinuous force of 100 g for 12 hours/day. Though the authors used the term continuous forces, but elastics provides intermittent forces according to the classical definition. So, the comparison in this study is basically between continuous intermittent force and interrupted intermittent force. Four included trials in this review compared heavy versus light force and found that heavy force (225 g) produced significantly higher RR than light force (25 g).

Roscoe/2015 [20]

Two included studies [25, 26], in this review, investigated the effect of continuous and interrupted forces on root resorption. One study [25] did not find a significant difference between different force systems on OIIRR. In contrast, another study [26] found a significant difference between stainless steel and superelastic archwire systems regarding OIIRR, with a significantly larger OIIRR in the superelastic group. Though the authors did not explain in which domain the two wires fall, but it is our understanding that stainless steel wires provide interrupted force due to its low working range while superelastic NiTi wires provide light continuous force.

Evidence Summary

In the Weltman systematic review [11], a comparison was made between continuous intermittent force and interrupted intermittent force of the same magnitude and it was found that continuous forces cause more OIIRR. However, when a comparison was made between heavy (225 g) versus light forces (25 g), heavy force provoked more RR. In the second review [20], continuous and interrupted forces were compared. One trial [25] did not report a significant influence of the force system on OIIRR. While another included trial [26] found that continuous force produced more OIRR than the interrupted force.

Evidence Interpretation

Continuous and heavy forces produce greater root resorption. From a clinical point, using a rest period between forces may avoid critical OIIRR. The clinician may consider a pause period during tooth movement, whether using continuous or intermittent force, to reduce the chances of resorption. Also, whatever force system is used the force magnitude should always be low.

Viewpoint

For the force continuity, Acar study [24] was judged at a high risk of bias in the systematic review of Weltman [11]. Hence, the evidence, regarding the effect of the continuity of the force on OIIRR, is from low-quality evidence, and the results should be interpreted with caution. Also, the authors reported the OIRR only in 9 weeks for both force regimes (24 versus 12 hours per day).

In clinical orthodontics, we mostly use light continuous forces. As the level of evidence for continuous force is low, and root resorption during orthodontic treatment is inevitable, the light continuous forces may still be used till further high-quality evidence is available.

Orthodontic Appliance Types

Clinical Question 8: What Is the Difference in Root Resorption Between Conventional and Self-Ligating Appliances?

Evidence

Systematic Review and Meta-Analysis
Yi/2016 [27]
This systematic review included seven studies: one was RCT, two were CCTs, and four were cohort studies. Five trials (1 RCT, 2 CCTs, and two cohort studies) were pooled in a meta-analysis. The five studies investigated root resorption in the upper

and lower incisors. Meta-analysis showed that self-ligating brackets (SLB) caused less root resorption in upper central incisors when compared with conventional brackets (CB) (SMD: −0.31, 95% CI: −0.60 to −0.01). In contrast, there were no statistically significant differences regarding root resorption between SLB and CB in maxillary lateral incisors (SMD; −0.14, 95% CI: −0.16 to 0.43), mandibular central incisors (SMD: 0.20, 95% CI: −0.05 to 0.45) and mandibular lateral incisors (SMD: −0.15, 95% CI: −0.45 to 0.14).

Evidence Summary

The best available evidence suggests that there is no difference between self-ligating and conventional brackets in regard to OIRR except for the upper central incisors. This difference was minor but statistically significant (SMD −0.31; 95% CI: −0.60 to −0.01), favoring the self-ligating brackets.

Evidence Interpretation

From the available evidence, there is no difference in RR when using different fixed appliances; conventional or self-ligating. Hence, OIIRR is more affected by the magnitude of the force and the applied mechanics, rather than the type of the fixed appliance.

Viewpoint

Most of the included studies in Yi review [27] were at moderate risk of bias. Most included studies were from cohort design and suffering from confounding. The authors included different study designs in the meta-analysis that reduced the quality of the evidence.

Clinical Question 9: What Is the Difference in Root Resorption Between Aligners and the Fixed Appliance?

Evidence

Systematic Reviews and Meta-Analyses
Gandhi/2020 [28]

This review included 16 studies, 4 were prospective, and 12 were retrospective studies, to compare the fixed appliance (FA) with clear aligners (CAT) regarding the root resorption in the upper four incisors. Seven included trials investigated RR in FA, while only 3 trials investigated RR in CAT. The authors found that the overall RR was less than 1 mm in the upper central and lateral incisors for all appliances (overall OIIRR, MD; 0.49 mm; 95%CI:0.24–0.75 mm). The difference in RR of the four incisors between the two appliances was not statically significant (MD; −0.19, 95%CI: −0.77 to 0.39, p = 0.524). There was a statistically significant difference between the FA and CAT only for the upper left lateral incisor (MD; −0.41, 95%CI: −0.67 to −0.15, p = 0.002) but not for other incisors.

Fang/2019 [29]

This study included 11 studies in the qualitative analysis. The authors pooled three cohort studies in meta-analysis to investigate the differences in RR between FA and CAT. All incisors exhibited a significantly lesser RR in CAT than FA (SMD; −0.65, 95% CI: −0.74 to −0.55, P < 0.01).

Systematic Reviews

Elhaddaoui/2017 [30]

This review included three studies to investigate root resorption after orthodontic treatment using clear aligners (CAT). One included study was a randomized controlled trial, and the other two studies were from retrospective design. In one included trial [31], there were no signs of RR in 54% of teeth after orthodontic treatment using CATs. For the rest, 27.75% of teeth had a mild reduction of root length (0%–10%), 12% of the teeth had moderate reduction (10%–20%), while 6.3% of teeth had severe resorption (> 20% reduction) after orthodontic treatment using CATs. However, an unpublished retrospective study [32] found that there was no RR in the CAT group, while it was 2–50% in the FA group. Another RCT [33] study found that the clear aligners presented root resorption similar to the FA group with light force (25 g).

Roscoe/2015 [20]

Only one included trial [33] evaluated the impact of appliance design on OIIRR. The authors found that patients treated using either CAT or conventional FA reported similar results regarding OIRR under a low-force system.

Evidence Summary

Looking into the available evidence collectively, the best evidence indicates no major difference in root resorption between aligners and fixed appliances. Gandhi et al. [28] reported that there is no difference between aligners and fixed appliances except for the upper left central incisor (0.36 mm and 0.74 mm, for CAT and FA, respectively). Other studies [20, 30], reported similar results regarding OIIRR between CAT and FA.

In contrast, Fang et al. [29] found that the CAT exhibited less OIIRR in the incisors (SMD = −0.65). Also, one unpublished retrospective study [32] reported that there was no root resorption in the clear aligners group.

Evidence Interpretation

There is no significant difference between CAT and FA in terms of RR. However, a slightly less RR was noted in CAT, but at the clinical level, the difference is not significant.

In general, it is an established fact that the root movement in aligners is limited, as most of these cases are simple cases of leveling and alignment, or need a minor tooth movement, which may be a major reason for decrease OIIRR in the aligner group.

Viewpoint

In Gandhi et al. review [28], most of the included studies were retrospective in nature with the absence of high-quality randomized trials. Also, confounding factors and conflict of interest may bias the findings.

Elhaddaoui et al. review [30] analyzed qualitatively three studies. Only one study was RCT, but with low sample size and a short follow-up period of 8 weeks. The authors did not assess the quality of the included studies. Also, the retrospective study that reported no RR in the aligner group was an unpublished thesis and had a lot of shortcomings due to selection and confounding bias, as well as the conflict of interest. So, the bias in the included trials may reduce the quality of the evidence.

In Fang review [29], the limitations were inclusion of only cohort studies and the lack of unified measurement of RR. In most included studies, only non-extraction cases were included, which means the cases were of mild to moderate crowding that may also cause bias of confounding factors. A related point to note is the suboptimal statistical methods to analyze the cluster data.

Expansion and OIIRR

Clinical Question 10: What Is the Effect of Expansion Appliances on Root Resorption?

Evidence

Systematic Review and Meta-Analysis
Samandara/2019 [13]

In this systematic review, three included studies that investigated RME effect on OIIRR found that the linear OIIRR average was 0.4 mm (95% CI; -1.0 to 1.7 mm) without any significant differences among teeth. However, the average volumetric OIIRR after RME was 25.7 mm^3 (95% CI; 6.9–44.5 mm^3;4 studies), and the differences among teeth were considerable; the first molar showed significantly greater OIIRR than first premolars; 40.2 and 14.8 mm^3, respectively. The evidence for these findings was low.

Systematic Review
Forst/2014 [34]

This review included three studies that investigated the effect of jackscrew maxillary expansion on root resorption. Two of the included studies were non-randomized trials, while one was a retrospective study. Two included studies assessed root resorption on 2D radiographs and found that there was no sign of root resorption post-expansion. In contrast, the same two studies evaluated the root resorption using either scanning electron or light microscopy after premolars extraction and found that all anchored premolars exhibited root resorption that could not be noticed on the 2D radiographs. The 3D radiographic (CBCT) assessment used in one included study revealed that there is a statistically significant root volume loss post-expansion.

Evidence Summary

Collectively the best available evidence showed consistency in the data regarding OIIRR post-expansion. One systematic review [13] assessed the impact of RME on root resorption and found that the linear OIIRR was 0.4 mm (95% CI;−1.0 to 1.7 mm), while the volumetric OIIRR was 25.7 mm^3 (95% CI; 6.9 to 44.5 mm^3;4 studies). The first molar showed a larger OIRR (40.2 mm^3) than the first premolars (14.8 mm^3). A systematic review [34] assessed the root resorption post-treatment by jackscrew maxillary expansion. This review found that all anchored premolars exhibited mild OIIRR, which is not noticeable on the 2D radiographs. In contrast 3D radiographic (CBCT) assessment used in one included study revealed that there is a statistically significant root volume loss post-expansion.

Evidence Interpretation

Maxillary expansion may induce root resorption of the expander-supporting teeth, especially the molars. Also, if the clinician wants to assess root resorption post-expansion, CBCT is a more reliable tool to detect root resorption than conventional 2-dimensional X-rays.

Viewpoints

The included studies in Forst's review [34] failed to calculate sample sizes or to report inter- or intra-rater reliability. Other weaknesses were present in the allocation concealment and blinding that reduced the quality of the evidence regarding the aforementioned outcome. Viewpoint about other evidence has already been discussed.

Tooth Vitality

Clinical Question 11: What Is the Difference in Root Resorption Between Vital and Endodontically Treated Teeth?

Evidence

Systematic Review and Meta-Analysis
Alhadainy/2019 [35]

This review included seven studies in meta-analysis to investigate the difference between vital teeth (VT) and endodontically treated teeth (ETT) regarding RR. Four included studies were retrospective, and three were prospective. The authors found that there is a statistically significant less OIIRR in ETT (MD;0.31 mm; 95% CI: 0.11–0.5 mm; P = 0.02; I^2 = 69%). The authors graded the evidence at very low level.

Systematic Review
Walker/2013 [36]

This systematic review included four split-mouth retrospective studies investigating the difference between VT and ETT regarding RR. There was a statistically significant RR in both groups. The authors found that there is no difference in RR between ETT and analogous VT during orthodontic treatment, with a slightly increased RR in VT with a range of (0.22–0.77 mm).

Evidence Summary

Collectively, the best available evidence showed that there is slightly more RR in VT than ETT. One review [36] revealed that there was no statistically significant difference in OIIRR between ETT and VT with a slightly increased OIIRR in VT, while another review [35] concluded that the OIIRR was statistically greater by 0.31 mm (0.11–0.5 mm; P = 0.002) in VT when compared with ETT. The difference between the two reviews [35, 36] findings could be due to the number and the design of included studies.

Evidence Interpretation

ETT exhibited less OIIRR than VT, but this difference was very minor. The clinical significance of the findings is that endodontically treated teeth can be moved by orthodontic force with less risk of OIIRR.

The evidence does not suggest doing endodontic treatment to vital teeth with a higher risk of root resorption.

Viewpoint

Methodological variations between included studies in both Walker and Alhadainy review [35, 36], lack of standardization of the radiographs (panoramic and periapical), and confounders are limitations of the aforementioned reviews. Also, the findings should be interpreted with caution as the included studies were retrospective and prone to confounders like a history of previous trauma, external root resorption prior to orthodontic treatment, and variation of orthodontic treatment mechanics.

Treatment Duration and OIIRR

Clinical Question 12: What Is the Effect of the Treatment Duration on Root Resorption?

Evidence

Systematic Reviews
Roscoe/2015 [20]

This systematic review concluded that there is a positive correlation between increased treatment time and increased RR. Included trials compared three experimental periods of force application (4, 8, and 12 weeks) and found that OIIRR was significantly higher in 12 weeks group. One included trial [37] reported that the depth of resorption lacunae increased significantly from the third week of the force application.

Samandara/2019 [13]

In this systematic review, meta-regression indicated that longer treatment duration was associated with higher root resorption by 0.36 mm/year.

Evidence Summary

The best available evidence suggests that the OIIRR increases when the treatment duration increases. One review [20] concluded that OIIRR was greater in the 12th week than fourth and eighth weeks. Likewise, it was reported that a higher root resorption by 0.36 mm for each extra year in the treatment duration [13].

Evidence Interpretation

The clinician should bear in mind the effect of orthodontic treatment duration on RR, and every effort should be made to keep the treatment duration to a realistic minimum.

Viewpoint

The limitations of the reviews are already being discussed.

Extraction and OIRR

Clinical Question 13: What Is the Effect of Extraction Pattern on OIRR?

Evidence

Systematic Reviews and Meta-Analyses
Samandara/2019 [13]

This review reported that the extraction may increase the OIRR; OIRR in extraction and non-extraction groups was 0.8 and 0.5 mm, respectively. The authors suggested that longer treatment in the extraction group might be the reason for increasing the OIRR.

Deng/2018 [38]

This review included 9 trials in meta-analysis to investigate the effect of extraction on OIRR. Subgroup analysis showed that OIRR in the extraction group was 1.03 mm (95%CI:0.77 to 1.30, p < 0.001), and it was 0.77 mm (95%CI:0.37 to 1.18, p < 0.001) in non-extraction group. The difference between the two groups was not statistically significant.

Evidence Summary

Looking into evidence collectively, the best available evidence suggests that the extraction may increase OIRR, but this did not reach a statistically significant difference. The average OIRR ranged from 0.5 to 0.77 mm in non-extraction group and from 0.8 mm to 1.03 mm in the extraction group due to different inclusion criteria between the systematic reviews [13, 38].

Evidence Interpretation

Extraction treatments are associated with a greater amount of root resorption than non-extraction treatments. The clinician should be aware of the OIRR in extraction treatments and should make this point clear to the patients and their parents.

Viewpoint

Deng et al. review [38] included non-randomized studies of moderate quality that may reduce the quality of the evidence. These studies lack a sample size calculation that may underpower the findings. Furthermore, many confounding factors such as the magnitude of force, alveolar shape, type of tooth movement, age, and gender play a vital role in OIRR.

Other studies have been discussed before.

Effect of Pause on RR

Clinical Question 14: What Is the Impact of Treatment Pause on Root Resorption?

Evidence

Systematic Review
Weltman/2010 [11]

In this systematic review, one included trial [39] found that the pause during active treatment significantly decreased the amount of RR (0.4 ± 0.7 mm) when compared with treatment using continuous forces without a pause (1.5 ± 0.8 mm). According to this systematic review, there is some evidence that a 2–3 months pause in treatment decreases the total root resorption.

Randomized Clinical Trial
Levander/1994 [39]

This RCT was included in the Weltman review [11]. The authors randomly assigned 28 patients into two groups; 32 teeth in a group without pause (WP) and 30 teeth in a group with pause (P) using a 0.018 edgewise appliance. The treatment continued in the WP group according to the treatment plan, while it was discontinued for 2–3 months in the P group during active treatment using passive wire. The mean duration of active treatment was 21 months in the WP group and 20 months in the P group. The radiographs were done using an individual film holder. The researchers found that the RR in the P group was statistically less than the RR in the WP group. In WP group, 23 teeth have RR more than 1.5 mm and 8 teeth more than 2.5 mm. While in P group, RR was equal or less than 0.5 mm in 23 teeth, and seven teeth exhibited more than 0.5 mm of RR.

Evidence Summary

Looking into evidence collectively, low-level evidence suggests that the pause after active treatment results in a significant decrease in RR. The amount of RR was (0.4 ± 0.7 mm) in P group, while it was (1.5 ± 0.8 mm) in the WP group.

Evidence Interpretation

A treatment pause of 2–3 months during active treatment can decrease iatrogenic root resorption.

In contemporary clinical practice, no treatment pause is given, but in cases with significant RR, a pause of 2–3 months in active orthodontic treatment may help the clinician to prevent further RR.

Viewpoint

Levander trial [39] provided the clinician with a piece of good information. The shortcomings of the study were the lack of sample size calculation that may under-power the study, the lack of proper randomization and blinding, and the confounding factors which result from the imbalance between groups regarding age, gender, and initial malocclusion. Weltman [11] systematic review has been already discussed.

Supplementation and OIIRR

Clinical Question 15: What Is the Effect of Supplementation on the OIIRR?

Evidence

Systematic Review and Meta-Analysis
Haugland/2018 [40]

This review included 9 human studies and 36 animal studies to investigate the effect of different adjunctive therapies on OIIRR. Meta-analysis showed that systemic supplements of fluoride decreased the OIRR (ES; -2.08, 95%CI: -3.02 to -1.14, $p < 0.05$). Other systemic supplements did not provide a significant effect on OIRR; prostaglandin (PGE) (ES; 0.26, 95%CI: -0.14 to 0.66, $p > 0.05$). Low-level laser therapy (LLLT) did not have a significant impact on OIRR in animals (ES; -0.35, 95%CI: -1.04 to 0.34, $p > 0.05$). Likewise, other interventions such as low-intensity pulsed ultrasound (LIPUS) and mechanical vibration have no effects on OIRR. In contrast, corticotomy increased the OIRR (ES;0.38, 95%CI:0.05, 0.71, $p < 0.05$).

For hormone administration in rats, thyroxine inhibited OIRR (ES: -1.91, 95%CI: -3.20 to-0.61, p < 0.05), while ovariectomy (OVX) increased OIRR (ES:1.90, 95%CI: -0.65 to 4.45, p > 0.05). Medications such as nonsteroidal anti-inflammatory drugs (NSAIDs) did not have a significant impact on OIRR in animal studies. In contrast, steroids inhibited OIIRR (ES = -2.79, 95%CI: -4.26 to -1.33).

Systematic Reviews
Kaklamanos/2020 [41]
This review included studies that assessed exposed participants (age: 12–28 years) to high and low amounts of fluoride intake from birth. Nabumetone administration seems to be effective in reducing OIIRR, whereas fluoride was not. Fluoride showed a protective effect during the period of the heavy force application.

Berry/2020 [42]
This review included 8 animal studies investigating the effect of thyroxine administration on OIRR. Three included trials reported that thyroxine administration decreased OIRR, while two trials found no significant effect of thyroxine administration on OIRR, and the evidence was of low quality.

Evidence Summary
Looking into evidence collectively, fluoride decreased the OIRR (ES;-2.08, 95%CI:-3.02, -1.14, p < 0.05) in animal studies [40] with contradictory data from human studies; as it seems that fluoride has no effect in human studies [41]. Likewise, thyroxine inhibited OIRR (ES: -1.91, 95%CI: -3.20, -0.61, p < 0.05) in animal studies. On the other hand, PGE, LLLT, LIPUS, and mechanical vibration have no effect on OIRR. While, OVX and corticotomy increased the OIIRR.

Evidence Interpretation
Most of the studies did not provide the adverse effects of adjunctive supplementation. Hence, increasing the uptake of fluoride seems to have no effect on OIRR and if there are adverse effects it should not be recommended, especially for teeth abnormalities in children. From a clinical point, thyroxine injections may be considered unethical due to its systematic effect. So, patients with thyroid hormone-related disorders should be assessed carefully. In regard to other medications and interventions, it appears that they are not effective to decrease RR and the evidence comes from animal and primary studies, so these interventions should not be used at present.

Viewpoint
Haugland et al. review [40] provided information on OIRR from both animal and humans studies. Hence, the findings cannot be directly extrapolated to humans. Most of the included studies were at unclear risk of bias that may lead to poor quality of the evidence.

Kaklamanos review [41] provided good information on the effects of fluoride on OIRR in humans. But the inclusion of non-randomized studies and the unclear risk of bias in the included studies may reduce the quality of the evidence. The comparison was made between two groups that received different concentrations of fluoride via drinking water with no zero-intake control group.

Berry et al. review [42] provide a useful information from prospective human trials. A high risk of bias was given to most trials due to the lack of randomization and blinding. Thyroxine injection may be an indicator of clinical malpractice due to its systematic effect.

Mobility and OIRR

Clinical Question 16: What Is the Relationship between Root Length and Mobility in Teeth with Severe OIRR?

Evidence

Ambidirectional Study
Levander/2000 [43]

This was a long-term follow up study for orthodontic-treated patients. The authors examined 73 maxillary incisors in 20 patients; 13 patients (age 24–32 years) were checked after 10–15 years of active treatment, and 7 patients (age 20–25 years) were checked after 5–10 years. Twenty-three incisors had fixed twist flex retainer. Researchers assessed tooth mobility using Miller's index (0–4) and Periotest method. The total root lengths of incisors ranged from 5.5 mm to 18.1 mm. Twenty-seven incisors had root lengths less than 9 mm. The intra-alveolar root lengths ranged from 4.1 mm to 16.6 mm. The authors found that a mobility rating of 1 was recorded in 15 teeth; 14 teeth with root lengths less than 9 mm, and one tooth with root lengths of 12.1 mm. Similarly, the value of Periotest (objective measurement of tooth mobility by measuring the damping characteristics of periodontium) higher than 10 was recorded in 19 teeth with root lengths less than 9 mm. A Periotest value of 10 was recorded only in one tooth with a root length 12.1 mm. Interestingly, 12 teeth out of 23 bonded teeth had Periotest $\geq$ 10 with no significant effect of bonding retainers on mobility.

Evidence Summary

The best available evidence suggests that a tooth with roots shorter than 9 mm has a mobility rating value of 1 and Periotest value higher than 10.

Evidence Interpretation

Teeth with severe root resorption that results in root length less than 9 mm had a higher risk of tooth mobility. As such, a long-term follow up is recommended for teeth with severe root resorption.

Viewpoint

Levander trial [43] was a small study without sample size calculation. Some patients refused to contribute to this study, and others moved to other places. The different follow-up periods and the wide age range may reduce the certainty in the findings.

Authors' Recommendation

1. There is always a small amount of root resorption associated with orthodontic treatment. This resorption is progressive and increases as the treatment duration increases.
2. Extraction treatments are associated with greater amount of root resorption than non-extraction treatments.
3. Predisposing factors for root resorption are:
   - Upper anterior teeth
   - Peg-shaped lateral incisors
   - Unusual root morphology
   - Increased length of teeth
   - Intrusion movement
   - Torque
   - Heavy forces and involved biomechanics
   - Lack of rest period in force application
   - Maxillary expansion
4. During orthodontic space closure, the clinicians can apply light continuous forces (NiTi springs) or light intermittent forces (elastics).
5. There is either no difference between CAT and FA in terms of RR and sometimes CAT appliances show slightly less RR than FA.
6. There is no difference in RR between conventional and self-ligating brackets.
7. OIIRR is less prevalent in ETT than VT.
8. In cases with significant RR, a pause of 2–3 months in active orthodontic treatment can help the clinician prevent further RR.
9. Supplementations seem to have no effect on OIRR, and they are still in the trial phase.
10. Long-term follow-up is recommended for teeth with severe root resorption.

References

1. Brezniak N, Wasserstein A. Root resorption after orthodontic treatment: part 2. Literature review. Am J Orthod Dentofac Orthop. 1993;103(2):138–46. https://doi.org/10.1016/s0889-5406(05)81763-9.
2. Ramanathan C, Hofman Z. Root resorption in relation to orthodontic tooth movement. Acta Med (Hradec Kralove). 2006;49(2):91–5.
3. Ketcham AH. A preliminary report of an investigation of apical root resorption of permanent teeth. Int J Orthod Oral Surg Radiogr. 1927;13(2):97–127. https://doi.org/10.1016/S0099-6963(27)90316-0.

4. Poumpros E, Loberg E, Engstrom C. Thyroid function and root resorption. Angle Orthod. 1994;64(5):389–93; discussion 94. https://doi.org/10.1043/0003-3219(1994)064<0389:tfarr>2.0.co;2.

5. Sameshima GT, Sinclair PM. Predicting and preventing root resorption: part I. diagnostic factors. Am J Orthod Dentofac Orthop. 2001;119(5):505–10. https://doi.org/10.1067/mod.2001.113409.

6. Hartsfield JK Jr, Everett ET, Al-Qawasmi RA. Genetic factors in external apical root resorption and orthodontic treatment. Crit Rev Oral Biol Med. 2004;15(2):115–22.

7. Tieu LD, Saltaji H, Normando D, Flores-Mir C. Radiologically determined orthodontically induced external apical root resorption in incisors after non-surgical orthodontic treatment of class II division 1 malocclusion: a systematic review. Prog Orthod. 2014;15:48. https://doi.org/10.1186/s40510-014-0048-7.

8. Linge L, Linge BO. Patient characteristics and treatment variables associated with apical root resorption during orthodontic treatment. Am J Orthod Dentofac Orthop. 1991;99(1):35–43.

9. Sameshima GT, Sinclair PM. Characteristics of patients with severe root resorption. Orthod Craniofacial Res. 2004;7(2):108–14.

10. Levander E, Bajka R, Malmgren O. Early radiographic diagnosis of apical root resorption during orthodontic treatment: a study of maxillary incisors. Eur J Orthod. 1998;20(1):57–63.

11. Weltman B, Vig KW, Fields HW, Shanker S, Kaizar EE. Root resorption associated with orthodontic tooth movement: a systematic review. Am J Orthod Dentofac Orthop. 2010;137(4):462–76; discussion 12A. https://doi.org/10.1016/j.ajodo.2009.06.021.

12. Levander E, Malmgren O. Evaluation of the risk of root resorption during orthodontic treatment: a study of upper incisors. Eur J Orthod. 1988;10(1):30–8.

13. Samandara A, Papageorgiou SN, Ioannidou-Marathiotou I, Kavvadia-Tsatala S, Papadopoulos MA. Evaluation of orthodontically induced external root resorption following orthodontic treatment using cone beam computed tomography (CBCT): a systematic review and meta-analysis. Eur J Orthod. 2019;41(1):67–79. https://doi.org/10.1093/ejo/cjy027.

14. Fernandes LQP, Figueiredo NC, Montalvany Antonucci CC, Lages EMB, Andrade I Jr, Capelli JJ. Predisposing factors for external apical root resorption associated with orthodontic treatment. Korean J Orthod. 2019;49(5):310–8. https://doi.org/10.4041/kjod.2019.49.5.310.

15. Brin I, Tulloch JFC, Koroluk L, Philips C. External apical root resorption in class II malocclusion: a retrospective review of 1- versus 2-phase treatment. Am J Orthod Dentofac Orthop. 2003;124(2):151–6. https://doi.org/10.1016/s0889-5406(03)00166-5.

16. Smale I, Artun J, Behbehani F, Doppel D, Van't Hof M, Kuijpers-Jagtman AM. Apical root resorption 6 months after initiation of fixed orthodontic appliance therapy. Am J Orthod Dentofac Orthop. 2005;128(1):57–67. https://doi.org/10.1016/j.ajodo.2003.12.030.

17. Kook YA, Park S, Sameshima GT. Peg-shaped and small lateral incisors not at higher risk for root resorption. Am J Orthod Dentofac Orthop. 2003;123(3):253–8. https://doi.org/10.1067/mod.2003.81.

18. Mirabella AD, Artun J. Risk factors for apical root resorption of maxillary anterior teeth in adult orthodontic patients. Am J Orthod Dentofac Orthop. 1995;108(1):48–55. https://doi.org/10.1016/s0889-5406(95)70065-x.

19. Bellini-Pereira SA, Almeida J, Aliaga-Del Castillo A, Santos C, Henriques JFC, Janson G. Evaluation of root resorption following orthodontic intrusion: a systematic review and meta-analysis. Eur J Orthod. 2020;43(4):432–41. https://doi.org/10.1093/ejo/cjaa054.

20. Roscoe MG, Meira JB, Cattaneo PM. Association of orthodontic force system and root resorption: a systematic review. Am J Orthod Dentofac Orthop. 2015;147(5):610–26. https://doi.org/10.1016/j.ajodo.2014.12.026.

21. Han G, Huang S, Von den Hoff JW, Zeng X, Kuijpers-Jagtman AM. Root resorption after orthodontic intrusion and extrusion: an intraindividual study. Angle Orthod. 2005;75(6):912–8. https://doi.org/10.1043/0003-3219(2005)75[912:Rraoia]2.0.Co;2.

22. Harris DA, Jones AS, Darendeliler MA. Physical properties of root cementum: part 8. Volumetric analysis of root resorption craters after application of controlled intrusive light and

heavy orthodontic forces: a microcomputed tomography scan study. Am J Orthod Dentofac Orthop. 2006;130(5):639–47. https://doi.org/10.1016/j.ajodo.2005.01.029.

23. Currell SD, Liaw A, Blackmore Grant PD, Esterman A, Nimmo A. Orthodontic mechanotherapies and their influence on external root resorption: a systematic review. Am J Orthod Dentofac Orthop. 2019;155(3):313–29. https://doi.org/10.1016/j.ajodo.2018.10.015.

24. Acar A, Canyürek U, Kocaaga M, Erverdi N. Continuous vs. discontinuous force application and root resorption. Angle Orthod. 1999;69(2):159–63; discussion 63-4. https://doi.org/10.1043/0003-3219(1999)069<0159:Cvdfaa>2.3.Co;2.

25. Owman-Moll P, Kurol J, Lundgren D. Continuous versus interrupted continuous orthodontic force related to early tooth movement and root resorption. Angle Orthod. 1995;65(6):395–401; discussion-2. https://doi.org/10.1043/0003-3219(1995)065<0395:Cvicof>2.0.Co;2.

26. Weiland F. Constant versus dissipating forces in orthodontics: the effect on initial tooth movement and root resorption. Eur J Orthod. 2003;25(4):335–42.

27. Yi J, Li M, Li Y, Li X, Zhao Z. Root resorption during orthodontic treatment with self-ligating or conventional brackets: a systematic review and meta-analysis. BMC Oral Health. 2016;16(1):125. https://doi.org/10.1186/s12903-016-0320-y.

28. Gandhi V, Mehta S, Gauthier M, Mu J, Kuo CL, Nanda R, et al. Comparison of external apical root resorption with clear aligners and pre-adjusted edgewise appliances in non-extraction cases: a systematic review and meta-analysis. Eur J Orthod. 2020;43(1):15–24. https://doi.org/10.1093/ejo/cjaa013.

29. Fang X, Qi R, Liu C. Root resorption in orthodontic treatment with clear aligners: a systematic review and meta-analysis. Orthod Craniofacial Res. 2019;22(4):259–69. https://doi.org/10.1111/ocr.12337.

30. Elhaddaoui R, Qoraich HS, Bahije L, Zaoui F. Orthodontic aligners and root resorption: a systematic review. Int Orthod. 2017;15(1):1–12. https://doi.org/10.1016/j.ortho.2016.12.019.

31. Krieger E, Drechsler T, Schmidtmann I, Jacobs C, Haag S, Wehrbein H. Apical root resorption during orthodontic treatment with aligners? A retrospective radiometric study. Head Face Med. 2013;9(1):21. https://doi.org/10.1186/1746-160X-9-21.

32. Fowler B. A comparison of root resorption between invisalign treatment and contemporary orthodontic treatment. [Thesis presented to the faculty of the USC graduate school uni- versity of Southern California]. 2010.

33. Barbagallo LJ, Jones AS, Petocz P, Darendeliler MA. Physical properties of root cementum: part 10. Comparison of the effects of invisible removable thermoplastic appliances with light and heavy orthodontic forces on premolar cementum. A microcomputed-tomography study. Am J Orthod Dentofac Orthop. 2008;133(2):218–27. https://doi.org/10.1016/j.ajodo.2006.01.043.

34. Forst D, Nijjar S, Khaled Y, Lagravere M, Flores-Mir C. Radiographic assessment of external root resorption associated with jackscrew-based maxillary expansion therapies: a systematic review. Eur J Orthod. 2014;36(5):576–85. https://doi.org/10.1093/ejo/cjt090.

35. Alhadainy HA, Flores-Mir C, Abdel-Karim AH, Crossman J, El-Bialy T. Orthodontic-induced external root resorption of endodontically treated teeth: a meta-analysis. J Endod. 2019;45(5):483–9. https://doi.org/10.1016/j.joen.2019.02.001.

36. Walker SL, Tieu LD, Flores-Mir C. Radiographic comparison of the extent of orthodontically induced external apical root resorption in vital and root-filled teeth: a systematic review. Eur J Orthod. 2013;35(6):796–802. https://doi.org/10.1093/ejo/cjs101.

37. Kurol J, Owman-Moll P, Lundgren D. Time-related root resorption after application of a controlled continuous orthodontic force. Am J Orthod Dentofac Orthop. 1996;110(3):303–10. https://doi.org/10.1016/s0889-5406(96)80015-1.

38. Deng Y, Sun Y, Xu T. Evaluation of root resorption after comprehensive orthodontic treatment using cone beam computed tomography (CBCT): a meta-analysis. BMC Oral Health. 2018;18(1):116. https://doi.org/10.1186/s12903-018-0579-2.

39. Levander E, Malmgren O, Eliasson S. Evaluation of root resorption in relation to two orthodontic treatment regimes. A clinical experimental study. Eur J Orthod. 1994;16(3):223–8. https://doi.org/10.1093/ejo/16.3.223.

40. Haugland L, Kristensen KD, Lie SA, Vandevska-Radunovic V. The effect of biologic factors and adjunctive therapies on orthodontically induced inflammatory root resorption: a systematic review and meta-analysis. Eur J Orthod. 2018;40(3):326–36. https://doi.org/10.1093/ejo/cjy003.
41. Kaklamanos EG, Makrygiannakis MA, Athanasiou AE. Does medication administration affect the rate of orthodontic tooth movement and root resorption development in humans? A systematic review. Eur J Orthod. 2020;42(4):407–14. https://doi.org/10.1093/ejo/cjz063.
42. Berry S, Javed F, Rossouw PE, Barmak AB, Kalogirou EM, Michelogiannakis D. Influence of thyroxine supplementation on orthodontically induced tooth movement and/or inflammatory root resorption: a systematic review. Orthod Craniofacial Res. 2020;24(2):206–13. https://doi.org/10.1111/ocr.12428.
43. Levander E, Malmgren O. Long-term follow-up of maxillary incisors with severe apical root resorption. Eur J Orthod. 2000;22(1):85–92. https://doi.org/10.1093/ejo/22.1.85.

White Spot Lesions

9

Contents

Abbreviations

CCP- ACP	CPP-amorphous calcium phosphate
CPP	Casein phosphopeptide
CPP-ACFP	CPP-amorphous calcium fluoride phosphate

© The Author(s), under exclusive license to Springer Nature Switzerland AG 2023   225
S. Mheissen, H. Khan, *Orthodontic Evidence*,
https://doi.org/10.1007/978-3-031-24422-3_9

FRM	Fluoride-releasing materials
IS	Incognito system
PE	Partial etching
QLF	Quantitative light-induced fluorescence
SBLs	sub-bracket lesions
TE	Total etching
WS	WIN DW Lingual System
WSLs	White spot lesions

Introduction

White spot lesions (WSLs) result from subsurface enamel demineralization due to acid attack by lactic acid products of plaque metabolism, thus changing the light scattering properties of enamel and giving the lesion an opaque white appearance. These lesions develop on any surface of the tooth where the plaque remains undisturbed for a sufficient time. The lesion develops in two stages. The first stage is surface softening, and the second stage is subsurface lesions. Mostly if the plaque remains undisturbed for 3–4 weeks, the WSLs become visible even with the naked eye [1]. In the case of fixed orthodontics, the underwings areas of brackets provides a suitable site for plaque accumulation, and if the patient is not motivated for oral hygiene care, there are increased chances to develop WSLs. WSLs around brackets become visible after a month of bonding in case fluoride substitution is not given [2]. WSLs also develop underneath the bracket base area and are called sub-bracket lesions (SBLs).

The prevalence of WSLs in non-orthodontic patients is 9–24% [3], while in orthodontic patients, it was reported from 2–97% [4–6]. A meta-analysis reported an overall prevalence of 68.5% in orthodontic patients, while the prevalence of a new white spot lesion in orthodontic patients was reported to be 45.8% [7]. Risk factors for WSLs include poor oral hygiene, poor diet control, long treatment duration, medications, low fluoride intake, microbial factors, the composition of saliva, and genetic predisposition.

Different techniques are used for detecting and measuring the severity of WSLs. These include subjective techniques such as visual inspection, which is based on the qualitative assessment of the lesion and varies according to personal perception. WSLs on visual inspection are classified [4] into; stage 0: no lesion, stage 1: slight rim, stage 2: broad rim, and stage 3: cavitation. The objective techniques involve noninvasive techniques such as quantitative light-induced fluorescence (QLF) in which enamel is exposed to visible light having a wavelength of 370 nm by an illumination lamp and a CCD micro camera captures the tooth image. The reasoning behind this technique is that the demineralized enamel fluoresce less. A modification of the QLF technique is the digital QLF. It involves taking two simultaneous images, one white light image and one QLF image. The rationale is that plaque is not visible in white light, so a change of filters and fluorescene with red light makes the plaque visible. Commercially available fluorescence devices are DIAGNODent Pen™ (uses a red laser beam at 655 nm) and VistaProof™ (uses violet light at 405 nm). Another objective technique for measuring the white spot lesions is transverse radiography which involves removing an 80 μm sample from the enamel surface, exposing it to a monochromatic X-ray beam, and comparing it with a standard.

Prevention and treatment of WSLs mostly involve oral hygiene measures such as the use of fluoride-containing products which include mouthwashes, varnishes, acidulated phosphate fluoride, and stannous fluoride. More recently Casein phosphopeptide (CPP) formulations which include CPP-amorphous calcium phosphate (CCP-ACP) and CPP-amorphous calcium fluoride phosphate (CPP-ACFP) have been used to treat white spot lesions. CPP formulations are dairy products used as a source of calcium and phosphate for the tooth. These products decrease the incidence of WSLs by reducing the binding of strep mutants to tooth surfaces, and have buffering action on plaque acid. It also promotes the diffusion of ions into the lesion [8]. Invasive treatment for WSLs comprises resin infiltration and microabrasion. Resin infiltration involves etching the enamel with 15% hydrochloric acid followed by drying with ethanol and applying a low-viscosity unfilled TEGDMA-based resin. Microabrasion involves the use of either 37% phosphoric acid and pumice or 6–18% hydrochloric acid mixed as a slurry with fine-powdered pumice and glycerin. The paste or slurry is applied to the tooth surface with rubber cups on a slow-speed handpiece.

Orthodontics and WSLs

Clinical Question 1: What Is the Prevalence of WSLs in Orthodontic Patients?

Evidence

Systematic Review and Meta Analysis
Sundararaj/ 2015 [7]
In this review, the authors included 14 cross-sectional studies to investigate the prevalence of WSLs. The authors found that 68.4% (850/1242) of patients undergoing orthodontic treatment had WSLs, and 45% (935/2041) developed WSLs during the course of the orthodontic treatment.

A Cross-sectional Clinical Studies
Lucchese/2013 [9]
This study was included in the previous review [7]. This cross-sectional study divided the participants into three groups: the control group without orthodontic treatment, 6-month fixed orthodontics treatment group, and the 12-months fixed orthodontic treatment group. The control group was comprised of 68 patients (36 girls and 32 boys) with an average age of 9 ± 1.5 years. The 6-month group consisted of 59 patients (28 girls and 31 boys) with a mean age of 9 ± 1.3 years. The 12 months group

comprised 64 patients (36 girls and 28 boys) with a mean age of 10 ± 1.4. The visual examination showed that only 13% had at least one WSL in the control group. However, in the 6 months group, 40% had at least one visible WSL, while 59% had no WSLs. In the 12 months group, 43% had at least one visible WSL, and 56% had no WSLs. The prevalence of WSLs was significantly greater in 6 and 12 months groups when compared with the control group. There was no statistically significant difference between the 6 and 12 months groups, with a greater proportion of patients having a score of 2. WSL covers more than one-third of the surface in the 12 months group.

Tufekci/2011 [10]

This study was included in the previous review [7]. In this study, the researchers visually investigated the presence of enamel demineralization in three groups of patients; The 6 months group, where the patients were examined at the end of six months, comprised 37 participants (16 females, 21 males) with a mean age of 17.4 ± 1.3 years. The 12 months group, in which the patients were examined at the end of 12 months, comprised 35 patients (18 females, 17 males) with an average age of 17.5 ± 1.4 years. The control group was examined for WSLs immediately after brackets' bonding, comprised 28 patients (13 females, 15 males) with an average age of 15.1 ± 1.5 years. At least one visible WSL was observed in 38% of the 6 months group and in 46% of the 12 months group. In the control group, only 11% of the sample showed at least one WSL, with a statistically significant difference from the 6 and 12 months groups ($p = 0.021$, $p = 0.005$, respectively).

Evidence Summary

The best available evidence suggests that patients with fixed orthodontic treatment had higher odds of developing WSL than untreated patients. The prevalence of WSLs was 68.4% in orthodontic patients [7]. In young patients aged 9 ± 1.5 years, the rate of WSLs by the visual inspection was 40% and 43% for the 6 months and 12 months, respectively, after orthodontic bonding, while the rate of untreated patients who developed WSLs was 13% [9]. On the other hand, the patients of older age 17.4 ± 1.3 with at least one WSL were 38% and 46% after 6- and 12-months of bonding, respectively, while in the untreated patients, it was 11% [10].

Evidence Interpretation

The prevalence of WSLs in orthodontic patients is 68.4% on average. Orthodontic treatment increases the chances of WSLs, and approximately 40% of adolescent and adult patients have at least one WSL after six months of brackets bonding. Also, there is a likelihood of an increase in WSLs prevalence over time. The patient should be informed about the probabilities of developing WSLs during the course of orthodontic treatment and written consent should be taken.

Viewpoint

Sundararaj et al. review [7] provided a quantitative estimate of the prevalence of WSLs in orthodontic patients. It is worth mentioning that the search was limited to two databases without using MeSH terms. The search was limited to the published articles, so it may miss some relevant studies. The authors provide the overall prevalence by pooling the incidence and the prevalence, which is suboptimal as the incidence accounts for the time while the prevalence does not.

The two studies [9, 10] did not correlate the effect of oral hygiene on the prevalence of WSLs, which may have a considerable impact on the outcome. Lucchese study [9] was conducted in the private practice of the author on a small Caucasian sample that may limit the applicability of the results to other patients from different ethnicities and patients who are seeking treatment in hospitals. Tufekci study [10] was done in university settings. The patients' ethnicity and the small sample size should be taken into account for generalizability.

Teeth and WSLs

Clinical Question2: Which Teeth Are More Affected by WSLs?

Evidence

Systematic Review and Meta-Analysis
Sundararaj/ 2015 [7]
In this review, three included trials [11–13] found that the maxillary anterior teeth were more affected by WSLs than mandibular anterior teeth; WSLs were 2.5 times more common in the upper teeth than in lower teeth [13]. The maxillary canine followed by the maxillary laterals were the most affected teeth [11, 14]. However, the upper lateral incisors were the most affected teeth in another trial [4].

In mandibular arch, the posterior teeth were the most affected teeth in the arch [11]. The sequence of the most affect lower teeth was the second premolar followed by the first premolar, the canine, and the incisors [9].

Evidence Summary
The best available evidence suggests that different distribution of WSLs was observed in different studies. Most of the included studies in this review [7]found that the maxillary anterior teeth were more prone to WSLs, sometimes by 2.5 times. There was no agreement regarding the most affected teeth in the maxilla; it was the canine in two studies and the lateral in another trial [7]. In the mandible, the most affected teeth were the second premolar and first molar, with more prevalence in the second premolars.

Evidence Interpretation
Maxillary anterior and mandibular posterior teeth are the most affected teeth by white spot lesions. In the maxillary arch, WSLs are mostly found on lateral incisors and canines, while in the mandibular arch the most affected teeth by WSLs are the second premolars.

A rigorous inspection and oral hygiene instruction should be given to the patient for meticulous care of the most susceptible teeth.

Viewpoint

The SR has already been discussed.

Factors Affecting WSLs

Clinical Question3: What Is the Effect of Age on WSLS?

Evidence

Systematic Review and Meta-Analysis
Sundararaj/ 2015 [7]

In this review, an included trial [11] found that adolescent patients are twice more likely to develop WSLs than adults. Another trial concluded that WSLs decrease by 0.59 for each year increase in the age of the patient [15]. On the other hand, a study [12] reported no impact of age on the prevalence of WSLs. Finally, oral hygiene seems to have a significant impact on the incidence of WSLs [16].

Evidence Summary

The best available evidence suggests that adolescent patients are two times more likely to develop WSLs than adults, and the WSLs decrease by 0.59 for each year increase in age. In contrast, one study [12] did not find any impact of age on WSLs prevalence. WSLs were associated with poor oral hygiene [16].

Evidence Interpretation

The evidence is not conclusive regarding the relationship between age and WSLs. However, it seems that patients with older age have less prevalence of WSLs. This might be related to poor oral hygiene which is a predictive factor in developing new WSLs. Orthodontic treatment should always be accompanied with a plaque preventive diet and good oral hygiene motivation, especially in adolescents.

Viewpoint

The systematic review has already been discussed.

Clinical Question 4: What Is the Effect of Treatment Duration on WSLS?

Evidence

Systematic Review and Meta-Analysis
Sundararaj/ 2015 [7]

One included trial [11] found that increasing the treatment duration from 24 months to 36 months or more increased the likelihood of WSL formation by 3.65 times. Similarly, three other studies [9, 10, 13] reported increase in the prevalence of WSLs from 38% to 40% in the first six months to 43–46% in 12 months. A multiple regression analysis found that the number of WSLs increased by 0.08 lesions per month for each month's increase in the treatment duration [15].

Evidence Summary

The best available evidence suggests that increasing the treatment duration may increase the likelihood of WSLs. Longer treatment duration, from 24 to more than 36 months, may increase the WSLs formation by 3.65 times. Also, there is a possibility of an increase of 0.08 lesions per month for each extra month increase in the treatment duration.

Evidence Interpretation

Longer treatment duration is associated with more WSLs. So, every effort should be made to make the treatment duration as minimal as possible. Also, preventive measures for WSLs should always be used in fixed orthodontic treatment.

Viewpoint

The systematic review has already been discussed.

Clinical Question 5: What Is the Effect of Partial or Total Etching Procedures on the Rate of WSLs Formation?

Evidence

Randomized Controlled Clinical Trial
Yagci/2019 [17]

The authors recruited 20 Class I patients, with satisfactory oral hygiene, in this split-mouth RCT. They randomly allocated the 40 maxillary quadrants into two groups; total etching (TE) or partial etching (PE) using blue high-viscosity gel etchant containing 37% phosphoric acid. They followed the patients for three-time points, 3 and 6 months after the start of treatment, and at debonding phase. WSLs parameters like lesion volume, lesion depth, and the greatest depth of the lesion were studied using light fluorescence images. With a treatment time of 10.33 ± 2.41 months, no difference was observed in different parameters of WSLs between the TE and PE groups at 3 months period and at debonding phase. But at the time point of 6 months, the TE group showed significantly higher lesion volume and lesion area scores than the PE group ($P < 0.05$). The lesion depth increased significantly in both groups after 6 months of treatment. The lesion volume decreased from 6 months point to the debonding phase in the TE group when compared with the PE group.

Evidence Summary

The best available evidence suggests that there is no difference between TE and PE regarding the WSLs parameters. There was a statistically significant increase in

WSLs depth over time. The WSL volume increased in the first 6 months in the TE group more than in the PE group and decreased after 6 months of treatment.

Evidence Interpretation

In a full orthodontic course of 12 months, there is no difference between partial or total etching regarding WSLs parameters. There is an increase in lesion volumes in the TE group over the first six months after bonding, so it is recommended to avoid total etching as it has no added benefit.

Viewpoint

In Yagci trial [17], the authors excluded the brackets accidentally debonded or needed re-bonding for any patients during the treatment, with a higher bracket failure rate in the TE group than the PE group that may confound the results due to the different number of included teeth in both groups. There was a lack of information regarding allocation concealment, which may increase bias in the randomization process. The sample calculation was based on a 0.9 effect size which is a large and would yield a small sample size. Interestingly, the study was from a longitudinal cluster design that may require different statistical methods from the reported methods [18, 19]. Finally, controlling individual oral hygiene is very difficult and may confound the results.

Prevention and WSLs

Clinical Question 6: What Is the Effectiveness of Preventive Procedures for WSLs During Active Orthodontic Treatment?

Evidence

Systematic Reviews and Meta-analyses
Benson/2019 [20]
Ten RCTs with 458 participants were included in this Cochrane review, investigating different interventions for WSLs prevention. The application of fluoride varnish (7700 or 10,000 parts per million (ppm) fluoride), every six weeks seems to have insignificant effect on preventing new WSLs (RR: 0.52, 95% CI: 0.14–1.93, 405 participants; low-certainty evidence). However, it may reduce the severity of the WSLs (RR: 0.46, 95%CI: 0.22–0.95, 148 participants, 1 trial). The application of fluoride foam (12,300 ppm) every two months reduced the risk of new WSLs (RR: 0.26, 95% CI: 0.11–0.57, 95 participants). The use of a high-concentration fluoride toothpaste (5000 ppm) reduced the risk of new WSLs when compared with conventional fluoride toothpaste (1450 ppm) (RR: 0.68, 95% CI 0.46–1.00, 380 participants). The evidence for the aforementioned procedures was low. A 250-ppm fluoride mouth rinse and amine fluoride gel have a similar effect to the control or placebo group. The intraoral fluoride-releasing glass bead device attached to the brace has a similar effect to the daily fluoride mouth rinse.

Likewise, an amine fluoride and stannous fluoride toothpaste/mouthrinse combination has a similar effect to a sodium fluoride toothpaste/mouthrinse.

Nascimento/2016 [21]

In this review, the authors pooled four studies comparing fluoride-releasing materials (FRM) in a meta-analysis. They found that the relative risk of developing WSLs was 0.42 (95% CI: 0.25–0.72) for the FRM group compared to the control group, which means that using FRMs decreased the risk of WSLs by 58%. For the extent of WSLs, there was no statistically significant difference between FRMs and control groups (mean reduction: 0.12, 95% CI: −0.29 to 0.04, $p < 0.16$, $I^2 = 51\%$).

Sardana/2019 [22]

The authors included four RCTs in this systematic review investigating preventive effects on WSLs using topical fluoride at different follow-ups. Three included trials were pooled in a meta-analysis. The authors found that the risk ratio of developing WSLs was 0.39 (95%CI: 0.26–0.59, $p = 0.005$, $I^2 = 81\%$), favoring the topical fluoride group, which means there is less risk by 61% of developing WSLs in the topical fluoride group when compared to the control group.

Tasios/2019 [23]

This systematic review included 23 trials. Five within-person randomized trials investigated the effectiveness of flat surface sealants on WSLs; the meta-analysis of the five RCTs found that using the flat surface sealants around the brackets was effective in reducing WSLs development (RR = 0.77; 95% CI: 0.63–0.95, $P = 0.01$, $I^2 = 50\%$). Two included RCTs indicated that the use of fluoride varnish was significantly associated with a smaller WSL area (MD; −0.32 mm^2, 95% CI: −0.44 to −0.21 mm^2, $P < 0.001$, $I^2 = 0\%$). The evidence was graded as low. Interestingly, patients' reminder was effective in reducing the number of patients with WSLs (RR; 0.44, 95% CI: 0.31–0.64, $P < 0.001$, $I^2 = 0\%$), fluoride-releasing adhesive and glass ionomer did not have a statistically significant impact on WSLs development when compared to conventional adhesive (RR: 0.86, 95%CI:0.70–1.07, $p = 0.18$, $I^2 = 4\%$, 5 trials) and (RR: 0.81, 95%CI: 0.47–1.39, $p = 0.44$, $I^2 = 73\%$, 3 trials), respectively. The evidence was low for reminders and sealants and moderate for fluoride-releasing adhesive.

Systematic Review
Pithon/2019 [24]

This review included eleven studies (9 were RCTs, and 2 were non-RCTs) estimating the effectiveness of casein phosphopeptide-amorphous calcium phosphate (CPP-ACP) materials in the prevention of WSLs. The most common method of CPP-ACP was the topical application of 1 g CPP-ACP cream for 1–3 minutes once a day at night for prevention. The researchers found that CPP-ACP has a similar effect to fluoride materials. A 12-week study [25] reported that the reduction of WSLs was 76.8% and 58.6% for CPP-ACP and placebo groups, respectively, and this was statistically significant.

Evidence Summary

Looking into the evidence collectively, the best available evidence suggests that using FRMs and topical fluoride for WSLs prevention decreases the risk of WSLs by 58% and 61%, respectively [21, 22]. Fluoride foam (12,300 ppm) every two months and high-concentration fluoride toothpaste (5000 ppm) reduced the risk of WSLs. Fluoride varnish did not show an impact on WSLs prevention, but it decreased the WSLs area by only 0.32 mm². Reminders were effective in reducing the number of patients with WSLs, and sealants around the bracket were effective in reducing WSLs development by 23%, A single short-term trial [25] reported a statistically significant difference between CPP-ACP and placebo groups in reducing WSLs [24].

Evidence Interpretation

For prevention of WSLs, CPP-ACP and fluoride-releasing materials, such as fluoride foam (12,300 ppm), fluoride toothpaste (5000 ppm), and fluoride oral rinse, may be effective methods in decreasing the risk of WSLs in patients undergoing orthodontic treatment. Applying sealants on the teeth surface around the brackets may decrease the chances of new WSLs. Also, reminders to patients for proper oral hygiene care decrease the risk of new WSLs.

Viewpoint

Benson et al. [20] was a well-conducted Cochrane review. There were some concerns about the blinding of assessors, patients, and operators in the included trials. The authors excluded the split-mouth studies due to cross-over contamination between the control and experimental sides, and this may affect the results.

In Nascimento review [21], all included studies were at high risk of bias that may reduce the quality of the evidence. Furthermore, the patient's oral hygiene, enamel surface, and race of the patients may confound the results. So, the evidence should be interpreted with caution.

In Sardana review [22], most of the included trials suffered from some concerns in the randomization that increased bias and reduced evidence quality. Interestingly, the authors did not provide enough details for the other included studies.

Most of the included studies in Tasios review [23] had a high risk of bias due to the lack of randomization, blinding, and selective outcome reporting. The vast majority of within-person randomized trials did not take clustering and data dependence into their account, which might affect their results. Also, small trials were included in the meta-analyses.

Pithon review [24] was a well-conducted review that included both RCTs and Non-RCTs. The authors assessed the quality of the included studies at low risk of bias. They aimed at assessing the effectiveness of CPP-ACP, but they compared this intervention with other interventions, not only the control. So, they decided not to pool the effect of this intervention in meta-analysis. Also, the authors combined methods for WSLs treatment with methods for WSLs prevention that may confound the findings.

Interventions and Post-orthodontic WSL

Clinical Question 7: What Is the Effectiveness of Post-orthodontic WSLs Treatment?

Evidence

Systematic Review and Meta-Analysis
Höchli/2017 [26]

This systematic review included 20 RCTs; 942 patients in total, with an average age of 16.1 years. The mean number of WSLs was 8.2 lesions per patient (range 2.2–45.4). The used supplement to treat WSLs varied between studies; CPP–ACP creams (with or without fluoride), external tooth bleaching, low- or high-concentration fluoride materials (FRMs in the form of film, gel, mouth rinse, toothpaste, or varnish), resin infiltration, miswak chewing sticks, or bioactive glass toothpaste. The follow-up period was from a couple of weeks to 6.5 months after the application of the supplemental material. The researchers found that the treatment interventions provide a small and insignificant improvement of lesion area (MD; −0.48, 95%CI: −0.98 to 0.0, 6 trials), enamel fluorescence (MD; −0.35, 95%CI: −0.75 to 0.05, 8 trials), and clinical evaluation (OR; 0.97; 95% CI: 0.60 to 1.56, $P > 0.05$, 3 trials) when compared with daily oral hygiene group. However, the evidence was judged as low to moderate.

Systematic Reviews
Borges/2017 [27]

Four non-randomized studies (NRS) and seven RCT studies investigating the effectiveness of resin infiltration (RI) in treating post-orthodontic WSLs were included in this systematic review. The included studies compared resin infiltration with no treatment, remineralization, bleaching, or the initial condition. For the whitish color masking efficacy, two included studies found a higher color variation in RI group; $\Delta E = 2.55$ for RI vs. 0.29 for control in one trial [28], $\Delta E = 5.53$ for RI vs. 2.53 for control in the another trial [29]. The reduction of the affected area was better in the RI group; 60.9% for RI group vs. 1% for the control group [30], 53.5% for RI group compared to 49.2% in the fluoride varnish group [31].

Sonesson/2017 [32]

This review included eight clinical trials. Different managements of post-orthodontic WSLs were used; five studies evaluated the remineralization agents CPP-ACP, one assessed the microabrasion, one assessed the remineralization agents and microabrasion, and two trials evaluated resin infiltration (RI). There was a lack of evidence on the effectiveness of remineralization agents. The microabrasion (hydrochloric acid and pumice powder) with normal tooth brushing was effective over 6 months study [33]. Two included studies [28, 30] found improvement in the esthetic appearance of WSLs in the RI group compared with untreated lesions. The evidence was graded as low.

Pithon/2019 [24]

In this review, the authors investigated the effectiveness of CPP-ACP materials in treating post-orthodontic WSLs. They found that the reduction rate of WSLs was 50%, 48%, 45% for CPP-ACP, fluoride rinse and brushing only, respectively. Better results were obtained with microabrasion; the reduction rate was 97% of WSLs area. Over 12 months, one included study [20] found that 64% of WSLs become invisible to visual inspection by using CPP-ACP while 23% of WSLs become invisible by using the fluoride-based rinse. Moreover, there was no difference in lesion depth between groups.

Evidence Summary

Looking into evidence collectively, the evidence is inconclusive regarding the best management of post-orthodontic WSLs. One review [26] concluded that the interventions for post-orthodontic WSLs have a small and insignificant effect on the lesion area (MD; −0.48, 95%CI: −0.98,0.0, 6 trials), the enamel fluorescence (MD; −0.35, 95%CI:−0.75 to 0.05, 8 trials), and the clinical evaluation (OR = 0.97; 95% CI: 0.60 to 1.56; 3 trials) compared with daily oral hygiene group. In contrast, two included studies [28, 29], in another review [27], reported a higher color variation in RI group (ΔE = 2.55 for RI vs 0.29 for control, ΔE = 5.53 for RI vs 2.53 for control) [27]. The reduction of the affected area was better in the RI group; 60.9% for RI group vs. 1% for the control group [30] and 53.5% for the RI group when compared to the fluoride varnish group that was 49.2% [31]. Also, the affected area reduction was better in RI group by 53.5% when compared to the reduction in the varnish group, that was 49.2% [27]. Microabrasion with normal tooth brushing was effective in treating post-orthodontic WSLs. Furthermore, a review [24] found that CPP-ACP has a similar effect to fluoride materials and may reduce the WSLs percentage by 50% when compared to fluoride rinse (48%) and fluoride brushing (45%). Interestingly, one trial [21] reported that 64% of WSLs became invisible to the visual inspection in CPP-ACP over 12 months, while this was 23% in the fluoride rinse group.

Evidence Interpretation

Microabrasion, resin infiltration, CPP-ACP, fluoride rinse, and daily brushing may be effective procedures in reducing post-orthodontic WSLs. Microabrasion and resin infiltration are invasive techniques and can camouflage severe WSLs in the short term.

Viewpoint

Höchli et al. review [26] was a well-conducted review with some limitations mostly in the primary studies; the 11 included studies were at high risk of bias and 9 were at unclear risk of bias due to blinding and reporting issues. The variety of interventions and follow-up period may reduce the quality of the evidence. Many of the included studies used inappropriate analyses methods that disregarded the correlation of multiple WSLs within each patient.

Borges et al. review [27] included RCTs and NRS that reduce the quality of the evidence. Also, most of these studies have unclear to high risk of bias with a short follow-up period. The outcome data was synthesized using the qualitative method.

Most of the studies included, in Sonesson et al. review [32], were at high risk of bias with no details regarding the design of these studies. The long-term effects of some procedures on WSLs are still unknown and prolonged follow-up is required.

Clinical Question 8: What Is the Effectiveness of Fluoride Varnishes for Post-orthodontic WSLs?

Evidence

Systematic Review and Meta-Analysis
Höchli/2017 [26]
This systematic review found that the monthly use of fluoride varnish was the best supplement to improve WSLs regarding the lesion area (MD; -0.80 mm^2; 95% CI: -1.10 to -0.50 mm^2; $P < 0.05$; high quality, 1 trial) and enamel fluorescence (SMD; -0.92; 95% CI: -1.32 to -0.52; $P < 0.05$, high quality, 3 trials), followed by the use of fluoride film.

Sardana/2019 [22]
Three RCTs were included in the meta-analysis to investigate the reversal of WSLs. The authors found that DIAGNOdent scores at three months were statistically less in the professional topical fluoride varnish group than in the control group (SMD: -0.57, 95% CI: -0.23 to -0.91, $p < 0.01$, $I^2 = 62.3\%$).

Evidence Summary
Looking into evidence collectively, the best available evidence suggests that fluoride varnish is effective in reducing the WSLs area. One systematic review [26] indicated that fluoride varnish reduced the WSLs area by 0.8 mm^2 and improved the fluorescence scores (SMD; 0.92). Similarly, another piece of evidence [22] indicated that the fluoride varnish has less DIAGNOdent scores (SMD; 0.57)

Evidence Interpretation
There is a level of uncertainty in using fluoride varnish for treating WSLs. Fluoride varnishes might reduce the area of WSLs and its severity, but it is not significantly effective when compared with daily oral hygiene measures.

Viewpoint
The reviews have been already discussed.

The Best Protocol

Clinical Question 9: What Is the Best Treatment Protocol for Fluoride Varnishes in Post-orthodontic WSLs?

Evidence

Systematic Review and Meta-Analysis
Höchli/2017 [26]
This review concluded that the monthly use of a 22,600-ppm fluoride varnish or a 5% sodium fluoride film seems to be the best viable protocol for reducing the WSL area and increasing the esthetic appearance (fluorescence; high quality of evidence).

Evidence Summary
The best available evidence suggests that the best protocol for reducing WSL area, as well as increasing the esthetic appearance, is the monthly use of 22,600 ppm fluoride varnish or a 5% sodium fluoride film.

Evidence Interpretation
Both fluoride varnish and sodium fluoride film can be used to treat WSLs effectively.

Viewpoint
The evidence has already been discussed.

Lingual Appliance and WSLs

Clinical Question10: Which Lingual Brackets Is Better Regarding WSLs and Sub-Bracket Lesions (SBLs)?

Evidence

Cohort Study
Knösel/2016 [34]
This trial recruited 630 consecutive patients into two groups for lingual orthodontic treatment; either WIN DW Lingual System (WS) or Incognito system (IS). The mean age of the patients was 17.47 ± 8.1 and 17.48 ± 7.3 for WS and IS groups, respectively. The treatment duration was 21.04 ± 7.31 and 24.71 ± 7.99 for WS and IS, respectively. The pre-existing WSLs were 28 in WS and 34 in IS groups, with 10,830 included teeth in WS group and 6076 teeth in IS group. The key finding was that IS has significantly more sub-bracket lesions (SBLs) than WS, while there was no difference in WSLs between the two groups. There was a positive correlation between treatment duration and WSLs and SBLs formation. Also, age has a negative impact on SBLs formation, which increased in pre-adolescents ≤ 16 years when

compared with adolescents >16 years. Gender has a significant effect on WSLs, with greater predominance in males.

Evidence Summary

The best available evidence is inconclusive and suggests that there is a higher statistically significant SBLs in IS group when compared to WS group, with no difference between the two appliances in regard to WSLs. However, there is a significant impact of different factors on WSLs; the longer the treatment duration, the younger the patient, more would be chances of WSLs with male predominance.

Evidence Interpretation

Lingual fixed appliances are associated with WSLs and SBLs. Longer treatment and younger male patients are more likely to have WSLs.

Viewpoint

Knösel trial [34] was a cohort study with many limitations; there was a lack of randomization with many confounding factors such as age, gender, and number of included teeth in each arm. The authors found a positive correlation between WSLs formation and treatment duration which may be another confounder. Nonetheless, the treatment duration was longer in IS group with more difficult cases and subsequently, the authors did not consider the number of bracket failures/re-bonding that may have a potential impact on a local increase or decrease of enamel demenralization. One of the authors declared that he is the inventor of WS, which may represent some conflict of interest. With the aforementioned factors, the available evidence is not crucial for the effect of fixed brackets type.

Authors' Recommendations

- Orthodontic treatment increases the chances of new WSLs development.
- Longer treatment duration and poor oral hygiene directly correlate with the development of new WSLs.
- Maxillary anterior teeth and mandibular posterior teeth are more likely to develop WSLs, so more active monitoring of these teeth should be implemented during orthodontic treatment.
- Partial etching is recommended while bonding orthodontic brackets as it is cost effective and is not associated with increased chances of WSLs.
- Reminders to patients for proper oral hygiene care decrease the risk of new WSLs.
- Prevention of WSLs during orthodontic treatment can be done by recommending fluoride toothpaste (5000 ppm), and fluoride mouthwashes to the patients. In patients who have increased chances of WSLs such as patients with pre-existing WSLs or having long comprehensive treatment, daily CPP-ACP use or fluoride foam (12,300 ppm) application can be effective. Furthermore, sealants on the teeth surface around the brackets may be an effective procedure.

- Post-orthodontic WSLs can be treated with routine brushing, fluoride mouthrinse, or CPP-ACP. If there is no improvement within 3–6 months, in-office fluoride varnishes can be given. Microabrasion and resin infiltration being invasive procedures should always be used as the last resort.

References

1. Fejerskov O, Kidd E. Dental caries: the disease and its clinical management. Oxford: John Wiley & Sons; 2009.
2. Ogaard B, Rølla G, Arends J. Orthodontic appliances and enamel demineralization. Part 1. Lesion development. American Journal of Orthodontics and Dentofacial Orthopedics: Official publication of the American Association of Orthodontists, its constituent societies, and the American Board of Orthodontics. 1988;94(1):68–73. https://doi.org/10.1016/0889-5406(88)90453-2.
3. Banks P, Burn A, O'Brien K. A clinical evaluation of the effectiveness of including fluoride into an orthodontic bonding adhesive. Eur J Orthod. 1997;19(4):391–5.
4. Gorelick L, Geiger AM, Gwinnett AJ. Incidence of white spot formation after bonding and banding. Am J Orthod. 1982;81(2):93–8.
5. Boersma J, Van der Veen M, Lagerweij M, Bokhout B, Prahl-Andersen B. Caries prevalence measured with QLF after treatment with fixed orthodontic appliances: influencing factors. Caries Res. 2005;39(1):41–7.
6. Sandvik K, Hadler-Olsen S, El-Agroudi M, Ogaard B. Caries and white spot lesions in orthodontically treated adolescents—a prospective study. Eur J Orthod. 2006;28:e258.
7. Sundararaj D, Venkatachalapathy S, Tandon A, Pereira A. Critical evaluation of incidence and prevalence of white spot lesions during fixed orthodontic appliance treatment: a meta-analysis. J Int Soc Prev Community Dent. 2015;5(6):433–9. https://doi.org/10.4103/2231-0762.167719.
8. Cochrane N, Saranathan S, Cai F, Cross K, Reynolds E. Enamel subsurface lesion remineralisation with casein phosphopeptide stabilised solutions of calcium, phosphate and fluoride. Caries Res. 2008;42(2):88–97.
9. Lucchese A, Gherlone E. Prevalence of white-spot lesions before and during orthodontic treatment with fixed appliances. Eur J Orthod. 2013;35(5):664–8. https://doi.org/10.1093/ejo/cjs070.
10. Tufekci E, Dixon JS, Gunsolley JC, Lindauer SJ. Prevalence of white spot lesions during orthodontic treatment with fixed appliances. Angle Orthod. 2011;81(2):206–10. https://doi.org/10.2319/051710-262.1.
11. Khalaf K. Factors affecting the formation, severity and location of white spot lesions during orthodontic treatment with fixed appliances. J Oral Maxillofac Res. 2014;5(1):e4. https://doi.org/10.5037/jomr.2014.5104.
12. Sagarika N, Suchindran S, Loganathan S, Gopikrishna V. Prevalence of white spot lesion in a section of Indian population undergoing fixed orthodontic treatment: an in vivo assessment using the visual International Caries Detection and Assessment System II criteria. J Conserv Dent. 2012;15(2):104–8. https://doi.org/10.4103/0972-0707.94572.
13. Julien KC, Buschang PH, Campbell PM. Prevalence of white spot lesion formation during orthodontic treatment. Angle Orthod. 2013;83(4):641–7. https://doi.org/10.2319/071712-584.1.
14. Geiger AM, Gorelick L, Gwinnett AJ, Griswold PG. The effect of a fluoride program on white spot formation during orthodontic treatment. Am J Orthod Dentofac Orthop. 1988;93(1):29–37. https://doi.org/10.1016/0889-5406(88)90190-4.
15. Richter AE, Arruda AO, Peters MC, Sohn W. Incidence of caries lesions among patients treated with comprehensive orthodontics. Am J Orthod Dentofac Orthop. 2011;139(5):657–64. https://doi.org/10.1016/j.ajodo.2009.06.037.

16. Akin M, Tazcan M, Ileri Z, Basciftci FA. Incidence of white spot lesion during fixed orthodontic treatment. Turk J Orthod. 2013;26(2):98–102. https://doi.org/10.13076/j.tjo.2013.26.02_98.

17. Yagci A, Seker ED, Demirsoy KK, Ramoglu SI. Do total or partial etching procedures effect the rate of white spot lesion formation? A single-center, randomized, controlled clinical trial. Angle Orthod. 2019;89(1):16–24. https://doi.org/10.2319/013018-84.1.

18. Mheissen S, Seehra J, Khan H, Pandis N. Do sample size calculations in longitudinal orthodontic trials use the advantages of this study design? Angle Orthod. 2022;92(3):402–8. https://doi.org/10.2319/091321-707.1.

19. Mheissen S, Khan H, Almuzian M, Alzoubi EE, Pandis N. Do longitudinal orthodontic trials use appropriate statistical analyses? A meta-epidemiological study. Eur J Orthod. 2021;44(3):352–7. https://doi.org/10.1093/ejo/cjab069.

20. Benson PE, Parkin N, Dyer F, Millett DT, Germain P. Fluorides for preventing early tooth decay (demineralised lesions) during fixed brace treatment. Cochrane Database Syst Rev. 2019; https://doi.org/10.1002/14651858.CD003809.pub4.

21. Nascimento PL, Fernandes MT, Figueiredo FE, Faria ESAL. Fluoride-releasing materials to prevent white spot lesions around orthodontic brackets: a systematic review. Braz Dent J. 2016;27(1):101–7. https://doi.org/10.1590/0103-6440201600482.

22. Sardana D, Zhang J, Ekambaram M, Yang Y, McGrath CP, Yiu CKY. Effectiveness of professional fluorides against enamel white spot lesions during fixed orthodontic treatment: a systematic review and meta-analysis. J Dent. 2019;82:1–10. https://doi.org/10.1016/j.jdent.2018.12.006.

23. Tasios T, Papageorgiou SN, Papadopoulos MA, Tsapas A, Haidich AB. Prevention of orthodontic enamel demineralization: a systematic review with meta-analyses. Orthod Craniofac Res. 2019;22(4):225–35. https://doi.org/10.1111/ocr.12322.

24. Pithon MM, Baião FS, Sant'Anna LID, Tanaka OM, Cople-Maia L. Effectiveness of casein phosphopeptide-amorphous calcium phosphate-containing products in the prevention and treatment of white spot lesions in orthodontic patients: a systematic review. J Investig Clin Dent. 2019;10(2):e12391. https://doi.org/10.1111/jicd.12391.

25. Bailey DL, Adams GG, Tsao CE, Hyslop A, Escobar K, Manton DJ, et al. Regression of post-orthodontic lesions by a remineralizing cream. J Dent Res. 2009;88(12):1148–53. https://doi.org/10.1177/0022034509347168.

26. Höchli D, Hersberger-Zurfluh M, Papageorgiou SN, Eliades T. Interventions for orthodontically induced white spot lesions: a systematic review and meta-analysis. Eur J Orthod. 2017;39(2):122–33. https://doi.org/10.1093/ejo/cjw065.

27. Borges AB, Caneppele TM, Masterson D, Maia LC. Is resin infiltration an effective esthetic treatment for enamel development defects and white spot lesions? A systematic review. J Dent. 2017;56:11–8. https://doi.org/10.1016/j.jdent.2016.10.010.

28. Knösel M, Eckstein A, Helms HJ. Durability of esthetic improvement following Icon resin infiltration of multibracket-induced white spot lesions compared with no therapy over 6 months: a single-center, split-mouth, randomized clinical trial. American Journal of Orthodontics and Dentofacial Orthopedics: official publication of the American Association of Orthodontists, its constituent societies, and the American Board of Orthodontics. 2013;144(1):86–96. https://doi.org/10.1016/j.ajodo.2013.02.029.

29. Gugnani N, Pandit I, Gugnani S, Gupta M, Soni S, Juneja V, et al. Evaluation of esthetic improvement of non-pitted fluorosis using CIELAB parameters and patient satisfaction, when treated with resin infiltration, bleaching and bleaching with resin infiltration. J Dent Res. 2015;94(A)

30. Senestraro SV, Crowe JJ, Wang M, Vo A, Huang G, Ferracane J, et al. Minimally invasive resin infiltration of arrested white-spot lesions: a randomized clinical trial. J Am Dent Assoc. 2013;144(9):997–1005. https://doi.org/10.14219/jada.archive.2013.0225.

31. Wang L, Jian J, Lu H. Efficiency of resin infiltration versus fluride varnish for treatment of post-orthodontic white spot lesions. J Clin Rehabil Tissue Eng Res. 2013;17(29):5303–8.

32. Sonesson M, Bergstrand F, Gizani S, Twetman S. Management of post-orthodontic white spot lesions: an updated systematic review. Eur J Orthod. 2017;39(2):116–21. https://doi.org/10.1093/ejo/cjw023.
33. Akin M, Basciftci FA. Can white spot lesions be treated effectively? Angle Orthod. 2012;82(5):770–5. https://doi.org/10.2319/090711.578.1.
34. Knösel M, Klang E, Helms HJ, Wiechmann D. Occurrence and severity of enamel decalcification adjacent to bracket bases and sub-bracket lesions during orthodontic treatment with two different lingual appliances. Eur J Orthod. 2016;38(5):485–92. https://doi.org/10.1093/ejo/cjv069.

Retention

10

Contents

© The Author(s), under exclusive license to Springer Nature Switzerland AG 2023   243
S. Mheissen, H. Khan, *Orthodontic Evidence*,
https://doi.org/10.1007/978-3-031-24422-3_10

Introduction

Orthodontic retention refers to holding the teeth in their final functional and aesthetic position. As orthodontic treatment involves moving the teeth to a new position by leveling and alignment or translation movement, time is required for reorganizing tooth neighboring structures. These structures involve bone, gingival and transseptal fibers. Also, neuromuscular and soft tissue adaption of neighboring structures is necessary to accommodate these teeth in their new positions. Reorganization and adaptation of these structures prevent relapse or moving back of the teeth to their original position. Reorganization of the different structures requires different times, such as PDL fibers reorganizing in 3–4 months, gingival collagenous fibers in 4–6 months and elastic fibers requiring up to 6 months. Furthermore in young patients retention is required till the patient is growing.

Removable and fixed retainers are used for orthodontic retention. These retainers work on the principle that they should not interfere with the physiological movement of the teeth so that reorganization of the gingival and periodontal fibers can easily take place. The most popular removable retainers are the Hawley retainer (HR), Begg or Wraparound retainer, Spring or Barrer retainers or clip-on retainers and Vacuum or pressure-formed retainers (VFR or PFR). In fixed retainers, 0.017-in. multistranded wire, 0.0195-in. coaxial wire, fiber-reinforced composite wires, polyethylene ribbon-reinforced resin retainers, twist flex, flex tech, Beta-titanium and NiTi or titanium-based CAD CAM retainers [1]. There is controversy in the literature about the selection of retainers and retention protocols. In contemporary orthodontics, the retention protocol depends upon patient preferences, clinician experience, type of malocclusion, type of tooth movement during treatment, final occlusal outcomes and cost of the retainers [2]. This chapter answers important questions related to the selection of orthodontic retainers, the retention protocol and potential problems associated with these retainers.

Retention Requirement

Clinical Question 1: Why Orthodontic Retainers Should Be Used?

Evidence

Systematic Review and Meta-Analysis

Littlewood/2016 [3]
This Cochrane systematic review included two RCTs investigating the stability of lower incisors by using Little's Irregularity Index. The average relapse was 0.43 mm and 1.03 mm using fixed and removable appliances after 1 year of retention in one trial, while this was 0.05–0.07 after 18 months in another trial.

Randomized Controlled Trial

Naraghi/2021 [4]
In this trial, the researchers recruited 63 impacted canine patients with a moderate irregularity index of the upper anterior six teeth. They randomly allocated 32 patients to the retention group and 31 patients to the non-retention group. In the retention group, the upper removable vacuum-formed retainer on the day of debonding was given to all the patients. The patients were told to wear the retainer 22–24 h/day for 4 weeks. After 4 weeks the patients were instructed to wear the VFR for 10–12 h/day. In the non-retention group, after active treatment, the archwires were removed while the brackets were left in place, and the patients were followed for 10 weeks. The mean treatment time was 29.7 ± 7.0 months in the retention group and 30.1 ± 9.1 months in the non-retention group, with no significant difference between groups. The researchers found that the change in irregularity index was statistically higher in the non-retention group (1.3 mm) when compared with the retention group (0.4 mm) in the follow up period. The maximum increase in the irregularity index was 2.5 mm in the retention group while it was 3.2 mm in the non-retention group. No statistically significant changes between the groups were found in arch length or intercanine and intermolar width. After the 1-year observation period, 93.5% of patients in the retention group and 80% of patients in the non-retention group had lower incisors irregularity index (LII) of less than 3 mm.

Evidence Summary

The best available evidence suggests that the relapse after 1 year of retention was 0.43 mm and 1.03 mm using fixed and removable retainers, respectively [3]. The irregularity index was higher in the non-retention group (1.3 mm), while it was 0.4 mm in the retention group in 10 weeks follow up [4]. The maximum increase in LII was up to 3.2 mm in the non-retention group and 2.5 mm in the retention group. After 1 year of follow up, 20% of the non-retention group patients had LII of more than 3 mm, while only 6.5% of the retention group got LII of more than 3 mm.

Evidence Interpretation

Retainers are used at the end of orthodontic treatment to maintain the treatment results. If retainers are not used after treatment, there is a great chance that teeth will relapse to their original positions. Even with retainers, some minor relapse is inevitable. In terms of the type of retention, fixed retainers are more efficient than removable retainers in maintaining lower incisors' alignment.

Viewpoint

Littlewood et al. review [3] was a Cochrane review that follow rigor methods in conducting and reporting. Most of the included trials were assessed as having a high risk of bias due to attrition bias and selective reporting, thus leading to reduce the quality of the evidence. As such, the authors acknowledge that the quality of evidence is not adequate to recommend any retention approach over another.

Naraghi trial [4] was a well-conducted trial. The authors used intention to treat analysis and tried to reduce the confounding factors to avoid selection bias. However, the cases were treated by one unblinded operator, which may be a source of bias. In the retention group, four patients had interdental spaces, and the researchers placed fixed retainers on them, while there was no information regarding spaces in the non-retention group, which may confound the results.

Common Retention Protocols

Clinical Question 2: Which Are the Most Commonly Used Retainers by Orthodontists?

Evidence

Systematic Review

Bahije/2018 [5]

This systematic review included seven studies to evaluate different retention protocols. Six studies reported that the common retention protocols were a vacuum-formed retainer (VFR) or a Hawley retainer (HR) in the upper arch and fixed retainers (FR) in the lower arch.

Cross-Sectional Study

Carneiro/2022 [6]

An online survey was distributed to 576 Canadian orthodontists. One hundred one orthodontists participated in this survey. Most of the respondents were males (74.3%) working in private practice (96%). The authors found that almost half of the participants preferred VFR in the maxilla (50.5%) and bonded retainers (BR) in the mandible (54.5%). The orthodontists preferred a combination between BR and VFR in the maxilla for re-treated cases, diastema, and impacted anterior teeth.

Singh/2009 [7]

This survey was distributed to 301 UK based orthodontists to investigate the retention regime in the crowded Class II division 1 cases. Two-hundred forty UK orthodontists completed the survey: 77 were females and 163 were males. Sixty-one percent of the participants were working in more than one practice setting. VFR was the most common retainer in both maxilla and mandible for NHS and hospitals. Likewise, VFR was the most common retainer in the maxilla in private practice, while the combination of bonded with VFR was the common retention regime in the mandible in private practice. In the maxilla, orthodontists working in NHS and hospitals were more likely to prefer removable retainers than those working in a private setting by 8.73 and 5.57 times, respectively. In the mandible, orthodontists working in NHS and hospitals were more likely to prefer removable retainers than those working in a private setting by 6.96 and 4.03 times, respectively.

The multivariable logistic regression showed no statistically significant difference between males and females regarding the retainer choice ($P = 0.11$ and 0.46 for maxilla and mandible, respectively). Likewise, there was no difference between younger and older orthodontists in regard to the retainer choice.

Evidence Summary

The best available evidence suggests that the most common retention protocols among orthodontists are vacuum-formed or a Hawley retainer in the upper arch and fixed retainers in the lower arch [5, 6]. In Class II division I cases, the most common retainer was VFR in both arches in NHS and hospital settings, and VFR in the maxilla and the combination of bonded and VFR in the mandible in the private setting.

Evidence Interpretation

There is no evidence for the selection of any specific type of retainers. So, the choice is retainers is mostly dependent on clinician experience, patients' choice, compliance, and the cost involved. Orthodontists commonly use removable retainers in the upper arch; VFR or HR and fixed retainers with or without combined VFR in the lower arch.

Viewpoint

Albeit Bahije review [5] provided us with good information, there were different shortcomings in it. The search was limited for 10 years, with no search for gray literature that may increase the publication bias. There was no risk of bias assessment of the included trials with a lack of clear description of these trials. Likewise, no clear PICO format was used. The authors included different designs of studies that may reduce the quality of the evidence. As such, this review [5] is not conclusive evidence in terms of retention protocols.

The response rate in Carneiro et al. survey [6] was low (18%), thus suggesting the sample does not adequately represent the population. No sample size calculation was reported that leave the study in concerns regarding statistical power. The table of the participants' characteristics was missing. The wide age range (19.7 ± 12 years) may influence and confound the findings. Furthermore, the authors did not provide information regarding the validity of the survey questions.

In Singh et al. study [7], the response rate (80%) was high, increasing the orthodontist's population representation in the findings. The results might be related to orthodontists working in the United Kingdom. Similarly, the specific type of malocclusion may limit the generalizability of the findings.

Removable and Fixed Retainers

Clinical Question 3: What Should Be the Choice of Orthodontic Retainers, Removable or Fixed Retainer?

Evidence

Systematic Review and Meta-Analysis

Littlewood/2016 [3]
This systematic review included two RCTs comparing the effectiveness of fixed retainers (multistrand) and removable thermoplastic retainer in the stability of lower anterior teeth. One included trial found a statistically significant higher relapse with VFR by 0.6 mm/year than the fixed retainer (MD; 0.6, 95% CI 0.17–1.03; $P = 0.0061$). Similarly another trial found a statistically significant of 0.05 mm, also favoring the fixed retainer. The quality of evidence was low.

Systematic Review

Bellini-Pereira/2022 [8]
This systematic review included five RCTs comparing the effectiveness of VFR and bonded retainers (BR) in maintaining treatment stability. Both retainers have similar retention capacity with a better result of BR in the lower arch, especially on long-term of follow up. However, two studies [9, 10] found that BR was associated with more plaque and calculus accumulation, and more gingival inflammation than VFR.

In the upper arch, both retainers showed the same failure rate after 1 year of retention in one trial [9], while after 2 years, the failure rate was higher in VFR (50%) compared to BR (23%) [11]. In the lower arch, two trials [9, 12] reported a higher failure rate with BR than VFR, while one study [13] did find a significant difference between both of them.

Randomized Controlled Trial

Naraghi/2021 [11]
The researchers recruited 90 subjects for this trial. They randomly allocated the subjects into three retention groups as follows: 0.0195 wire bonded retainer 13–23 (six-teeth group), 0.0195-in bonded retainer 12–22 (four-teeth group), and removable VFR with 1.5 mm thickness covering the maxillary teeth including the second molars. LII and contact point discrepancy (CPD) increased slightly in all [8] groups with no statistically significant differences between the three groups. The six-teeth group showed statistically significantly less rotational changes than the VFR group ($P = 0.036$). Furthermore, the intercanine width increased only in the VFR group, which was statistically significant ($P = 0.023$). There were minor changes in over-bite, overjet, intermolar width, and arch length without any significant differences between groups. Fourteen VFR patients with poor adherence had an increase in LII when compared to the patients with suspected good adherence.

Evidence Summary
Looking into evidence collectively, the best available evidence suggests that VFR and FR are effective for orthodontic retention with a higher statistically but not clinically significant relapse in VFR when compared to FR. This difference in relapse ranged from 0.05 to 0.6 mm between VFR and FR for 1 year of retention [3]. FR and VFR have similar retention capacities with a better retention result in the lower arch when FR was used, especially for the long-term follow-up. However, after 1 year of retention, FR was associated with more gingival inflammation and calculus accumulation. The failure rate was higher with BR than VFR in the lower arch, while it was a controversy between studies in the upper arch.

One trial [11] found that six-upper anterior teeth FR provide less rotational changes than the VFR group ($P = 0.036$), with an increase of intercanine width in VFR. Interestingly, 14/30 (46%) of the VFR group has poor adherence that increased the LII.

Evidence Interpretation
Fixed retainer provided slightly better retention than VFR, which might be not clinically significant with some differences between them in the failure rate. On the downside, fixed retainers are associated with more gingival inflammation and calculus accumulation. As such, there is no high level of evidence for any choice of any specific type of retainer and the choice of retainer is largely dictated by clinician experience, cost and patient compliance.

In the maxilla, FR and VFR provide good stability results with a minor relapse in the first year of retention.

In the mandible, FR is more effective than VFR but the difference between FR and VFR was not clinically significant.

Viewpoint

Bellini-Pereira et al. review [8] was a well-conducted review. However, the clinical and methodological heterogeneity such as the wide age range between studies (13.8 ± 1.5 and 21.5 ± 3.0 years) and the different retention protocols with different wires for FR, hindered undertaking the meta-analysis.

Naraghi trial [11] was a well-conducted trial. However, there was no blinding for the operator or the patients. The number of non-adherent participants (47%) in the VFR group was high and may confound the results. The patients were adolescents (mean age 14 years), with a mean CPD of 3.3 mm in bonded retainers and 2.7 mm in VFR groups, with less extraction and bimaxillary cases in the VFR group, which may suggest that only mild cases were included in the VFR group. As such, the findings of the study have limited generalizability to adolescent patients with mild crowding.

The included studies have already been discussed in previous questions.

Fixed Retainers

Clinical Question 4: Which Is the Best Fixed Retainer?

Evidence

Systematic Review and Meta-Analyses

Liu/2022 [14]

In this review, 10 RCTs and 1 CCT were included to compare the effectiveness of fiber-reinforced composite (FRC) and multistranded stainless steel wire (MSW) retainers. Less relapse was found in FRC when compared to MSW in 12 month follow-up period (MD; -0.39 mm, 95% CI: -0.41 to -0.37; $P < 0.00001$). There was no statistically significant difference between the both retainers in terms of the whole retainer failure rate (RR; 1.76, 95% CI, 0.86–3.58; $P = 0.12$, 5 trials) or the failure rate per tooth (RR; 0.85, 95% CI, 0.47–1.52; $P = 0.58$, 3 trials). Only one trial [15] investigated the patients' satisfaction and found that polyethylene ribbon-reinforced resin retainers were more acceptable to wear than MSW (MD; 1.49, 95% CI: 0.80–2.18; $P < 0.0001$). The evidence was of low quality.

Randomized Controlled Trials

Gunay/2018 [16]

The authors randomly assigned 120 patients (60 without extraction and 60 with first premolar extraction) into two lingual fixed retainers' groups. They used 0.0175-in. six-stranded stainless steel wire (Ortho Technology, Lutz, Fla) for the first group (SS) and 0.0195-in. dead-soft coaxial wire (Respond; Ormco, Orange, Calif) for the second group (Cox). They followed the patients for 3, 6, 9 and 12 months. The total orthodontic treatment duration was 17 months for the SS group and 19 months for the Cox group. There was a statistically significant difference in the mean irregularities of the post-treatment models between groups and this was 1.88 mm and 1.56 mm for SS and Cox groups, respectively. The irregularities increased over time of retention in both groups. The researchers found that the mean irregularity measurement differences between post-treatment and the 12-month retention period were 0.82 mm in the SS group and 1.97 mm in the Cox group. The amount of mandibular arch irregularity was significantly higher in the Cox group than in the SS group after 12 months. There was no statistically significant difference in the SS group over time regarding the intercanine distance, while there was a statistically significant decrease in the Cox group over time regarding intercanine distance. On the other hand, there was a significant difference in the arch length measurements in the SS group but not in the Cox group.

The failure rates were 13.2% for the SS group and 18.9% for the Cox group. The difference between the groups was not statistically significant ($P > 0.05$).

Naraghi/2021 [11]

The researchers recruited 90 subjects (54 females and 36 males) with a mean age of 13.9 years in this trial. They randomly allocated the subjects into three retention groups as follows: bonded retainer 13–23 (six-teeth group), bonded retainer 12–22 (four-teeth group), and removable VFR covering the maxillary teeth, including the second molars. Fixed retainers were manufactured from Penta-One 0.0195-in. in a laboratory. After a follow-up of 2 years of retention, LII and contact point discrepancy (CPD) increased slightly in all three groups without any statistically significant differences between the three groups. The six-teeth group showed statistically less rotational changes than four-teeth group ($P = 0.014$) and VFR group ($P = 0.036$). Furthermore, the intercanine width decreased in the six-teeth group and remained unchanged in the four-teeth. The difference in intercanine width was statistically significant between bonded retainer 13–23 and VFR ($P = 0.023$). There were minor changes in overjet, overbite, intermolar width and arch length without any significant inter-group differences.

Evidence Summary

Looking at the evidence collectively, the best available evidence suggests that different types of fixed retainers are effective in retention after orthodontic treatment. FRC has less relapse when compared to MSW by 0.39 mm in LLI, which is not clinically significant. However, FRC was more acceptable by the patients.

0.0175-in. six-stranded stainless steel wire has significantly less mean irregularity measurement after a 12 months retention period (0.82 mm) when compared to the Cox (1.97 mm). The failure rate was higher but insignificant in coaxial wire 18.9% compared to 13.2% in the six-stranded wire. The intercanine distance decreased in the Cox group with no significant change in the SS group. Regarding arch length measurements, a significant difference was found in the SS group but not in the Cox group. In terms of the number of teeth involved in the fixed retainers, when the six-teeth fixed retainer was compared with the four-teeth retainer in the maxilla, the six-teeth retainer showed statistically significant less rotational changes than four-teeth group after 2 years of retention. The intercanine width decreased in the six-teeth retainer group and remained unchanged in the four-teeth group but this was not clinically significant. However, the changes in LII, overjet, overbite, intermolar width and arch length were not statistically significant.

Evidence Interpretation

The fiber-reinforced composite retainers seem slightly better than multistranded retainers which in turn are superior to coaxial retainers.

Fixed retainers in the maxillary arch, either on six or four teeth, prevent a significant relapse after 2 years of retention with no clinically significant difference between six- and four-teeth retainers.

Viewpoint

In Liu et al. review [14], the electronic search yielded only 99 records and 49 records, before and after removing the duplicates. This could be due to the sensitive search strategy. Most of the included trials were rated as having some concerns to a high risk of bias that may reduce the quality of the available evidence. The follow-up period in the included studies was different and one average short. Finally, the clinical heterogeneity between the included trials in the age, gender, and initial malocclusion may affect the findings.

There was a lack of information regarding the allocation concealment and the blinding in Gunay trial [16]. However, the wire was fabricated on the model in the SS group while it was adapted in the mouth for the Cox group, which may confound the results as the retainer might be not fully passive in the Cox group. Patients with rotation of the mandibular anterior teeth were excluded from the study which may restrict the results' generalizability. The treatment time was higher in the Cox group that also may confound the findings.

Removable Retainers

Clinical Question 5: Which Is a Better Removable Retainer?

Evidence

Systematic Reviews

Outhaisavanh/2020 [17]
This systematic review included 15 RCTs. Five included trials compared Hawley and vacuum-formed retainers. They found that there is no statistically significant difference between the two types of retainers in both maxillary and mandibular arches. Two included trials reported that there is no significant difference in the arch length when wearing full-time HR and VFR. In contrast, one trial [18] found that

VFR was more effective than HR in terms of the maxillary arch length ($P = 0.007$). likewise, two studies found that VFR is more effective than HR in both arches regarding Little's Irregularity Index (LII).

Al Rahma/2018 [19]

This systematic review included ten RCTs investigating the performance of HR and VFR. One trial [20] found a greater change in the LII in the Hawley group in the 6-month period. Likewise, another trial found more rotation in maxillary teeth in the Hawley group than VFR after 9 months of debonding [21]. Regarding overjet and overbite, no statistically significant difference between the two retainers was found. The authors graded the evidence as low.

Mai/2014 [22]

This systematic review included seven studies; five RCTs and two CCTs. Four studies compared VFR and HR regarding the stability of orthodontic patients' teeth. Three studies found no significant differences in the intercanine and intermolar widths between HRs and VFRs. Also, two studies reported no significant differences in arch length between the two retainers.

Randomized Controlled Trial

Ashari/2022 [23]

In this multi-center RCT, the authors randomly assigned 35 patients, with at least 3 mm of expansion using quadhelix, into two groups: 18 patients in the modified VFR group and 17 patients in the HR group. They modified the VFR by adding a palatal coverage. After a follow-up for 24 months, only 26 patients' data were analyzed. There was no statistically significant difference in the arch width relapse between the modified VFR and HR.

Evidence Summary

Looking into the evidence collectively, the best available evidence suggests that VFR and HR are effective in terms of teeth stability during the retention period. Regarding arch length, no significant difference was found between HR and VFR in the two reviews [17, 22]. On the other hand, one trial [18] found that VFR is more effective than HR in terms of the maxillary arch length. Two reviews [17, 19] found more LII change in the HR group than in the VFR group, with more rotation in the HR group. No statistically significant difference between the two retainers was found in overjet, overbite, intercanine and intermolar width.

Evidence Interpretation

Vacuum formed and Hawley retainers are effective in the retention phase after orthodontic treatment. But with low certainty, VFR may provide more stability in arch length, teeth rotation and LII than HR.

Viewpoint

In Outhaisavanh review [17] six studies were classified as having a high risk of bias. Although the author followed a rigorous methodology, the limited number of RCTs which was clinically heterogeneous regarding the retention protocol and the type of retainers hindered pooling the results in meta-analysis. As such, the authors included one or two trials in each outcome which may reduce the quality of the evidence.

Al Rahma review [19] included only RCTs which are considered the highest quality evidence. The limitation in this review arises from the nature of the included studies and the lack of evidence in terms of the same outcome that may reduce the quality of the evidence.

Mai review [22] outcomes should be interpreted with caution because of the poor quality of the included studies and the clinical heterogeneity.

Ashari et al. trial [23] was a well-conducted trial. However, the sample size was small and was calculated based on the arch meaningful expansion difference rather than the relapse. Also, the calculation did not consider data dependence as the design was longitudinal [24]. The age range was wide in both groups that may lead to different relapse degrees between growing and non-growing patients. Likewise, this may affect the reported outcomes.

Wearing Schedules

Clinical Question 6: What Should be The Wearing Schedule for Removable Retainers?

Evidence

Systematic Reviews

Outhaisavanh/2020 [17]

Five included trials compared full versus part-time wear of removable retainers. There was no statistically significant difference between the two-duration wear of the removable retainers in both maxillary and mandibular arches. One study [25] investigated using VFR for two-duration wear and found that there was no statistically significant difference between full-time wear and night-time wear regarding overjet and overbite. In contrast, another study [26] found a statistically significant difference between both wearing schedule regarding the overbite ($P = 0.02$), but the difference was only 0.6 mm, which seems to be not clinically significant.

Al Rahma/2018 [19]

Only one included trial (Shawesh et al. [27]) compared full-time wear with part-time wear of Hawley retainers. In the full-time group, the patients were instructed to wear the retainer 24/day for 6 months and at night only for the next 6 months, while the part-time group was asked to wear the retainer at night only for 1 year. No statistically significant differences were observed between the two retention regimens regarding maxillary and mandibular LLI or labial segment crowding.

Evidence Summary

Looking into evidence collectively, the best available evidence suggests that there is no statistically significant difference between part and full-time wearing of removable retainers. Only one trial found a statistically but not clinically significant difference in the overbite changes (0.6 mm) between full and part-time wear of removable retainers.

Evidence Interpretation

There is no difference between part-time and full-time wear of orthodontic retainers. So, part-time wear of retainers can be recommended to the patients.

Viewpoint

The review [19] authors assessed Shawesh et al. trial [27] at low risk of bias. The study investigated the change in the orthodontic outcome after 1 year regarding LLI/labial segment crowding, so longer studies are needed to investigate more outcomes that may be related to the initial malocclusion. Considering other confounding factors is important as this study is limited to mild and moderate crowded cases.

Outhaisavanh review [17] has been already discussed in this chapter.

Cost-Effectiveness

Clinical Question 7: What Is the Cost-Effectiveness of Removable Retainers?

Evidence

Systematic Reviews

Outhaisavanh/2020 [17]
One included RCT [20] evaluated the cost-effectiveness of the Hawley retainer and vacuum-formed retainer and found that the VFR costs less than HR over 6 months of retention period, based on the patients attending an unscheduled appointment. The authors analyzed the cost in the United Kingdom and National Health Service (NHS). The authors found the cost of HR is higher than VFR (41.22 € and 33.83 €, respectively) in private practice settings. Likewise, the cost in NHS was 152.42 € for HR and 121.08 € for VFR.

Al Rahma/2018 [19]
Two included trials [20, 28] were done in the United Kingdom and analyzed the cost of HR and VFR. The authors found that VFR was more cost-effective than HR from the perspectives of the NHS in the United Kingdom, the orthodontic practice and

the individual patients, but the evidence for the comparison of individual patients was deemed to be weak.

Mai/2014 [22]

One included trial [28] investigated the cost for NHS, private practice, and patients. Sixty-two subjects (HR: 41, VFR: 21) were analyzed for attending extra appointments regarding problems with their retainers (travel costs, childcare costs, patient fees and lost income). The HR patients had statistically greater costs than the VFR patients (MD; 2.15 €, 95% CI: −2.90, 7.57). National Health Service and the orthodontic practices reported greater costs for HR than VFR, with a statistically significant mean difference of 31.35 € (95% CI; 28.06, 34.68) and 32.60 € (95% CI; 30.58, 34.67), respectively. As such, the cost-effectiveness analysis of the retainers showed that VFRs were more cost-effective than HRs over a 6-month retention period.

Evidence Summary

Looking into available evidence collectively, the best evidence suggests that VFR is more cost-effective than HR in the United Kingdom, with different cost values due to the inclusion criteria and date of search of the aforementioned systematic reviews. For instance, the mean cost difference was 31.35 € (95% CI: 28.06, 34.68) and 32.60 € (95% CI: 30.58, 34.67) for NHS and private practice, respectively [22]. Another review reported these values for private practice (41.22 € and 33.83 €, HR and VFR, respectively) and NHS (152.42 € for HR and 121.08 € for VFR) [17]. Furthermore, the additional cost was considered for HR patients rather than VFR patients due to extra appointments for retainer problems.

Evidence Interpretation

The VFR is more cost-effective than HR in the United Kingdom. The place of residency may play a vital role in the cost of the retainers. So, the clinician can estimate the retainers' cost due to his practice.

Viewpoint

The three included reviews which answered this question, provided the cost analysis in the United Kingdom that limit the generalizability of the finding of this outcome.

The Survival Rate of FR

Clinical Question 8: What Is the Survival Rate of Fixed Retainers?

Evidence

Systematic Reviews and Meta-Analyses

Jedliński/2021 [29]

This review included 21 studies from different designs to investigate the failure rate of fixed retainers. The study found that the failure rate ranged from 3.7% to 50%, with more failure rate in the upper arch. Seven studies were pooled in meta-analysis and found that there is no difference in the failure rate between (fiber-reinforced composite) FRC retainers and multistranded SS wire retainers. The type of wire has no effect on the failure rate.

Iliadi/2015 [30]

This review included 27 studies; 9 were RCTs, 6 were prospective studies and 12 were retrospective studies. In general, the quality of the evidence was low. This study found that the failure rate for glass-fiber reinforced retainers ranged from 11% to 71%. One included retrospective study found that Cr–Ni retainer (0.6 mm wire bonded only to the mandibular canines) bond failure was 34.9%. Another prospective trial found 11.6% failures for Co-based alloy retainers which were bonded to all lower anterior teeth with a chemically cured adhesive over a mean period of 15.7 months. Twenty studies reported that bond failure of multistranded wire retainer ranged from 8.8% to 46%.

Two included trials compared polyethylene weaved ribbon retainer with 0.0175 in. multistranded wire retainer in terms of failure (breakage, detachment, and bond failure incidents). The same light-cured adhesive was used for all retainers. The meta-analysis showed no statistically significant difference in the risk of failure between the two retainers (RR: 1.74; 95% CI: 0.45, 6.73; $P = 0.42$, 2 trials).

Randomized Controlled Trials

Gunay/2018 [16]

The investigators used 0.0175-in. six-stranded stainless steel wire (Ortho Technology, Lutz, Fla) for the first group (SS) and 0.0195-in. dead-soft coaxial wire (Respond; Ormco, Orange, Calif) for the second group (Cox). They followed the patients for 3, 6, 9, and 12 months. The failure rates were 13.2% for the SS group and 18.9% for the Cox group. The difference between the groups was not statistically significant ($P > 0.05$).

Naraghi/2021 [11]

This RCT randomly assigned 90 patients into three groups: 13–23 bonded retainer (six-teeth group), 12–22 bonded retainer (four-teeth group), and VFR group. During the 2-year period, seven patients in six-teeth group, and six in the four-teeth group lost their retainer.

Evidence Summary

Looking into available evidence collectively, the best evidence suggest that the FR failure rate ranged from 3.7% to 50%, with more failure rate in the upper arch. The failure rate ranged from 11 to 71% in Glass-fiber reinforced retainers, while it ranged from 8.8 to 46% in multistranded wire retainers, and it was 34.9% for Cr–Ni retainers and 11.6% for Co-based alloy retainers. No statistically significant difference was found between ribbon retainer and multistranded wire retainer regarding the failure rate. Interestingly, no agreement concerning the optimal type of wire was reported. The failure rate was 13.2% for the 0.0175-in. six-stranded stainless steel wire group and 18.9% for the 0.0195-in. dead-soft coaxial wire group with no statistically significant intergroup difference ($P > 0.05$).

Evidence Interpretation

The fixed retainers have a survival rate of 50–96% with more failures in the upper arch. Upper arch retainers' failure can be explained by the fact that these retainers interfere with incisor occlusion and are difficult to place in a good finished Class I incisor relationship. Wire type of retainer has no significant effect on the failure rate but more failures were reported on thicker 0.0195-in. dead-soft coaxial wire than on 0.0175-in. six-stranded stainless steel wire.

Multiple factors may play a vital role in the failure rate of fixed retainers. For instance, occlusal interferences for maxillary retainers, the experience and preferences of the clinician, bonding materials, and patient compliance.

Viewpoint

Jedliński [29] systematic review has some limitations due to the differences in design between included studies, different types of wire used, different outcomes measures, the experience of the clinician and bonding materials. Many studies have also included growing patients. Growth inevitably has an impact on the stability outcome in the retention phase. Another limitation is the period of follow-up and different frequencies of check-ups in the included studies.

Most of the included studies, in Iliadi review [30], were of low quality due to the high risk of bias. Likewise, including different study designs may reduce the quality of the evidence. As such the true effect may be substantially different from the present estimate of the effect.

The Survival Rate of RR

Clinical Question 9: What Is the Survival Rate of Removable Retainers?

Evidence

Systematic Reviews

Outhaisavanh/2020 [17]

Three included studies investigated the survival rate of HR and VFR. One trial [31] found that there is no statistically significant difference between the two retainers over 1 year of follow-up, while another trial [32], in which a comparison was made between HR and VFR from two thicknesses 1 mm and 1.5 mm, reported that the breakage was the main reason for changing the retainer within 6 months and the highest breakage retainer was for 1 mm thickness of VFR. There was no significant difference in the loss and discoloration of the three removable retainers, with perforations found only in the VFR. In contrast, another trial [20] estimated the rate of loss and breakage within 6 months of wear and found a statistically significant lower rate of breakage in VFR compared to HR ($P < 0.001$).

One trial [33] compared the survival time for two different thicknesses of VFR (0.75 and 1 mm) and did not find a statistically significant difference in both maxillary and mandibular arches.

Mai/2014 [22]

In this review, one included study [31] randomly assigned 120 adolescent patients into two intervention groups to investigate the survival time of HRs and VFRs over a 1-year of follow-up. The authors found that there was no statistically significant difference between the HR and VFR groups for either the maxilla ($P = 0.254$) or the mandible ($P = 0.188$). Another included study [28] investigated the rates of retainer breakage and loss of both retainers for a 6-month retention period. The broken retainers were statistically higher in the HR group than in the VFR group ($P < 0.001$). However, there was no difference in the loss rates of the retainers between the groups.

Randomized Controlled Trials

Naraghi/2021 [11]

This RCT randomly assigned 90 patients into three groups: 13–23 fixed retainer, 12–22 fixed retainer and VFR group. 15 patients in the VFR group either lost the retainer or had a breakage of the retainer. Also, a poor adherence to the wearing instructions was found in 14 patients (47%) according to the notes.

Ashari/2022 [23]

In this multi-center RCT, the authors randomly assigned 35 patients into two groups: 18 patients in modified VFR group and 17 patients in HR group. The VFR modification was by adding palatal coverage. After a follow-up of 2 years, only 26 patients' data were analyzed. In regard to the survival analysis, loss rate was 6% in HR group only and breakage rate was 6% in HR and 22% in modified VFR.

Evidence Summary

The best available evidence suggests that there is no consensus regarding the breakage and loss of removable retainers. One trial [31] reported that there is no significant difference between HR and VFR in terms of the failure rate over 1 year. In contrast, another trial [20, 28] found more breakage in HR rather than VFR over 6 months. The follow-up period and the settings of the trial [28, 31] may explain the difference between the findings. In VFR, more breakage rate was reported in 1 mm thickness VFRs than 1.5 mm VFRs. It is worth noting that there were perforations [17, 22] in VFRs. Modification of VFRs like palatal coverage may increase the breackage rate to 22%.

Interestingly, 50% (15/30) of patients had either loss or breakage of the VFR in an RCT [11], which reported poor adherence to the wearing instructions in 47% of the patients.

Evidence Interpretation

The evidence for the survival rate difference between VFR and HR is still inconclusive. With low certainty, VFR and HR have similar breakage and loss rates within 1 year of retention.

Breakage rate has a negative association with the thickness of the VFR, as more breakage rate was noticed in 1 mm VFR compared to 1.5 mm VFR. The breakage rate and poor adherence to VFR were substantial for the maxilla and by adding palatal coverage. However, occlusal forces, overbite, patients' age, and patients adherence should be taken into account for the survival rate of VFR and HR.

Viewpoint

The included studies have already been discussed in previous questions.

Factors Related to Retention

Clinical Question 10: What Is the Impact of Different Factors on Relapse of Orthodontic Alignment?

Evidence

Systematic Review and Meta-Analysis

Swidi/2019 [34]

This systematic review included one randomized control trial (RCT) and 29 observational studies in meta-analysis. The pooled estimate reported that the mandibular anterior teeth irregularity in the extraction group was significantly higher than that in non-extraction group ($P=0.026$) between post-orthodontic treatment and post-retention time points; SMD was 1.22 (95% CI: 1.04–1.40) and 0.85 (95% CI: 0.63–1.07) for extraction and non-extraction groups, respectively. There was a significant influence of follow-up duration (1–10 vs. 10–20 years) and study design (interventional versus observational studies) on the irregularity changes. The SMD of the 1–10 years follow-up group was significantly lesser 0.89 (95% CI: 0.73–1.05), when compared to the 10–20 years follow-up group 1.39 (95% CI: 1.18–1.60). The SMD was 1.90 (95% CI: 1.13–2.67) and 1.05 (95% CI: 0.91–1.19) for the interventional and observational studies, respectively. The evidence was graded as low to moderate.

Evidence Summary

The best available evidence suggests that the irregularity of the lower anterior teeth was statistically higher in the extraction group when compared to the non-extraction group (SMD was 1.22 and 0.85 for extraction and non-extraction groups, respectively). The irregularity of teeth increases over time after orthodontic treatment; SMD of 1–10 years follow-up was 0.89, while it was 1.39 for 10–20 years follow-up. Interventional studies reported a statistically higher SMD than observational studies due to robust methods.

Evidence Interpretation

With low certainty, extraction treatment is associated with a higher teeth irregularity post-orthodontics than non-extraction treatment. Orthodontic retention is required for both extraction and non-extraction cases.

If the orthodontist or the patient wishes no relapse, long-term retention is required as relapse was even observed 20 years post-orthodontic treatment.

Viewpoint

Most of the included studies in the Swidi review [34] were from a retrospective design that may reduce the quality of the evidence and increase the selection and recall bias. The quality of the included studies was fair due to the used risk of bias tool. Multiple factors may affect the alignment of the lower teeth, which may be considered as confounding factors and should be addressed. A significant risk of publication bias was found, which may suggest only studies with larger sample sizes and significant findings were published. As such, unpublished studies could have affected the irregularity estimates reported in this review.

Expansion and Retention

Clinical Question 11: What Should be The Duration of Retention After Maxillary Expansion, and Is It Effective?

Evidence

Systematic Review

Costa/2017 [35]
This systematic review included six trials; two RCTs, and four non-randomized studies that investigated the relapse of corrected crossbite. The patients were of different ages and they were treated using different appliances. The researchers found that the relapse of the maxillary expansion ranged from 0% [36] to 27% [37] in a follow-up period of 6–60 months. The relapse of the intermolar distance was 3.2% [36] and 1.2% [38] when the removable appliances were used as retainers for 6 months.

Evidence Summary

The best available evidence suggests that the relapse in intermolar distance after maxillary expansion ranged from 0% to 27%. This distance decreased to 3.2% and 1.2% when the removable appliance was used for 6 months as a retainer.

Evidence Interpretation

Orthodontic retention should be given for at least 6 months post-expansion to decrease the risk of relapse. Retention can be provided by fixed lingual arches if a second phase of orthodontic treatment is required. If no further orthodontic treatment is needed, removable retainers are given to maintain the outcomes of expansion.

Viewpoint

Most of the included trials in Costa review [35] were non-randomized trials that reduced the quality of this evidence. The included trials were assessed as having a moderate to high risk of bias. Interestingly, no study assessed or compared different periods of retention with different protocols in patients wearing the same kind of appliance.

Patient Satisfaction

Clinical Question 12: Which Removable Retainer Is More Acceptable by the Patients?

Evidence

Systematic Reviews

Outhaisavanh/2020 [17]
One includes trial reporting that HR is more embarrassed than the VFR ($P = 0.005$). Likewise, another trial [39] found that VFR was more acceptable than HR in speech, appearance, self-confidence, and comfort over 6 months of retention. Another trial [33] compared two different thicknesses of VFRs (0.75 and 1.00 mm) and found no statistically significant difference in either thickness regarding patients' comfort.

Mai/2014 [22]
One included trial [28] randomly assigned 397 participants into two intervention groups (HR: 196, VFR: 201). 350 participants completed a survey in terms of satisfaction (Hawley: 168, VFR: 182) at 6 months. There was more embarrassment in the HR group than in the VFR group ($P = 0.005$) and this was statistically significant. More patients felt better with the VFR than HR when the retainers were compared with fixed appliances ($P < 0.001$). However, there was no statistically significant difference in the amount of time a retainer was worn away from home.

Randomized Controlled Trials

Ashari/2022 [23]
In this multi-center RCT, the authors analyzed data of 26 patients with VFR or HR, 13 patients each. For patient-reported outcomes, no differences between HR and VFR were reported regarding fitting, speech, comfort, durability and oral hygiene after 24-month wear. However, the patient gave higher scores for the appearance of VFR compared to HR.

Saleh/2017 [39]
The authors randomly assigned 94 patients in parallel arm RCT to investigate the performance and acceptability of VFR and HR in the first 6 months of retention. The participants were asked to fill out a questionnaire on three occasions: 1 week, 3 months, and 6 months after fitting the retainer. The authors analyzed data for 86 patients (41 in the HR group and 45 in the VFR group). After 1-week, higher scores

were given to VFR in all parameters, but this was not significant for biting, fitting, and durability. After 3 months, the appearance also becomes insignificant. After 6 months, HR was statistically better in biting and durability, while hygiene became insignificant.

Evidence Summary

Looking into evidence collectively, the best available evidence suggests that the embarrassment was statistically higher in patients wearing HR than those wearing VFR. Likewise, VFR was more acceptable for patients than HR in terms of speech, appearance, self-confidence, and comfort over 6 months of retention. No influence of the VFR thickness on patients' comfort was found.

Evidence Interpretation

VFRs are more acceptable by patients than HR in terms of many perspectives. As such, the preferences of the patients should be taken into account when the clinician makes a related decision.

Viewpoint

In Saleh et al. [39] study, a lack of information regarding random generation may increase the randomization bias. Six patients in the HR group and two patients in the VFR group were lost to follow-up with no analysis to deal with this missing data. Also, higher missingness happened in the HR group. Although the authors used repeated measure ANOVA in their statistical analyses, but they reported the results using t-test and did not report the interaction between time and response, which may increase the selective reporting and p-hacking. The authors declared that they used Biostar machine to fabricate VFR, but this machine produced only pressure-formed retainers (PFR).

Breakage and loss of retainers were higher in VFR, but authors did not assess the effect of these failures on the findings. Finally, the sample size calculation did not take the longitudinal design into account [24].

Occlusal Settling

Clinical Question 13: What Is the Effect of Different Removable Retainers on Occlusal Contacts?

Evidence

Systematic Reviews

Outhaisavanh/2020 [17]

In this systematic review, one included trial [40] investigated the stability of occlusal contacts in modified VFR and full coverage VFR after 6 months. The investigators modified the VFR by opening the posterior occlusal surfaces. They found a significant increase of posterior contacts at 3 months after nightwear in the modified VFR group ($P < 0.01$) and a significant increase of anterior contacts after 3 months of nightwear in the full coverage VFR group, as well.

Mai/2014 [22]
One included trial [41] compared the changes in the number of occlusal contacts between VFR and HR after 3 months of retention. The trial found that the numbers of total contacts and posterior contacts were significantly higher in the HR than in the VFR.

Evidence Summary
The best available evidence suggests that the total and posterior occlusal contacts are statistically higher in HR when compared to VFR. Also, full coverage VFR significantly increases the anterior contacts after 3 months of nightwear, while modified VFR increases the posterior contacts.

Evidence Interpretation
Hawley retainers provide better occlusal contacts and subsequently better occlusal settling post-debonding than the vacuum-formed retainers. In VFR, there is a tendency for posterior open bite and less occlusal contact posteriorly. If the clinician wants to improve his posterior occlusal settling, modified VFRs with open posterior contacts should be used. However, in open bite cases, full coverage VFR may be favored.

Viewpoint
Both reviews have already been discussed.

Adverse Effect

Speech

Clinical Question 14: What Is the Impact of Removable Retainers on Speech?

Evidence

Systematic Review
Outhaisavanh/2020 [17]
One included trial [42], in this review, investigated the effect of HR and VFR on speech performance using spectral and temporal parameters. They found that HR was more affected by articulatory movement in consonant-vowel combinations than VFR. Likewise, another trial [43] found severe impairments in sounds as /3:/,/i:/,/f/,/ʊ/,/s/,/ʃ/ for the HR and /i:/,/ʊ/,/s/,/ʃ/ for the VFR. Both HR and VFR have sound distortions, but the changes in articulation were clearer in HR.

Al Rahma/2018 [19]

Two included trials [42, 43]evaluated different aspects of speech and found no statistically significant differences in the number of sound distortions at 3 months postdebonding. Various effects on the formant frequencies of four sustained vowels [a, e, i, u] and combinations of the vowel [a] with consonants were found in both groups at end of the 3-month evaluation period. The most apparent changes were for vowel [a] in HR group, [e] in VFR group, and [u] in both groups. However, Voice Onset Time values did not differ between individuals.

Evidence Summary

The best available evidence suggests that both HR and VFR have sound distortions, but the changes in articulation were more evident in HR. Also, HR was more affected by articulatory movement in consonant–vowel combinations than VFR.

Evidence Interpretation

Both HR and VFR cause sound distortions. Patients should be informed of these distortions and their potential effect on their quality of life. In some professions, such as patients having a specific career, patients' preferences should be taken into account. As retainers can be given for part-time in most patients, speech difficulty in some sounds only would not affect their daily life a great deal.

Viewpoint

Both reviews have already been discussed.

Periodontium and Retainers

Clinical Question 15: What Is the Effect of Different Retainers on Periodontal Health?

Evidence

Systematic Reviews
Arn/2020 [44]

This systematic review included 29 studies: 11 RCTs, 4 prospective cohort studies, 1 retrospective cohort study, and 13 cross-sectional studies. The evidence was of low quality. Ten included studies compared individuals having fixed retainers (FR) with a control group without retainers. Three studies found poor periodontal conditions in the FR group compared to the control group. In contrast, seven studies found no periodontal complications related to the fixed retainers, with a minor lingual gingival inflammation in FR group [45]. One included trial [46] found no difference in marginal bone levels between the two groups.

Eleven trials compared removable and fixed retainers: five trials found an increased accumulation of deposits in the FR group, while one trial [47] found more gingival inflammation in the FR group.

Five trials compared different types of fixed retainers. There was no difference between spiral and plain wires regarding periodontal health. However, four RCTs compared fiber-reinforced composite retainers to multistranded wire retainers. Two of them found no difference, and two studies found that multistranded wires were better in terms of gingival inflammation. Two studies found that the position of the fixed retainer (more incisally or more gingivally) does not affect periodontal health.

Outhaisavanh/2020 [17]

In this systematic review, one included trial investigated the gingival index scores (GI) in HR and VFR for 6 months and found that GI scores of thick VFR (1.5 mm) were higher than the 1 mm and HR; 1.19 ± 0.44; 1.13 ± 0.39; 1.04 ± 0.46, respectively.

Evidence Summary

Looking into evidence collectively, the best available evidence suggests that no periodontal or bone complications related to the fixed retainer were found. However, poor periodontal conditions in the FR group were reported compared to the control group. When FR was compared with removable retainers, more accumulation of deposits was found in the FR group with more gingival inflammation. The type of wire (spiral or plain) and the position of the retainer does not affect periodontal health. The multistrand retainer was statistically associated with less gingival inflammation than the fiber-reinforced composite retainer. For removable appliances, thick VFR was associated with slightly more gingival scores than HR.

Evidence Interpretation

In patients requiring orthodontic retainers following points should be considered when prescribing a retainer:

- Fixed retainers may complicate oral hygiene care and increase the accumulation of deposits that may yield poor periodontal health, so these retainers should be avoided in patients who already have poor oral hygiene at the end of treatment.
- The fiber-reinforced composite retainer is associated with more gingival inflammation than multistrand wire due to material characteristics.
- Thick VFR is associated with slightly more gingival inflammation than Hawley retainer and thin VFR.

Viewpoint

Arn review [44] included many trials from a different design that may reduce the quality of the evidence and increases bias. Most of the included trials were graded as having a high risk of bias. The included trials were heterogeneous in the clinical aspects leading to not feasible quantitative synthesis. As such, this review does not provide a robust clinical guidance for the retainers in terms of periodontal health.

Unexpected Complications

Clinical Question 16: What Are the Potential Complications of Fixed Retainers?

Evidence

Retrospective Study
Kucera/2016 [48]
This study included 3500 consecutive patients (1423 males, 2077 females) who finished their fixed orthodontic treatment followed by mandibular bonded flexible spiral wire fixed retainers. The multistrand wires were either a 0.0215-in. gold-plated five-stranded spiral wire (Penta-One; Gold'n Braces, Palm Harbor, Fla) or a 0.0175-in. six-stranded coaxial wire (Ortho Organizers). The patients also were instructed to wear lower VFR. The investigators recruited the patients with complications in a group and chose a random group as a control.

Thirty-eight (1.1%) patients experienced unexpected complications with the lower fixed retainer. Twenty-one had a twist effect (opposite inclination of the contralateral canines and increased the buccal inclination), 12 patients had X effect (torque difference between two adjacent incisors), and 5 had a non-specific complication such as spacing. The lower left canine inclined buccally in 89.5% of the patients who have a twist effect.

The patients with complications were significantly younger and had retainers for a shorter time than the control group; the retention period was 4.0 ± 2.8 years and 9.3 ± 2.0 years for complication and control groups, respectively. Also, the pre-treatment incisors' position and the mandibular angle were significantly larger in the complication group compared to the control group; 1-APog: 2.9 ± 2.3 and 1.9 ± 2.9, NS-ML: 36.4 ± 5.2 and 31.4 ± 6.7, for the complication and control groups, respectively.

Evidence Summary

The available evidence suggest that flexible spiral retainers may have some complications that may lead to unpredicted and unwanted tooth movements. Patients with younger ages are more prone to these complications. These complications mostly appear in the first 5 years after depending. Greater pre-treatment mandibular angle and longer pre-treatment linear incisors retrusion may increase these complications.

Evidence Interpretation

Fixed retainers might remain active and cause unwanted tooth movement, which was found while using spiral wire retainers. Spiral retainers might be active in some cases due to mechanical changes which may happen if the retention wires are coupled with anatomic conditions. Furthermore, patient characteristics such as high angle and increased lower incisors retraction may contribute to these iatrogenic effects. As such, the clinician should keep a long follow-up of their patients to ensure that these retainers are passive.

Viewpoint

The study of Kucera and Marek [48] was from a retrospective design that may have some inherent limitations. However, the large number of patients may provide a better estimation of the risk of fixed retainers complications. The authors chose a random sample as a comparison group but unfortunately it was not matched group regarding age and retention period. The sample size calculation was based on the inclination of the lower incisors with no clear rationale, and reported only the needed number of control groups. As such, the inferential statistics might be misleading.

Authors' Recommendations

- Orthodontic retainers should be used at the end of treatment to minimize relapse. Even with retainers, some minor relapse is inevitable.
- There is no clear evidence for the selection of fixed and removable retainers, but a fixed retainer is slightly better if the patient is able to maintain his/her oral hygiene. Mostly removable retainer is preferred in upper arch, while a fixed retainer alone in combination with a removable retainer is given in the lower arch. The choice is retainers are also dependent on clinician experience, patients' choice, compliance, and the cost involved.
- In fixed retainers, fiber-reinforced composite retainers are better than multi-stranded retainers which in turn are superior to coaxial retainers. Fixed retainer can be bonded to four or six anterior teeth with no significant difference between the two. Fixed retainers have a greater failure rate in the upper arch than in the lower arch.
- In removable retainers, vacuum-formed retainers are better than Hawley retainers in terms of cost, speech, and patient acceptability. Hawley retainers provide better occlusal settling post-treatment than VFR. For failure rate, both types of retainers have almost equal failure rate. Removable retainers are preferred for retention in cases where maxillary expansion has been done.
- There is a greater relapse in extraction cases than in non-extraction cases, but this subject is still controversial.
- The bonded retainers have a risk of unwanted tooth movement, so post-treatment follow-up is required.

References

1. Kravitz ND, Grauer D, Schumacher P, Jo YM. Memotain: a CAD/CAM nickel-titanium lingual retainer. American Journal of Orthodontics and Dentofacial Orthopedics: Official publication of the American Association of Orthodontists, its constituent societies, and the American Board of Orthodontics. 2017;151(4):812–5. https://doi.org/10.1016/j.ajodo.2016.11.021.
2. Littlewood SJ, Kandasamy S, Huang G. Retention and relapse in clinical practice. Aust Dent J. 2017;62(Suppl 1):51–7. https://doi.org/10.1111/adj.12475.

3. Littlewood SJ, Millett DT, Doubleday B, Bearn DR, Worthington HV. Retention procedures for stabilising tooth position after treatment with orthodontic braces. Cochrane Database Syst Rev. 2016;1:CD002283. https://doi.org/10.1002/14651858.CD002283.pub4.

4. Naraghi S, Ganzer N, Bondemark L, Sonesson M. Comparison of post-treatment changes with and without retention in adolescents treated for maxillary impacted canines-a randomized controlled trial. Eur J Orthod. 2021;43(2):121–7. https://doi.org/10.1093/ejo/cjaa010.

5. Bahije L, Ennaji A, Benyahia H, Zaoui F. A systematic review of orthodontic retention systems: the verdict. Int Orthod. 2018;16(3):409–24. https://doi.org/10.1016/j.ortho.2018.06.023.

6. Carneiro NCR, Nobrega MTC, Meade MJ, Flores-Mir C. Retention decisions and protocols among orthodontists practicing in Canada: a cross-sectional survey. Am J Orthod Dentofacial Orthop. 2022;162(1):51–7. https://doi.org/10.1016/j.ajodo.2021.02.022.

7. Singh P, Grammati S, Kirschen R. Orthodontic retention patterns in the United Kingdom. J Orthod. 2009;36(2):115–21. https://doi.org/10.1179/14653120723040.

8. Bellini-Pereira SA, Aliaga-Del Castillo A, Dos Santos CCO, Henriques JFC, Janson G, Normando D. Treatment stability with bonded versus vacuum-formed retainers: a systematic review of randomized clinical trials. Eur J Orthod. 2022;44(2):187–96. https://doi.org/10.1093/ejo/cjab073.

9. Forde K, Storey M, Littlewood SJ, Scott P, Luther F, Kang J. Bonded versus vacuum-formed retainers: a randomized controlled trial. Part 1: Stability, retainer survival, and patient satisfaction outcomes after 12 months. Eur J Orthod. 2018;40(4):387–98. https://doi.org/10.1093/ejo/cjx058.

10. Al-Moghrabi D, Johal A, O'Rourke N, Donos N, Pandis N, Gonzales-Marin C, et al. Effects of fixed vs removable orthodontic retainers on stability and periodontal health: 4-year follow-up of a randomized controlled trial. American Journal of Orthodontics and Dentofacial Orthopedics: Official publication of the American Association of Orthodontists, its constituent societies, and the American Board of Orthodontics. 2018;154(2):167–74.e1. https://doi.org/10.1016/j.ajodo.2018.01.007.

11. Naraghi S, Ganzer N, Bondemark L, Sonesson M. Stability of maxillary anterior teeth after 2 years of retention in adolescents: a randomized controlled trial comparing two bonded and a vacuum-formed retainer. Eur J Orthod. 2021;43(2):152–8. https://doi.org/10.1093/ejo/cjaa077.

12. O'Rourke N, Albeedh H, Sharma P, Johal A. Effectiveness of bonded and vacuum-formed retainers: a prospective randomized controlled clinical trial. American Journal of Orthodontics and Dentofacial Orthopedics: Official publication of the American Association of Orthodontists, its constituent societies, and the American Board of Orthodontics. 2016;150(3):406–15. https://doi.org/10.1016/j.ajodo.2016.03.020.

13. Kramer A, Sjostrom M, Hallman M, Feldmann I. Vacuum-formed retainer versus bonded retainer for dental stabilization in the mandible-a randomized controlled trial. Part I: Retentive capacity 6 and 18 months after orthodontic treatment. Eur J Orthod. 2020;42(5):551–8. https://doi.org/10.1093/ejo/cjz072.

14. Liu S, Silikas N, Ei-Angbawi A. Analysis of the effectiveness of the fiber-reinforced composite lingual retainer: a systematic review and meta-analysis. Am J Orthod Dentofacial Orthop. 2022; https://doi.org/10.1016/j.ajodo.2022.07.003.

15. Scribante A, Sfondrini MF, Broggini S, D'Allocco M, Gandini P. Efficacy of esthetic retainers: clinical comparison between multistranded wires and direct-bond glass fiber-reinforced composite splints. Int J Dent. 2011;2011:548356. https://doi.org/10.1155/2011/548356.

16. Gunay F, Oz AA. Clinical effectiveness of 2 orthodontic retainer wires on mandibular arch retention. Am J Orthod Dentofacial Orthop. 2018;153(2):232–8. https://doi.org/10.1016/j.ajodo.2017.06.019.

17. Outhaisavanh S, Liu Y, Song J. The origin and evolution of the Hawley retainer for the effectiveness to maintain tooth position after fixed orthodontic treatment compare to vacuum-formed retainer: a systematic review of RCTs. Int Orthod. 2020;18(2):225–36. https://doi.org/10.1016/j.ortho.2020.02.008.

18. Ramazanzadeh B, Ahrari F, Hosseini Z-S. The retention characteristics of Hawley and vacuum-formed retainers with different retention protocols. J Clin Exp Dent. 2018;10(3):e224–e31. https://doi.org/10.4317/jced.54511.

19. Al Rahma WJ, Kaklamanos EG, Athanasiou AE. Performance of Hawley-type retainers: a systematic review of randomized clinical trials. Eur J Orthod. 2018;40(2):115–25. https://doi.org/10.1093/ejo/cjx036.

20. Rowland H, Hichens L, Williams A, Hills D, Killingback N, Ewings P, et al. The effectiveness of Hawley and vacuum-formed retainers: a single-center randomized controlled trial. American Journal of Orthodontics and Dentofacial Orthopedics: Official publication of the American Association of Orthodontists, its constituent societies, and the American Board of Orthodontics. 2007;132(6):730–7. https://doi.org/10.1016/j.ajodo.2006.06.019.

21. Rohaya MAW, Shahrul Hisham ZA , Doubleday B. Randomised clinical trial: comparing the efficacy of vacuum-formed and Hawley retainers in retaining corrected tooth rotations. Malay Dent J. 2006;27:38–44.

22. Mai W, He J, Meng H, Jiang Y, Huang C, Li M, et al. Comparison of vacuum-formed and Hawley retainers: a systematic review. Am J Orthod Dentofacial Orthop. 2014;145(6):720–7. https://doi.org/10.1016/j.ajodo.2014.01.019.

23. Ashari A, Nik Mustapha NM, Yuen JJX, Saw ZK, Lau MN, Xian L, et al. A two-year comparative assessment of retention of arch width increases between modified vacuum-formed and Hawley retainers: a multi-center randomized clinical trial. Prog Orthod. 2022;23(1):40. https://doi.org/10.1186/s40510-022-00424-5.

24. Mheissen S, Seehra J, Khan H, Pandis N. Do sample size calculations in longitudinal orthodontic trials use the advantages of this study design? Angle Orthod. 2022; https://doi.org/10.2319/091321-707.1.

25. Gill DS, Naini FB, Jones A, Tredwin CJ. Part-time versus full-time retainer wear following fixed appliance therapy: a randomized prospective controlled trial. World J Orthod. 2007;8(3):300–6.

26. Thickett E, Power S. A randomized clinical trial of thermoplastic retainer wear. Eur J Orthod. 2010;32(1):1–5. https://doi.org/10.1093/ejo/cjp061.

27. Shawesh M, Bhatti B, Usmani T, Mandall N. Hawley retainers full- or part-time? A randomized clinical trial. Eur J Orthod. 2010;32(2):165–70. https://doi.org/10.1093/ejo/cjp082.

28. Hichens L, Rowland H, Williams A, Hollinghurst S, Ewings P, Clark S, et al. Cost-effectiveness and patient satisfaction: Hawley and vacuum-formed retainers. Eur J Orthod. 2007;29(4):372–8. https://doi.org/10.1093/ejo/cjm039.

29. Jedlinski M, Grocholewicz K, Mazur M, Janiszewska-Olszowska J. What causes failure of fixed orthodontic retention? – Systematic review and meta-analysis of clinical studies. Head Face Med. 2021;17(1):32. https://doi.org/10.1186/s13005-021-00281-3.

30. Iliadi A, Kloukos D, Gkantidis N, Katsaros C, Pandis N. Failure of fixed orthodontic retainers: a systematic review. J Dent. 2015;43(8):876–96. https://doi.org/10.1016/j.jdent.2015.05.002.

31. Sun J, Yu YC, Liu MY, Chen L, Li HW, Zhang L, et al. Survival time comparison between Hawley and clear overlay retainers: a randomized trial. J Dent Res. 2011;90(10):1197–201. https://doi.org/10.1177/0022034511415274.

32. Moslemzadeh SH, Sohrabi A, Rafighi A, Ghojazadeh M, Rahmanian S. Comparison of survival time of Hawley and Vacuum-formed retainers in orthhodontic patients – a randomized clinical trial. Adv Biosci Clin Med. 2017;5(1). https://doi.org/10.7575/aiac.abcmed.17.05.01.02.

33. Zhu Y, Lin J, Long H, Ye N, Huang R, Yang X, et al. Comparison of survival time and comfort between 2 clear overlay retainers with different thicknesses: a pilot randomized controlled trial. American Journal of Orthodontics and Dentofacial Orthopedics: Official publication of the American Association of Orthodontists, its constituent societies, and the American Board of Orthodontics. 2017;151(3):433–9. https://doi.org/10.1016/j.ajodo.2016.10.019.

34. Swidi AJ, Griffin AE, Buschang PH. Mandibular alignment changes after full-fixed orthodontic treatment: a systematic review and meta-analysis. Eur J Orthod. 2019;41(6):609–21. https://doi.org/10.1093/ejo/cjz004.

35. Costa JG, Galindo TM, Mattos CT, Cury-Saramago AA. Retention period after treatment of posterior crossbite with maxillary expansion: a systematic review. Dental Press J Orthod. 2017;22(2):35–44. https://doi.org/10.1590/2177-6709.22.2.035-044.oar.

36. Godoy F, Godoy-Bezerra J, Rosenblatt A. Treatment of posterior crossbite comparing 2 appliances: a community-based trial. Am J Orthod Dentofacial Orthop. 2011;139(1):e45–52. https://doi.org/10.1016/j.ajodo.2010.06.017.

37. Lagravère MO, Carey J, Heo G, Toogood RW, Major PW. Transverse, vertical, and anteroposterior changes from bone-anchored maxillary expansion vs traditional rapid maxillary expansion: a randomized clinical trial. Am J Orthod Dentofacial Orthop. 2010;137(3):304.e1–12; discussion -5. https://doi.org/10.1016/j.ajodo.2009.09.016.

38. Petrén S, Bjerklin K, Bondemark L. Stability of unilateral posterior crossbite correction in the mixed dentition: a randomized clinical trial with a 3-year follow-up. Am J Orthod Dentofacial Orthop. 2011;139(1):e73–81. https://doi.org/10.1016/j.ajodo.2010.06.018.

39. Saleh M, Hajeer MY, Muessig D. Acceptability comparison between Hawley retainers and vacuum-formed retainers in orthodontic adult patients: a single-centre, randomized controlled trial. Eur J Orthod. 2017;39(4):453–61. https://doi.org/10.1093/ejo/cjx024.

40. Aslan BI, Dinçer M, Salmanli O, Qasem MA. Comparison of the effects of modified and full-coverage thermoplastic retainers on occlusal contacts. Orthodontics: The art and practice of dentofacial enhancement. 2013;14(1):e198–208. https://doi.org/10.11607/ortho.990.

41. Sauget E, Covell DA Jr, Boero RP, Lieber WS. Comparison of occlusal contacts with use of Hawley and clear overlay retainers. Angle Orthod. 1997;67(3):223–30. https://doi.org/10.104 3/0003-3219(1997)067<0223:Coocwu>2.3.Co;2.

42. Atik E, Esen Aydinli F, Kulak Kayikçi ME, Ciger S. Comparing the effects of Essix and Hawley retainers on the acoustics of speech. Eur J Orthod. 2017;39(4):440–5. https://doi.org/10.1093/ejo/cjw050.

43. Wan J, Wang T, Pei X, Wan Q, Feng W, Chen J. Speech effects of Hawley and vacuum-formed retainers by acoustic analysis: a single-center randomized controlled trial. Angle Orthod. 2017;87(2):286–92. https://doi.org/10.2319/012716-76.1.

44. Arn ML, Dritsas K, Pandis N, Kloukos D. The effects of fixed orthodontic retainers on periodontal health: a systematic review. Am J Orthod Dentofacial Orthop. 2020;157(2):156–64 e17. https://doi.org/10.1016/j.ajodo.2019.10.010.

45. Booth FA, Edelman JM, Proffit WR. Twenty-year follow-up of patients with permanently bonded mandibular canine-to-canine retainers. Am J Orthod Dentofacial Orthop. 2008;133(1):70–6. https://doi.org/10.1016/j.ajodo.2006.10.023.

46. Westerlund A, Oikonomou C, Ransjö M, Ekestubbe A, Bresin A, Lund H. Cone-beam computed tomographic evaluation of the long-term effects of orthodontic retainers on marginal bone levels. Am J Orthod Dentofacial Orthop. 2017;151(1):74–81. https://doi.org/10.1016/j.ajodo.2016.06.029.

47. Gökçe B, Kaya B. Periodontal effects and survival rates of different mandibular retainers: comparison of bonding technique and wire thickness. Eur J Orthod. 2019;41(6):591–600. https://doi.org/10.1093/ejo/cjz060.

48. Kucera J, Marek I. Unexpected complications associated with mandibular fixed retainers: a retrospective study. Am J Orthod Dentofacial Orthop. 2016;149(2):202–11. https://doi.org/10.1016/j.ajodo.2015.07.035.